CLASSIFICATION OF CHRONIC PAIN

IASP Subcommittee on Taxonomy 1986

*Harold Merskey, DM (Canada, Chair)
*Michael R. Bond, PhD, MD (UK)
John J. Bonica, MD, DSc (USA)
*David B. Boyd, MD (Canada)
Amiram Carmon, MD, PhD (Israel)
A. Barry Deathe, MD (Canada)
Henri Dehen, MD (France)
Ulf Lindblom, MD (Sweden)
James M. Mumford, PhD, MSc (UK)
William Noordenbos, MD, PhD (The Netherlands)
Ottar Sjaastad, MD, PhD (Norway)
Richard A. Sternbach, PhD (USA)
Sydney Sunderland, MD, DSc (Australia)

*Subcommittee on Classification

IASP Task Force on Taxonomy 1994

Harold Merskey, DM (Canada, Chair)
Robert G. Addison, MD (USA)
Aleksandar Beric, MD, DSc (USA)
Helmut Blumberg, MD (Germany)
Nikolai Bogduk, MD, PhD (Australia)
Jorgen Boivie, MD (Sweden)
Michael R. Bond, PhD, MD (UK)
John J. Bonica, MD, DSc (USA)
David B. Boyd, MD (Canada)
A. Barry Deathe, MD (Canada)
Marshall Devor, PhD (Israel)
Martin Grabois, MD (USA)
Jan M. Gybels, MD, PhD (Belgium)
Per T. Hansson, MD, DMSc, DDS (Sweden)
Troels S. Jensen, MD, PhD (Denmark)
John D. Loeser, MD (USA)
Prithvi P. Raj, MB BS (USA)
John W. Scadding, MD, MB BS (UK)
Ottar M. Sjaastad, MD, PhD (Norway)
Erik Spangfort, MD (Sweden)
Barrie Tait, MB ChB (New Zealand)
Ronald R. Tasker, MD (Canada)
Dennis C. Turk, PhD (USA)
Arnoud Vervest, MD (The Netherlands)
James G. Waddell, MD (USA)
Patrick D. Wall, DM, FRS (UK)
C. Peter N. Watson, MD (Canada)

CLASSIFICATION OF CHRONIC PAIN

DESCRIPTIONS OF CHRONIC PAIN SYNDROMES AND DEFINITIONS OF PAIN TERMS

Second Edition

prepared by the

Task Force on Taxonomy
of the
International Association for the Study of Pain

Editors

Harold Merskey, DM
Department of Psychiatry
The University of Western Ontario
Department of Research
London Psychiatric Hospital
London, Ontario, Canada

Nikolai Bogduk, MD, PhD
Faculty of Medicine
The University of Newcastle
Newcastle, New South Wales, Australia

IASP PRESS • SEATTLE

© 1994 IASP Press,
International Association for the Study of Pain

No responsibility is assumed by IASP for any injury and/or damage to persons or property as a matter of product liability, negligence, or from any use of any methods, products, instruction, or ideas contained in the material herein. Because of the rapid advances in the medical sciences, the publisher recommends that there should be independent verification of diagnoses and drug dosages.

Library of Congress Cataloging-in-Publication Data

Classification of chronic pain : descriptions of chronic pain syndromes and
    definitions of pain terms / prepared by the International Association for the
    Study of Pain, Task Force on Taxonomy ; editors, Harold Merskey,
    N. Bogduk. — 2nd ed.
            p.   cm.
        Includes bibliographical references and index.
        ISBN 0-931092-05-1
        1. Chronic pain—Classification. 2. Pain—Terminology.
    I. Merskey, Harold. II. Bogduk, Nikolai. III. International Association for
    the Study of Pain. Task Force on Taxonomy.
        [DNLM: 1. Pain—classification. 2. Chronic Disease—classification.
    WL 704 C614 1994]
    RB127.C58   1994
    616′.0472′012—dc20
    DNLM/DLC
    for Library of Congress   94-8062

IASP Press
International Association for the Study of Pain
909 NE 43rd St., Suite 306
Seattle, WA 98105 USA
Fax: 206-547-1703

Printed in the United States of America

CONTENTS

COMBINED LIST OF CONTRIBUTORS
TO FIRST AND SECOND EDITIONS

D.C. Agnew
Pasadena, CA, USA

M. Backonja
Madison, WI, USA

H.J.M. Barnett
London, ON, Canada

P. Barton
Calgary, AL, Canada

R.W. Beard
London, England, UK

W.E. Bell *
Dallas, TX, USA

J.N. Blau
London, England, UK

L.M. Blendis
Toronto, ON, Canada

R.A. Boas
Auckland, New Zealand

N. Bogduk
Newcastle, NSW, Australia

J. Boivie
Linköping, Sweden

M.R. Bond
Glasgow, Scotland, UK

J.J. Bonica
Seattle, WA, USA

D.B. Boyd
London, ON, Canada

R.I. Brooke
London, ON, Canada

G.W. Bruyn
Leuven, Belgium

J.G. Cairncross
London, ON, Canada

A. Carmon
Jerusalem, Israel

J.E. Charlton
Newcastle upon Tyne, England, UK

M.J. Cousins
St. Leonards, NSW, Australia

A.B. Deathe
London, ON, Canada

S. Diamond
Chicago, IL, USA

M.B. Dresser
Chicago, IL, USA

R.J. Evans
Toronto, ON, Canada

T. Feasby
London, ON, Canada

C. Feinmann
London, England, UK

W. Feldman
Halifax, NS, Canada

H.L. Fields
San Francisco, CA, USA

N.L. Gittleson
Sheffield, England, UK

J.M. Gregg
Blacksburg, VA, USA

M. Grushka
Toronto, ON, Canada

J.M. Gybels
Leuven, Belgium

A. Hahn
London, ON, Canada

P. Hansson
Stockholm, Sweden

P.A.J. Hardy
Gloucester, England, UK

M. Harris
London, England, UK

M. Inwood
London, ON, Canada

G.W. Jamieson
London, ON, Canada

F.W.L. Kerr *
Rochester, MN, USA

I. Klineberg
Sydney, NSW, Australia

T. Komusi
St. John's, NF, Canada

D.W. Koopman
Leiden, The Netherlands

L. Kudrow
Encino, CA, USA

P.L. LeRoy
Wilmington, DE, USA

U. Lindblom
Stockholm, Sweden

S. Lipton
Liverpool, England, UK

J.D. Loeser
Seattle, WA, USA

D.M. Long
Baltimore, MD, USA

D.G. Machin
Liverpool, England, UK

G. Magni
Paris, France

A. Mailis
Toronto, ON, Canada

J. Marbach
New York, NY, USA

G. J. Mazars
Paris, France

P. McGrath
Halifax, NS, Canada

M. Mehta
Norwich, England, UK

J. Miles
Liverpool, England, UK

N. Mohl
Buffalo, NY, USA

F. Mongini
Turin, Italy

D. Moulin
London, ON, Canada

J.A. Mountifield
Toronto, ON, Canada

J.M. Mumford
Liverpool, England, UK

W. Noordenbos *
Amsterdam, The Netherlands

C. Pagni
Turin, Italy

I. Papo
Ancona, Italy

C.W. Parry
London, England, UK

P. Procacci
Florence, Italy

A. Rapoport
Stamford, CT, USA

M. Renaer
Leuven, Belgium

W.J. Roberts
Portland, OR, USA

J.W. Scadding
London, England, UK

B. Sessle
Toronto, ON, Canada

J. Shennan
Liverpool, England, UK

F. Sicuteri
Florence, Italy

O. Sjaastad
Trondheim, Norway

A.E. Sola
Seattle, WA, USA

E. Spangfort
Huddinge, Sweden

F.G. Spear
Sheffield, England, UK

R.H. Spector
Chicago, IL, USA

D.M. Spengler
Nashville, TN, USA

J. Spierdijk
Leiden, The Netherlands

E.L.H. Spierings
Boston, MA, USA

R.A. Sternbach
La Jolla, CA, USA

L.-J. Stovner
Trondheim, Norway

A. Struppler
Munich, West Germany

Sir S. Sunderland *
Melbourne, VIC, Australia

M. Swerdlow
Manchester, England, UK

W.H. Sweet
Boston, MA, USA

B. Tait
Christchurch, New Zealand

R.R. Tasker
Toronto, ON, Canada

M. Trimble
London, England, UK

E. Tunks
Hamilton, ON, Canada

F. Turnbull
Baltimore, MD, USA

G.S. Tyler
Scottsdale, AZ, USA

J. Van Hees
Leuven, Belgium

A.C.M. Vervest
Sneek, The Netherlands

A.P.E. Vielvoye-Kerkmeer
Leiden, The Netherlands

P. Walker
Toronto, ON, Canada

H. Wallach
London, ON, Canada

C.P.N. Watson
Toronto, ON, Canada

M.V. Wells
Campbell River, BC, Canada

F. Wolfe
Wichita, KS, USA

K.J. Zilkha
London, England, UK

D. Zohn
McLean, VA, USA

* *Deceased*

INTRODUCTION

"You are not obliged to complete the work,
but neither are you free to desist from it."

—Rabbi Tarphon, Talmud, Avot, 2:21

"לֹא עָלֶיךָ הַמְּלָאכָה לִגְמוֹר, וְלֹא
אַתָּה בֶן חוֹרִין לְהִבָּטֵל מִמֶּנָּה."

(רַבִּי טַרְפוֹן, פִּרְקֵי אָבוֹת, ב׳ כ״א)

The first two, and largest, parts of this volume contain explanatory material and a collection of descriptions of syndromes. These parts have been updated from the first edition. In the third part, the opportunity has been taken now, as before, to present some definitions of pain terms that were published previously in *Pain* and revised in 1986. Two new terms have been added to these definitions—Neuropathic Pain and Peripheral Neuropathic Pain—and the definition of Central Pain has been altered accordingly. Small changes have also been made in the notes on Allodynia and Hyperalgesia. Notes on the terms Sympathetically Maintained Pain and Sympathetically Independent Pain have also been introduced in a separate section, in connection with revised descriptions of what were formerly called Reflex Sympathetic Dystrophy and Causalgia and are now called Complex Regional Pain Syndromes, Types I and II, respectively.

The list of those who have contributed with drafts or with revisions of drafts precedes this introduction. Some have provided descriptions of a syndrome or comments on it; others have described a whole group or groups of syndromes. Some have also made theoretical contributions in working out how we should proceed. Dr. John J. Bonica, in particular, was instrumental in providing ideas from which the present volume has grown. Many contributors gave substantial portions of their time to the work. The range of contributions was such that it would be impossible to set up a precise scale of gratitude in proportion to the different amounts of help given, but the editors believe they can express thanks to all contributors, not only from the Task Force on Taxonomy of the International Association for the Study of Pain (IASP), but on behalf of the association as a whole.

In addition, Ms. Louisa E. Jones, Executive Officer, IASP, Mrs. J. Duncan, Mrs. C. Hanas, Ms. G. Hudson, and Ms. P. Serratore have been unfailingly patient and helpful in the production of the manuscript and in the associated correspondence over several years. Ms. Mai Why, M.L.S., provided much biblio-graphical assistance. Mr. Bryan Urakawa undertook the difficult task of merging the old and new material in an updated text. The production editor, Ms. Leslie Nelson Bond, has made detailed improvements to the wording and helped to establish the new format.

In the first edition it was observed that the volume was provisional. It contained gaps and, no doubt, some inaccuracies and inconsistencies. Its printing and distribution, however, marked the end of a stage in what is fundamentally a continuous process or sequence of scientific endeavor. It was offered as a provisional compilation for scrutiny and correction by all who have the expertise and the will to devote some effort to developing this statement of our existing knowledge of pain syndromes. Everyone who read it was invited to check it within his or her own field of knowledge for completeness and accuracy and to send any recommendations for additions or corrections to the chairperson of the Subcommittee on Taxonomy (now the Task Force on Taxonomy). The same invitation accompanies this edition, which in its turn should undergo development and modification.

THE NEED FOR A TAXONOMY

The need for a taxonomy was expressed in 1979 by Bonica, who observed: "The development and widespread adoption of universally accepted definitions of terms and a classification of pain syndromes are among the most important objectives and responsibilities of the IASP. It is possible to define terms and develop a classification of pain syndromes which are acceptable to many, albeit not all, readers and workers in the field; even if the adopted definitions and classifications are not perfect they are better than the Tower of Babel conditions that currently exist; adoption of such classification does not mean that it is 'fixed' for all time and cannot be modified as we acquire new knowledge; and, the adoption of such taxonomy with the condition that it can be modified will encourage its use widely by those who may disagree with some part of the classification. This in fact has been the experience and chronology of such widely accepted classifications as those pertaining to heart disease, hypertension, diabetes, toxemia of pregnancy, psychiatric disorders, and a host of others. I hope therefore that all IASP members will cooperate and use the classification of pain syndromes after this is adopted by IASP to improve our communications systems. This will require that they be incorporated in the spoken and written transfer of information, particularly scientific papers, books, etc., and in the development of research protocols, clinical records, and data banks for the storage and retrieval of research and clinical data."

It calls for very little special knowledge, actually, to recognize that we could benefit from a classification of chronic pain syndromes. The need arises because specialists from different disciplines all require a framework within which to group the conditions that they are treating. This framework should enable them to order their own data, identify different diseases or syndromes, and compare their experience and observations with those of others. Studies of epidemiology, etiology, prognosis, and treatment all depend upon the ability to classify clinical events in an agreed pattern. The delivery of medical services is also facilitated if both the type and number of conditions and patients to be treated can be established in a systematic fashion. In some centers, payment by insurance companies for medical care of the insured creates a demand for a classification system.

In regard to chronic pain, it is important to establish such a system of classification that goes beyond what is available in the general international systems such as the International Classification of Diseases. The need is not to replace but to supplement the new ICD-10. Specialist workers in various fields usually require a more detailed structure for classification than is provided by the overall system. The Ad Hoc Committee on Headache of the American Medical Association developed such an extensive system for one set of pain syndromes (Friedman et al. 1962), and the International Headache Society has now replaced that with another for headache disorders, cranial neuralgias, and facial pains (IHS 1988). Stroke has brought forth a schedule of its own (Capildeo et al. 1977), the American Rheumatism Association (1973) has produced its own system with criteria for diagnosis, hematologists have continuously developed the numbering of clotting factors, and so forth. In the field of chronic pain, two requirements spring readily to mind. The first is that we should be able to identify all the chronic pain syndromes we encounter. The second is that we should have as good a description of each as can be obtained, at least with respect to the pain. It would be expecting too much and also would probably be unnecessary to hope for a complete textbook description. But the members of the IASP should obviously be the most suitable experts to describe in full the pains of the syndromes we so often seek to relieve. Accordingly, a classification system for pain syndromes has been attempted which, without being a textbook, will provide standard descriptions of all the relevant pain syndromes and a means toward codifying them.

The present descriptions and coding systems have been developed in the light of the above considerations. They should allow the standardization of observations by different workers and the exchange of information. In the first edition it was remarked that when articles began to appear that used them as a point of reference, they would have achieved their first aim, and that if other articles emerged that revised or criticized them, they would be achieving their second aim, which was to stimulate a continuing effort at updating and improvement. Both these developments occurred, but more revisions have been generated internally within the Task Force on Taxonomy, or in response to communications from members of the IASP. In the spirit of the quotation at the head of this introduction, the work will still not be complete and it will not be interrupted.

THE NATURE OF CLASSIFICATION

Reassurance may be needed for those who feel that the classification should reflect some sort of ultimate truth and universal consistency. It is indeed correct that classifications should be true, at least so far as we know, but complete consistency is beyond the hopes of any medical system of classification. In an ideal system of classification, the categories should be mutually exclusive and completely exhaustive in regard to the data to be incorporated. The classification should also use one principle alone. No classification in medicine has achieved such aims, nor can it be expected to do so (Merskey 1983). Classification in medicine is a pragmatic affair, and we may consider briefly how classifications can be devised. Classifications may be natural if they reflect or presume to reflect an order of nature. Alternatively, they may be artificial but convenient. The simplest type of classification into animate or inanimate objects is a natural one. An extreme example of an artificial classification is provided by a telephone directory (Galbraith and Wilson 1966). The sequence of letters of the alphabet is used as the criterion for classification. That sequence bears little or no relation to the contents that it arranges, namely the people, their addresses, and their telephone numbers. By contrast, a phylogenetic classification by evolutionary relationships is a very superior form of classification. Impressive natural and phylogenetic classifications exist in chemistry, botany, and zoology.

Things are very different in medicine. In the ICD-10, conditions are classified by causal agent, e.g., infectious diseases or neoplasm; by systems of the body, e.g., gastrointestinal or genito-urinary; by system pattern and type of symptom, as in psychiatric illnesses; and by whether or not they are related to the artificial intervention of an operation. They may be grouped by time of occurrence, such as congenital anomalies or conditions originating in the perinatal period, or even grouped as symptoms, signs, and abnormal clinical and laboratory findings. There is a code (O80) for delivery in a completely normal case, including spontaneous breech delivery. Within major groups there are subdivisions by (a) symptom pattern, such as epilepsy or migraine; (b) the presence of hereditary or degenerative disease, e.g., Huntington's disease and hereditary ataxia; (c) extrapyramidal and movement disorders, e.g., Parkinson's disease and dystonia; (d) location, e.g., polyneuropathies and other disorders of the peripheral nervous system; and (e) infectious causes, e.g., meningitis. Overlapping occurs repeatedly in such approaches to categorization. Pain appears in the group of symptoms, signs, and abnormal clinical and laboratory findings as R52 Pain Not Elsewhere Classified. This code excludes some 19 other labels that reflect pain in different parts of the body and also "psychogenic" pain (F45.4) and renal colic (N23). Thus pain occurs at various levels of diagnosis and categorization in the ICD-10. In a sense this is inevitable. There must always be some provision for conditions that are not well described and which will overlap with others that are well described.

Operational considerations often have to be employed in classification, and indeed operational definitions are implicit in most classification activities in medicine. These definitions will suit one purpose and not another. Thus, in psychiatry we may diagnose operationally from biochemistry (phenylketonuria), serology (general paresis), genetics (Huntington's chorea), symptom pattern (schizophrenia, depression), mechanisms and site (tension headache), and even the presence or absence of irrationality (psychosis, neurosis). With regard to internal medicine, the same applies. It has been said that "acute nephritis" may be diagnosed on the basis of etiology, pathogenesis, histology, or clinical presentation (Houston et al. 1975). Pain syndromes are distinguished particularly often on the basis of duration, site, and pattern, some of which are frequently similar to different conditions. Accordingly, we can aim only at practical categories, largely defined operationally, but these can nevertheless be very useful. For some further consideration of this see Merskey (1983). Here we have aimed especially at describing chronic pain syndromes and at coding them.

THE PRESENT CLASSIFICATION

It has been mentioned that the present volume is not a textbook. Instead it deals with syndromes of chronic pain. Chronic pain has gradually emerged as a distinct phenomenon in comparison with acute pain. First, studies were undertaken that explored the special features of patients with persistent pain. Later, specific emphasis was given to the distinction between the two situations (Sternbach 1974). Chronic pain has been recognized as that pain which persists past the normal time of healing (Bonica 1953). In practice this may be less than one month, or more often, more than six months. With nonmalignant pain, three months is the most convenient point of division between acute and chronic pain, but for research purposes six months will often be preferred. Those who treat cancer pain find that three months is sometimes too long to wait before regarding a pain as chronic. Moreover, the definition related to the time of normal healing is not sufficient, nor is it honored consistently. Many syndromes are treated as examples of chronic pain although normal healing has not occurred. Pain that persists for a given length of time would be a simpler concept. This length of time is determined by common medical experience. In the first instance it is the time needed for inflammation to subside, or for acute injuries such as lacerations or incisions to repair with the union of separated tissues. A longer period is required if we wait for peripheral nerves to grow back after trauma. In these circumstances, chronic pain is recognized when the process of repair is apparently ended. Some repair, for example, the thickening of a scar in the skin and its changing color from pink (or dark) to white (or less dark), may be painless. Other repair may never be complete; for example, neuromata in an amputation stump constitute a permanent failure to heal that may be a site of persistent pain. Scar tissue around a nerve may be fully healed but can still act as a persistent painful lesion.

Many syndromes are treated as examples of chronic pain although it is well recognized that normal healing has not occurred. These include rheumatoid arthritis, osteoarthritis, spinal stenosis, nerve entrapment syndromes, and metastatic carcinoma. Others, such as persistent migraine, remit or heal and then recur. Moreover, the increasing knowledge about plasticity of the nervous system (Wall 1989) in response to injury indicates that CNS changes may prolong and maintain pain long after the usual time of response to acute lesions. Such changes can make it difficult to say that normal healing has taken place. Other less obvious failures to heal can last indefinitely (Macnab 1964, 1973); some of these lesions are not detectable even by modern imaging techniques (Taylor and Kakulas 1991) but will still give rise to persistent chronic pain. Chronic pain thus remains important, even if we must understand it slightly differently as a persistent pain that is not amenable, as a rule, to treatments based upon specific remedies, or to the routine methods of pain control such as non-narcotic analgesics. Given that there are so many differences in what may be regarded as chronic pain, it seems best to allow for flexibility in the comparison of cases and to relate the issue to the diagnosis in particular situations. As it happens, the coding system has always allowed durations to be entered as less than one month, one month to six months, and more than six months. This is probably the best solution for the purpose of comparing data within a diagnostic category, or even between some diagnoses.

In this volume only a small number of acute pain syndromes is included. Some are of theoretical importance or are helpful in pointing out a contrast (e.g., acute tension headache versus chronic tension headache) or are recurrent. Conditions have been selected where pain is prominent and pain management is also a leading problem—for example, causalgia. Sometimes, as with spinal stenosis, the main problem with the chronic syndrome is to recognize it reasonably early. After that, the treatment is specific and not one of pain management per se. Syndromes or states that do not meet one of the above characteristics are omitted. Thus, thyroiditis, which can be very painful, is not included, because its recognition and treatment are not usually problems for pain experts and do not present a major problem in acute pain management. Similarly, cerebral tumor is excluded because pain associated with it is not a focus of attention once the patient has consulted a physician or surgeon and the condition has been properly diagnosed. Other conditions, like facet tropism, are included because they reflect the existence of a condition that may or may not be painless.

After quite protracted discussion and correspondence, it was agreed that there were a number of pain syndromes that were best seen as generalized conditions, for example, peripheral neuropathy or radiculopathy, causalgia and reflex dystrophies (now called complex regional pain syndromes), central pain, stump pain and phantom pain, and pain purely of psychological origin. The majority of pain conditions, even including some of the foregoing, have a fairly specific localization, albeit such localization may be in different parts of the body at different times. A root lesion may be anywhere along the spinal column, and postherpetic neuralgia may affect any dermatome. Nevertheless, it seemed worthwhile to divide the descriptions of pain into two groups. First a smaller one, in which there is recognition of a general phenomenon that can affect various parts of the body, and second, a very much larger group, in which the syndromes are described by location. As a result, there is some repetition and redundancy in descriptions of syndromes in the legs which appear also in the arms, or in descriptions of syndromes in abdominal nerve roots which appear in cervical nerve roots.

The present arrangement has been adopted because it offers a particular advantage. That advantage stems from the fact that the majority of pains of which patients complain are commonly described first by the physician in terms of region and only later in terms of etiology. An arrangement by site provides the best practical system for coding the majority of pains dealt with by experts in the field. After thorough discussion, the original Subcommittee on Taxonomy therefore agreed that the majority of syndromes would be described in this fashion.

The descriptions were elicited by sending out requests to appropriate colleagues, of whom enough replied to get this work underway. The pattern of descriptions requested was systematic. Although initially it did not begin with a request for a definition, this was added later. Each syndrome then was to be described in terms of the following items: definition; site; system involved; main features of the pain including its prevalence, age of onset, sex ratio if known, duration, severity, and quality; associated features; factors providing relief; signs characteristic of the condition; usual course; complications; social and physical disabilities; specific laboratory findings on investigations; pathology; treatment where it was very special to the case; the diagnostic criteria if possible; differential diagnosis; and finally, the code. For this edition criteria have been sought for a variety of the conditions.

Emphasis was placed on the description of the pain. By contrast, this volume cannot provide a guide to treatment, but where the results of treatment may be relevant to description or diagnosis they are noted. Each colleague approached was asked to exchange his or her descriptions with others who were looking at the same topics. Accordingly, the majority of descriptions—but not quite all of them—have been scrutinized by colleagues in the same field. The descriptions vary in length. This reflects the decisions of the individual contributors. The senior editor's function was to seek relevance, adequate information, agreed positions, and clarity, and he has been content, within broad limits, to leave the judgment of the amount of detail required in the hands of the authors.

In this edition, as in the first, there are probably still some omissions. Some have occurred, as before, because the conditions in question either have been overlooked by the senior editor or do not seem to be important. In one or two cases help was not obtained in time and it was felt better to proceed with the published volume than to wait indefinitely. It must be emphasized, however, that the editors cannot decide on their own which conditions to incorporate and which to reject. They have had to reach conclusions on the basis of advice from others in most instances. Full descriptions of some conditions are not included, but codes are given. Referred pain from the chest to the abdomen provides an example. At the point where it is mentioned, a reference back to the chest is provided because the main features are to be found in the descriptions of chest conditions. The new sections on spinal and radicular pain, discussed later, provide only titles and codes for many conditions.

SOME CONTROVERSIAL ISSUES

Occasionally terms that are quite popular have been deliberately rejected. One such term is Atypical Facial Pain. The senior editor believes that this term does not describe a definite syndrome but is used variously by different writers to cover a variety of conditions. Some, but not all, of his advisors have accepted this position. It is suggested that what is often called Atypical Facial Pain may better be diagnosed under terms like Temporomandibular Pain Syndrome, Atypical Odontalgia, or Odontalgia Not Associated with Lesions. Some cases may even be variants of the primary headache syndromes such as Classical Migraine. Others should be diagnosed as pain of psychological origin. Alternatively, pain in the face, or anywhere else, for which a diagnosis has not yet been determined can be given a regional code in which the second digit will be 9 and the fifth digit 8, as follows: Code: X9X.X8.

The myofascial pain syndromes have presented obvious difficulties. In this field we are short of properly validated information with agreed criteria and repeatable observations. The amount of well-established knowledge is small compared with the frequency and troublesome quality of the disorders. Accordingly, the material offered on soft tissue pain in the musculoskeletal system is based on views which seem to have empirical justification but which are not necessarily proven. Overall, it has been accepted that there are some general phenomena, described as fibromyalgia, fibrositis, or generalized myofascial pain. These have been grouped together (Group I-9), while some but not all of the more localized phenomena have been given individual identities, under the spinal categories of trigger point syndromes. Sometimes also a prominent regional category such as acceleration-deceleration injury (cervical sprain) may be used, covering several individual muscle sprains, some of which are also described separately.

It is common in North America to find that patients are described as having "Chronic Pain Syndrome." In this case the words are being used as a diagnosis that usually implies a persisting pattern of pain that may have arisen from organic causes but which is now compounded by psychological and social problems in behavioral changes. The Task Force was asked to adopt such a label, particularly for use in billing in the United States. There was general agreement that this would not be desirable. Such a category evades the requirement for accurate physical and psychiatric diagnoses. It was considered that where both physical and psychological disorders might occur together, it was preferable to make both physical and psychiatric diagnoses and to indicate the contribution, if any, of each diagnosis to the patient's pain. In this approach pain is seen as a unitary phenomenon experientially, but still one that may have more than one cause; and of course the causes may all vary in importance. It was also noted that the term *Chronic Pain Syndrome* is often, unfortunately, used pejoratively.

CHANGES IN THE SECOND EDITION

This edition contains a number of additional descriptions in various sections. These include scattered descriptions, e.g., recurrent abdominal pain in children and proctalgia fugax, which represent an effort to include some chronic painful syndromes that were not described in the first edition. This approach is particularly evident in the section on headache, which has been substantially revised and enlarged. This section has been much influenced by recent advances in the identification and description of different types of headache. We have not, however, adopted the classification of the International Headache Society, for three main reasons. The first is that the IHS classification is more extensive in one respect, since it covers acute headaches comprehensively, whereas our focus is much more on chronic headache and is more detailed. Second, it was necessary, or at least highly desirable, that the IASP coding system be used throughout the whole classification. Third, some of the categories of the IHS classification require further attention. It is hoped however, that nearly all the categories we have used will be translatable into IHS codes for those who require that facility. In fact, a crosswalk has been provided from the IASP codes to the IHS codes where possible, and we hope for increased agreement in time.

Among the new conditions described in the headache sections and elsewhere, the following may be noted: Guillain-Barré Syndrome; Tolosa-Hunt Syndrome; SUNCT Syndrome; Raeder's Syndrome; Chronic Paroxysmal Hemicrania: Remitting Form; Syndrome of Jabs and Jolts; Headache Associated with Low CSF Pressure; Post Lumbar Puncture Headache; Hemicrania Continua; Cervicogenic Headache; Brachial Neuritis; Cubital Tunnel Syndrome; Internal Mammary Syndrome; Recurrent Abdominal Pain in Children; Proctalgia Fugax; and Peroneal Muscular Atrophy. Reflex Sympathetic Dystrophy and Causalgia are now described as Complex Regional Pain Syndromes, Types I and II, respectively, and the description of the former reflex sympathetic dystrophy has been substantially revised.

The largest changes have been made in the sections on spinal pain and radicular pain. The least satisfactory aspect of the first edition, acknowledged at the time, was the lack of an adequate way to organize the musculoskeletal syndromes related to spinal or radicular dysfunction and pain, particularly in the low back. The regional arrangement of pain was a start in this direction, but back pain remained amorphous, and we had not found a satisfactory approach to describing it comprehensively and in detail, according to the contributions of spinal features, radicular effects, and myofascial changes.

Within the Task Force on Taxonomy, a Subcommittee on Back Pain adopted schedules for back pain and root pain, which were originally drawn up by Dr. Nikolai Bogduk. These schedules provide a systematic and comprehensive organization of the phenomena of spinal and root pain and have been incorporated in the overall scheme. As in the rest of the classification, they require recognition of the site, system of the body, and features on all the existing five axes (see Scheme for Coding Chronic Pain Diagnoses, (pp. 3–4). However, the descriptions of the pain are relatively limited, for these are taken to be similar for spinal pain in most locations, and for root pain likewise. Further, not all the categories are described, simply because many are rarely responsible for chronic pain. On the other hand, those descriptions that are given are accompanied by criteria for the diagnosis. As with all criteria, the aim is to improve reliability and validity in diagnosis, which is particularly desirable for conditions where loose standards of diagnosis can lead to wide divergences in the meaning of terms in common use. A more detailed discussion of the principles employed in this revision of spinal and back pain is provided on pages 11–16 in the list of Topics and Codes, but that discussion applies to pain arising throughout the vertebral column.

The development of criteria has also been followed in other locations. This process has not been comprehensive, but with the updating and revision of many descriptions, the opportunity has been taken to incorporate criteria when possible. The most notable example of this is the revised description of fibromyalgia (fibrositis) by Dr. Fred Wolfe, which followed the criteria of the American College of Rheumatology, developed on the basis of an exceptional multicenter study.

THE CODING SYSTEM

The coding system is shown in the Scheme for Coding Chronic Pain Diagnoses (pp. 3–4). Particular thanks are due to Dr. Arnoud Vervest for his assistance with the coding system. In order to ensure that there was no overlap between codes, it was necessary to enter all the codes, provide a computer challenge between them, and identify all cases of overlap. Because of the use of variable axes, particularly the first and fourth axes, where as many as ten different entries were possible per diagnosis, there were numerous cases of overlap which required reconciliation before the codes could be adopted, and Dr. Vervest undertook the very demanding work of identifying these problems.

CONCLUSION

The purpose of this chapter has been first to introduce the reader to the considerations which led to the development of the present set of descriptions and codes. Second, the rationale is offered for the pattern chosen for the descriptions in the main body of the text. Third, the ideas behind the present coding system and its details are elucidated. In all this the positions taken are provisional—although of course some of them will not be lightly changed. Members of the Task Force on Taxonomy, those who have contributed so far, and anyone else who has the necessary skill and interest are all earnestly entreated to review the material provided and offer additions or improvements for later editions by writing to the editors (see Future Revisions).

REFERENCES

American Rheumatism Association, Primer on the Rheumatic Diseases, 7th ed. Prepared by a committee of the American Rheumatism Association Section of the Arthritis Foundation. Reprinted from G.P. Rodnam, C. McEwan and S.L. Wallace (Eds.), JAMA, 224, 5 (Suppl.) (1973).

Bonica, J.J., The Management of Pain, Lea & Febiger, Philadelphia, 1953.

Bonica, J.J., The need of a taxonomy (editorial), Pain, 6 (1979) 247–252.

Capildeo, R., Haberman, S. and Rose, F.C., New classification of stroke: preliminary communication, Br. Med. J., 2 (1977) 1578–1580.

Friedman, A.P., Finley, K.H., Graham, J.R., Kunkle, C.E., Ostfeld, M.O. and Wolff, H.G., Classification of headache. Special report of the Ad Hoc Committee. Arch. Neurol., 6 (1962) 173–176.

Galbraith, D.I. and Wilson, D.G., Biological Science: Principles and Patterns of Life, Holt, Rinehart & Winston, Toronto, 1966.

Houston, J.C., Joiner, C.C. and Trounce, J.P. A Short Textbook of Medicine, 5th ed., English Universities Press, London, 1975.

ICD-10 (International Statistical Classification of Diseases and Related Health Problems, 10th rev.), Vol. 1, World Health Organization, Geneva, 1992.

IHS (International Headache Society), Classification and diagnostic criteria for headache disorders, cranial neuralgias and facial pain, Cephalalgia, 8, Suppl. 7 (1988).

Macnab, I., Acceleration injuries of the cervical spine, J. Bone Joint Surg., 46A (1964) 1797–1799.

Macnab, I., The whiplash syndrome, Clin. Neurosurg., 20 (1973) 232–241.

Merskey, H., Development of a universal language of pain syndromes. In: J.J. Bonica, U. Lindblom and A. Iggo (Eds.), Proceedings of the Third World Congress on Pain. Advances in Pain Research and Therapy, Vol. 5. Raven Press, New York, 1983, pp. 37–52.

Sternbach, R.A., Pain Patients: Traits and Treatment, Academic Press, New York, 1974.

Taylor, J.R. and Kakulas, B.A., Neck injuries, Lancet, 338 (1991) 1343.

Wall, P.D., Introduction. In: P.D. Wall and R. Melzack (Eds.), Textbook of Pain, 2nd ed., Churchill Livingstone, Edinburgh, 1989, pp. 9–16.

FUTURE REVISIONS

It is expected that corrections, additions, and other possible revisions will occur to different readers and users of this volume. Anyone who wishes to offer suggestions for improvements is warmly invited to submit these suggestions to the editors for consideration. In doing so, please use the following arrangement. Identify yourself and your address and discipline at the head of a sheet of paper. Then identify the topic, its page in this volume, and the group number and coding. Then offer any or all suggestions on the specific topic on that page and any subsequent pages that may be necessary.

For a fresh topic please provide a new page identified in the same fashion as for the first one.

The senior editor's mailing address is:

Professor Harold Merskey
Department of Research
London Psychiatric Hospital
850 Highbury Avenue
P.O. Box 2532
London, ON, Canada N6A 4H1

ABBREVIATIONS

CPK	creatine phosphokinase
CT	computerized tomography
ECG	electrocardiogram
EEG	electroencephalogram
EMG	electromyogram
ESR	erythrocyte sedimentation rate
GI	gastrointestinal
LDH	lactate dehydrogenase
SGOT	serum glutamic acid oxaloacetic transaminase
TENS	transcutaneous electrical nerve stimulation

PART I

TOPICS AND CODES

SCHEME FOR CODING CHRONIC PAIN DIAGNOSES

The digital portion of the codes is explained first, followed by the letters used as suffixes.

The first digit (Axis I), concerned with the regions, has generally not been difficult to complete. If a patient has pain in more than one region, two codes should be completed for that patient.

The second digit (Axis II) also has generally not been difficult to complete, but the details in this area are open to debate. For example, migraine has been coded, in accordance with the belief of some specialists, as a disorder of the central nervous system, but others might think that it should be coded as a disorder of the vascular system. Again, we should emphasize the practical aspect of the matter: provided that the code is available and useful to those who accept criteria for migraine in accordance with the descriptions provided, the theoretical position adopted in regard to the second digit is not necessarily important.

The third digit (Axis III) deals with the characteristics of the pain episode. It is not controversial, but some judgment is required in deciding whether a condition is continuous with exacerbations or merely continuous.

The fourth digit (Axis IV) has to be filled in for each patient according to his or her particular report as to the severity or chronicity of his or her illness. Accordingly, it is shown as an X throughout the tabulation of codes in association with descriptions here.

The fifth digit (Axis V) is open to most argument because there is a great uncertainty about many of the mechanisms involved in the production of pain in different conditions. Again, it should be said that provided that the coding arrangements give each syndrome a specific and individual number or code, it is not important whether the ultimate truth of the cause of the syndrome be expressed in that code or not. In any case, since some syndromes have the same final code for the five digits, it has become necessary to distinguish them by adding a letter—a, b, c, etc.—in the sixth place. In certain instances the letter " a " has been used to indicate acute conditions compared with chronic conditions that share the same five digits. The leading example of this is acute tension headache. For the most part, however, the letter " a " in the sixth place merely indicates the first of several conditions to be described with the same five digits.

The letters S and R are used after the digits for the codes that identify spinal and radicular pain, respectively. Where both occur *in the same location,* the letter C, for combined spinal and root pain, is preferred.

A full list of those codes allocated so far is provided below. Before examining the value of the coding system, the reader may find it helpful to look at descriptions of conditions with which he or she is familiar and to consider if the codes do justice, or in his or her view any sort of injustice, to them. After that it may be worthwhile to compare the codes for the general syndromes with each other, and then compare with each other those where the same condition affects different parts of the body.

Give priority to the main site of the pain.

Axis I: Regions: Record main site first; record two important regions separately. If there is more than one site of pain, separate coding will be necessary. More than three major sites can be coded, optionally, as shown.

Head, face, and mouth	000
Cervical region	100
Upper shoulder and upper limbs	200
Thoracic region	300
Abdominal region	400
Lower back, lumbar spine, sacrum, and coccyx	500
Lower limbs	600
Pelvic region	700
Anal, perineal, and genital region	800
More than three major sites	900

Axis II: Systems

Nervous system (central, peripheral, and autonomic) and special senses; physical disturbance or dysfunction	00
Nervous system (psychological and social)*	10
Respiratory and cardiovascular systems	20
Musculoskeletal system and connective tissue	30
Cutaneous and subcutaneous and associated glands (breast, apocrine, etc.)	40
Gastrointestinal system	50
Genito-urinary system	60
Other organs or viscera (e.g., thyroid, lymphatic, hemopoietic)	70
More than one system	80
Unknown	90

Note: The system is coded whose abnormal functioning produces the pain, e.g., claudication = vascular. Similarly, the nervous system is to be coded only when a pathological disturbance in it produces pain. Thus pain from a pancreatic carcinoma = gastrointestinal; pain from a metastatic deposit affecting bones = musculoskeletal.

* To be coded for psychiatric illness without any relevant lesion.

Axis III: Temporal Characteristics of Pain: Pattern of Occurrence

Not recorded, not applicable, or not known	0
Single episode, limited duration (e.g., ruptured aneurysm, sprained ankle)	1
Continuous or nearly continuous, nonfluctuating (e.g., low back pain, some cases)	2
Continuous or nearly continuous, fluctuating severity (e.g., ruptured intervertebral disc)	3
Recurring irregularly (e.g., headache, mixed type)	4
Recurring regularly (e.g., premenstrual pain)	5
Paroxysmal (e.g., tic douloureux)	6
Sustained with superimposed paroxysms	7
Other combinations	8
None of the above	9

Axis IV: Patient's Statement of Intensity: Time Since Onset of Pain*

Not recorded, not applicable, or not known		.0
Mild	— 1 month or less	.1
	— 1 month to 6 months	.2
	— more than 6 months	.3
Medium	— 1 month or less	.4
	— 1 month to 6 months	.5
	— more than 6 months	.6
Severe	— 1 month or less	.7
	— 1 month to 6 months	.8
	— more than 6 months	.9

* Decide the time at which pain is recognized retrospectively as having started, even though the pain may occur intermittently. Grade for intensity in relation to the level of current pain problem.

Axis V: Etiology

Genetic or congenital disorders (e.g., congenital dislocation)	.00
Trauma, operation, burns	.01
Infective, parasitic	.02
Inflammatory (no known infective agent), immune reactions	.03
Neoplasm	.04
Toxic, metabolic (e.g., alcoholic neuropathy, anoxia, vascular, nutritional, endocrine), radiation	.05
Degenerative, mechanical*	.06
Dysfunctional (including psychophysiological)†	.07
Unknown or other	.08
Psychological origin (e.g., conversion hysteria, depressive hallucination).	.09

Note: No physical cause should be held to be present, nor any pathophysiological mechanism

* For example, biliary colic or lumbar puncture headache would be mechanical.
† For example, migraine, irritable bowel syndrome, tension headache. *Note:* Include syndromes where a pathophysiological alteration is recognized. Emotional causes may or may not be present.

Examples:

Mild postherpetic neuralgia of T5 or T6 6 months' duration	303.22e
Severe tension headache More than 6 months' duration	033.97c
Severe primary dysmenorrhea Duration not recorded	765.07b

TOPICS AND CODES

The arrangement of topics and codes follows the plan that was adopted in the first edition. Relatively generalized syndromes are presented first, followed by regional ones. Appropriate codes are provided. Because of the substantial changes in the treatment of spinal pain and radicular pain, it has been necessary to alter some of the numbering of the groups—for example, placing cervical spinal pain, thoracic spinal pain, and associated radicular syndromes together in Group IX, whereas lesions of the brachial plexus, which used to occupy Group X, have been placed with pain in the shoulder, arm, and hand as Group XI. Groups XXVI–XXIX are used for the revised versions of lumbar and sacrococcygeal and diffuse spinal pain and associated radicular pains. Inevitably some of the numbering within groups has also been changed, but as far as possible the original numbering has been retained so as to require the minimum of adaptation from existing data banks based upon the first edition.

Many new codes have been provided, mostly without description, and a number of old codes have been somewhat revised for greater accuracy and to make each code specific and individual. The following use of codes is particularly noteworthy.

In the case of spinal and radicular pains, the additional suffixes S and R are used. Where one is used it indicates that only spinal or only radicular pain is evident. Where both additional suffixes might be used because both phenomena are present, the letter C (for Combined spinal and root pain) is preferred. Many spinal codes will be usable with radicular codes. A few spinal codes theoretically should never give rise to radicular pain, e.g., fracture of a spinous process. A number more rarely give rise to radicular pain but theoretically could do so, e.g., infection of a vertebral body. In these circumstances the R codes have been provided for relative completeness but will rarely, if ever, be required.

Note: X = to be completed individually in each case

If there is no code:
(a) check the introduction to see if the item has been rejected, e.g., atypical facial pain;
(b) construct your own code or use the miscellaneous category 99X.X8; or
(c) code as undiagnosed: X9X.X8.

Note that construction of a new code will require a complete challenge because of the existence of many possible overlapping codes. The editors will be pleased to advise on the possibility of assistance in this respect.

The first part of the list of topics and codes follows. The second part begins on p. 17 after the discussion on radiculopathy.

A. RELATIVELY GENERALIZED SYNDROMES

I. Relatively Generalized Syndromes	
1. Peripheral Neuropathy	203.X2a (arms, infective) 203.X3a (arms, inflammatory or immune reactions) 203.X5a (arms, toxic, metabolic, etc.) 203.X8a (arms, unknown or other) 603.X2a (legs, infective) 603.X3a (legs, inflammatory or immune reactions) 603.X5a (legs, toxic, metabolic, etc.) 603.X8a (legs, unknown or other) X03.X4d (Von Recklinghausen's disease)
2. Stump Pain	203.X1a (arms) 603.X1a (legs)
3. Phantom Pain	203.X7a (arms) 603.X7a (legs)
4. Complex Regional Pain Syndrome, Type I (Reflex Sympathetic Dystrophy)	203.X1h (arms) 603.X1h (legs)
5. Complex Regional Pain Syndrome, Type II (Causalgia)	207.X1h (arms) 607.X1h (legs)
6. Central Pain If three or more major sites are involved, code first digit as 9: If only one or two sites are involved, code according to specific site or sites (e.g., for head or face, code 003.X5c, etc.).	903.X5c (vascular) 903.X1c (trauma) 903.X2c (infection) 903.X3c (inflammatory) 903.X4c (neoplasm) 903.X8c (unknown)
7. Syndrome of Syringomyelia (when affecting head or limb; code additional entries for other areas)	007.X0 (face) 207.X0 (arm) 607.X0 (leg)
8. Polymyalgia Rheumatica	X32.X3a
9. Fibromyalgia (Fibrositis)	X33.X8a
10. Rheumatoid Arthritis	X34.X3a
11. Osteoarthritis	X38.X6a
12. Calcium Pyrophosphate Dihydrate Deposition Disease (CPPD)	X38.X0 or X38.X5a
13. Gout	X38.X5b
14. Hemophilic Arthropathy	X34.X0a
15. Burns	X42.X1 or X82.X1
16. Pain of Psychological Origin 16.1. Muscle Tension 16.2. Delusional or Hallucinatory 16.3. Hysterical, Conversion, or Hypochondriacal 16.4. Associated with Depression	 X33.X7b X1X.X9a X1X.X9b X1X.X9d
17. Factitious Illness and Malingering	No code: see note in text

18.	Regional Sprains or Strains (code only)	X33.X1d
19.	Sickle Cell Arthropathy (code only)	X34.X0c
20.	Purpuric Arthropathy (code only)	X34.X0d
21.	Stiff Man Syndrome (code only)	934.X8
22.	Paralysis Agitans (code only)	902.X7
23.	Epilepsy (code only)	X04.X7
24.	Polyarteritis Nodosa (code only)	X5X.X3
25.	Psoriatic Arthropathy and Other Secondary Arthropathies (code only)	X34.X8c
26.	Painful Scar (code only)	X4X.X1b
27.	Systemic Lupus Erythematosis, Systemic Sclerosis and Fibrosclerosis, Polymyositis and Dermatomyositis (code only)	X33.X3b
28.	Infective Arthropathies (code only)	X33.X3c
29.	Traumatic Arthropathy (code only)	X33.X1a
30.	Osteomyelitis (code only)	X32.X2f
31.	Osteitis Deformans (code only)	X32.X5b
32.	Osteochondritis (code only)	X32.X5c
33.	Osteoporosis (code only)	X32.X5d
34.	Muscle Spasm (code only)	X37.X7
35.	Local Pain, No Cause Specified (code only)	X7X.XXa or X3X.X8e
36.	Guillain-Barré Syndrome	901.X3

B. RELATIVELY LOCALIZED SYNDROMES OF THE HEAD AND NECK

II. Neuralgias of the Head and Face	
1. Trigeminal Neuralgia (Tic Douloureux)	006.X8a
2. Secondary Neuralgia (Trigeminal) from Central Nervous System Lesions Arnold-Chiari Syndrome (code only)	006.X4 (tumor) 006.X0 (aneurysm) 002.X2b (congenital)
3. Secondary Trigeminal Neuralgia from Facial Trauma	006.X1
4. Acute Herpes Zoster (Trigeminal)	002.X2a
5. Postherpetic Neuralgia (Trigeminal)	003.X2b
6. Geniculate Neuralgia (VIIth Cranial Nerve): Ramsay Hunt Syndrome	006.X2
7. Neuralgia of the Nervus Intermedius	006.X8c
8. Glossopharyngeal Neuralgia (IXth Cranial Nerve)	006.X8b
9. Neuralgia of the Superior Laryngeal Nerve (Vagus Nerve Neuralgia)	006.X8e
10. Occipital Neuralgia	004.X8 or 004.X1 (if subsequent to trauma)
11. Hypoglossal Neuralgia (code only)	006.X8
12. Glossopharyngeal Pain from Trauma (code only)	003.X1a
13. Hypoglossal Pain from Trauma (code only)	003.X1b
14. Tolosa-Hunt Syndrome (Painful Ophthalmoplegia)	002.X3a
15. SUNCT Syndrome (Shortlasting, Unilateral, Neuralgiform Pain with Conjunctival Injection and Tearing)	006.X8j
16. Raeder's Syndrome (Raeder's Paratrigeminal Syndrome) Type I Type II	002.X4 (tumor) 002.X1a (trauma) 002.X3b (inflammatory, etc.) 002.X8 (unknown)

III. Craniofacial Pain of Musculoskeletal Origin	
1. Acute Tension Headache	034.X7a
2. Tension Headache: Chronic Form (Scalp Muscle Contraction Headache)	033.X7c
3. Temporomandibular Pain and Dysfunction Syndrome (also called Temporomandibular Joint Disorder)	034.X8a
4. Osteoarthritis of the Temporomandibular Joint (code only)	033.X6
5. Rheumatoid Arthritis of the Temporomandibular Joint	032.X3b
6. Dystonic Disorders, Facial Dyskinesia (code only)	003.X8
7. Crushing Injury of Head or Face (code only)	032.X1

IV. Lesions of the Ear, Nose, and Oral Cavity	
1. Maxillary Sinusitis	031.X2a
2. Odontalgia: Toothache 1. Due to Dentino-Enamel Defects	034.X2b
3. Odontalgia: Toothache 2. Pulpitis	031.X2c
4. Odontalgia: Toothache 3. Periapical Periodontitis and Abscess	031.X2d

5. Odontalgia: Toothache 4. Tooth Pain Not Associated with Lesions (Atypical Odontalgia)	034.X8b
6. Glossodynia and Sore Mouth (also known as Burning Tongue or Oral Dysesthesia)	051.X5 (if known) 051.X8 (alternative)
7. Cracked Tooth Syndrome	034.X1
8. Dry Socket	031.X1
9. Gingival Disease, Inflammatory (code only)	034.X2
10. Toothache, Cause Unknown (code only)	034.X8f
11. Diseases of the Jaw, Inflammatory Conditions (code only)	033.X2
12. Other and Unspecified Pain in Jaws (code only)	03X.X8d
13. Frostbite of Face (code only)	022.X1

V. Primary Headache Syndromes, Vascular Disorders, and Cerebrospinal Fluid Syndromes	
1. Classic Migraine (Migraine with Aura)	004.X7a
2. Common Migraine (Migraine without Aura)	004.X7b
3. Migraine Variants	004.X7c
4. Carotidynia	004.X7d
5. Mixed Headache	003.X7b
6. Cluster Headache	004.X8a
7. Chronic Paroxysmal Hemicrania (CPH) 7.1. Unremitting Form or Variety 7.2. Remitting Form or Variety	006.X8k 006.X8g
8. Chronic Cluster Headache	004.X8b
9. Cluster-Tic Syndrome	006.X8h
10. Post-traumatic Headache	002.X1b
11. The Syndrome of "Jabs and Jolts"	006.X8i
12. Temporal Arteritis (Giant Cell Arteritis)	023.X3
13. Headache Associated with Low Cerebrospinal Fluid Pressure	023.X1a
14. Post–Dural Puncture Headache	023.X1b
15. Hemicrania Continua	093.X8
16. Headache Not Otherwise Specified (code only)	00X.X8f

Note: A Headache Crosswalk follows this group in Part II, Detailed Descriptions of Pain Syndromes.

VI. Pain of Psychological Origin in the Head, Face, and Neck (code only)	
1. Delusional or Hallucinatory Pain (code only)	01X.X9e (head or face) 11X.X9e (neck)
2. Hysterical, Conversion, or Hypochondriacal Pain (code only)	01X.X9f (head or face) 11X.X9f (neck)
3. Associated with Depression (code only)	01X.X9g (head or face) 11X.X9g (neck)

See also: I-16, Pain of Psychological Origin; III-1, Acute Tension Headache; and III-2, Tension Headache: Chronic Form

VII. Suboccipital and Cervical Musculoskeletal Disorders	
1. Stylohyoid Process Syndrome (Eagle's Syndrome)	036.X6
2. Cervicogenic Headache	033.X6b

3. Superior Pulmonary Sulcus Syndrome (Pancoast Tumor)	102.X4a
4. Thoracic Outlet Syndrome	133.X6d or 233.X6a
5. Cervical Rib or Malformed First Thoracic Rib (*see* VII-4, Thoracic Outlet Syndrome)	133.X6d or 233.X6a
6. Pain of Skeletal Metastatic Disease of the Neck, Arm, or Shoulder Girdle	133.X4j or 233.X4

Note: For Cervical Sprain, see IX-8, Acceleration-Deceleration Injury of the Neck (Cervical Sprain)

VIII. Visceral Pain in the Neck	
1. Carcinoma of Thyroid	172.X4
2. Carcinoma of Larynx	122.X4
3. Tuberculosis of Larynx	123.X2
4. Chronic Pharyngitis (code only)	151.X5 (if known) 151.X8 (alternative)
5. Carcinoma of Pharynx (code only)	153.X4

C. SPINAL PAIN, SECTION 1: SPINAL AND RADICULAR PAIN SYNDROMES

Note on Arrangements

In this section, both spinal pain and radicular pain are considered. Definitions of spinal pain and related phenomena are offered first, followed by principles related to spinal pain and a comment on radicular pain and radiculopathy. Next there follows a detailed schedule of classifications of spinal pain affecting the cervical and thoracic regions. This schedule is intended to be comprehensive and includes numerous categories and coded items that are not described. Other elements, the more common and chronic with respect to pain, are described in detail later in the body of the text according to the usual pattern.

The coding system and schedules provide categories for both spinal pain and radicular pain when they are associated with each other or when they occur separately. A diagnosis for each should be made as required with the suffix S or R as appropriate, and C when both occur.

Subsequent to the schedule of classifications for the cervical and thoracic regions a more detailed description of radicular pain and radiculopathy is provided.

The schedule of classifications relating to lumbar, sacral, and coccygeal, spinal, and radicular pains is presented later in the text, after the incorporation of material dealing with other syndromes in the upper limbs, thorax, abdomen, and perineum.

Definitions of Spinal Pain and Related Phenomena

SPINAL PAIN

Spinal pain is pain perceived as arising from the vertebral column or its adnexa. The location of the pain can be described in terms similar to those used to describe the five regions of the vertebral column, i.e., cervical, thoracic, lumbar, sacral, and coccygeal. However, this relates only to the perceived location of the pain and, in the first instance, does not imply a direct relationship between the location of the pain and the location of its source. The following descriptions therefore apply only to the description of symptoms and not to their cause.

Wherever a pain is specified as coming from a particular region, it should be understood that this means that it is "perceived substantially" within that region. Thus a cervical pain which extended to a small portion of the upper arm may simply be regarded as a cervical pain. Similarly a lumbar pain which extended to the sacrum or a sacral pain which extended to a minor portion of the lower limb above the knee would be adequately qualified by the principal area in which it is felt. If two areas are substantially involved, then both areas are required to be identified and diagnoses listed for both areas.

Cervical Spinal Pain: Pain perceived as arising from anywhere within the region bounded superiorly by the superior nuchal line, inferiorly by an imaginary transverse line through the tip of the first thoracic spinous process, and laterally by sagittal planes tangential to the lateral borders of the neck.

Cervical pain may be subdivided into *upper cervical pain* and *lower cervical pain* by subdividing the above region into two equal halves by an imaginary transverse plane. Additionally, pain located between the superior nuchal line and an imaginary transverse line through the tip of the second cervical spinous process can be qualified as *suboccipital pain*.

Thoracic Spinal Pain: Pain perceived as arising from anywhere within the region bounded superiorly by an imaginary transverse line through the tip of first thoracic spinous process, inferiorly by an imaginary transverse line through the tip of the last thoracic spinous process, and laterally by vertical lines tangential to the most lateral margins of the erectores spinae muscles.

Pain located over the posterior chest wall but lateral to the above region is best described as *posterior chest wall pain* to distinguish it from thoracic spinal pain.

If required, thoracic spinal pain can be further qualified by dividing the above region into thirds from the top down, to establish regions of *upper thoracic, mid thoracic,* and *lower thoracic* spinal pain.

Lumbar Spinal Pain: Pain perceived as arising from anywhere within a region bounded superiorly by an imaginary transverse line through the tip of the last thoracic spinous process, inferiorly by an imaginary transverse line through the tip of the first sacral spinous process, and laterally by vertical lines tangential to the lateral borders of the lumbar erectores spinae.

Pain located over the posterior region of the trunk but lateral to the erectores spinae is best described as *loin pain* to distinguish it from lumbar spinal pain.

If required, lumbar spinal pain can be divided into *upper lumbar* spinal pain and *lower lumbar* spinal pain by subdividing the above region into equal halves by an imaginary transverse line.

Sacral Spinal Pain: Pain perceived as arising from anywhere within a region bounded superiorly by an imaginary transverse line through the tip of the first sacral spinous process, inferiorly by an imaginary transverse line through the posterior sacrococcygeal joints, and laterally by imaginary lines passing through the posterior superior and posterior inferior iliac spines.

Coccygeal Pain: Pain perceived as arising from the region defined by the location of the coccyx.

Cervico-Occipital Pain: Pain perceived as arising in the cervical region and extending over the occipital region of the skull.

Cervico-Thoracic Pain: Pain perceived as arising from a region encompassing or centered over the lower quarter of the cervical region as defined above and the upper quarter of the thoracic region as defined above.

Thoraco-Lumbar Pain: Pain perceived as arising from a region encompassing or centered over the lower quarter of the thoracic region as described above and the upper third of the lumbar region as described above.

Lumbosacral Pain: Pain perceived as arising from a region encompassing or centered over the lower third of the lumbar region as described above and the upper third of the sacral region as described above.

Combined States: Spinal pain not satisfying either the primary or conjunctional descriptors defined above but otherwise encompassing more than one spinal region should be described in composite forms, e.g., lumbar and thoracic spinal pain.

REFERRED PAIN

In clinical terms, referred pain may be defined as pain perceived as occurring in a region of the body topographically distinct from the region in which the actual source of pain is located. This definition, however, becomes ambiguous in situations where it is unclear where one region of the body ends and an adjacent region begins. Consequently, without detracting from the intent of the above definition, referred pain can be defined more strictly in neurological terms as pain perceived as arising or occurring in a region of the body innervated by nerves or branches of nerves other than those that innervate the actual source of pain. Referred pain may thus occur in a region that is either remote from or directly contiguous with the source of pain, but the two locations are distinguishable on the basis of their different nerve supply.

In the context of spinal pain, referred pain may occur in the head (Campbell and Parsons 1944; Feinstein et al. 1954; Ehni and Benner 1984; Bogduk and Marsland 1986, 1988; Dwyer et al. 1990), the upper limb girdle and upper limb (Kellgren 1938, 1939; Feinstein et al. 1954; Cloward 1959; Bogduk and Marsland 1988; Dwyer et al. 1990), the posterior or anterior chest wall (Kellgren 1938, 1939; Feinstein et al. 1954; Hockaday and Whitty 1967; Booth and Rothman 1976), the abdominal wall (Kellgren 1938, 1939; Feinstein et al. 1954; Hockaday and Whitty 1967), the lower limb girdle and the lower limb (Kellgren 1938, 1939; Feinstein et al. 1954; Mooney and Robertson 1976; McCall et al. 1979).

The distribution of referred pain in the **head** can be described in terms of the region encompassed based on the underlying bones of the skull or regions of the skull, viz., occipital, parietal, frontal, temporal, orbital, auricular, maxillary, and mandibular.

Referred pain to the **upper limb girdle** may encompass all or only part of the girdle. The following descriptors apply to various patterns that may occur.

Scapular Pain: Pain perceived as arising substantially within the area encompassed by the borders of the scapula.

Upper Scapular Pain: Pain perceived as arising substantially within a region bounded medially by an imaginary line in a parasagittal plane coincident with the medial border of the scapula, laterally by the glenohumeral joint, superiorly by the upper border of trapezius, and inferiorly by the spine of the scapula.

Lower Scapular Pain: Pain perceived as arising substantially within the area encompassed by the borders of the scapula but below its spine.

Shoulder Pain: Pain focused over the top of the glenohumeral joint, centered over the lateral margin of the acromion.

Anterior Shoulder Pain: Pain focused over the anterior fibers of the deltoid muscle.

Posterior Shoulder Pain: Pain focused over the posterior fibers of the deltoid muscle.

Referred pain in the **upper limb** can be qualified according to the topographic segment encompassed using standard anatomical definitions, viz., arm, forearm, hand, digits I–V, medial, lateral, anterior, posterior, ulnar, radial, etc.

Referred pain to the **thoracic wall** may be focused over the anterior, lateral, or posterior chest wall and should be described in such terms. Its exact topographic location can be specified by enunciating the ribs that it spans.

Referred pain to the **abdominal wall** can be qualified using established terminology describing the regions of the abdomen, viz., hypochondrial, epigastric, lumbar, umbilical, and suprapubic.

Referred pain located between the thighs may be described as **perineal** pain, unless it is perceived more specifically as occurring in the penis, scrotum, or testis, in which case those descriptions should apply. **Scrotal pain** and **testicular pain** should be distinguished on the basis that the former is perceived principally as being superficial and in the skin of the scrotum while the latter is perceived as being deep and related to the contents of the scrotum.

Referred pain over the **lower limb girdle** posteriorly may be described as **gluteal** pain. For this purpose the gluteal region may be defined as a sector central on the greater trochanter and spanning from the posterior inferior iliac spine to the anterior superior iliac spine. Referred pain immediately below this region posteriorly should be qualified as **posterior hip** pain; pain immediately below this region anteriorly should be qualified as **anterior hip** pain. Pain focused over the inguinal ligament may be qualified as **groin** pain.

Referred pain in the **lower limb** may be qualified using standard anatomical terms that describe its topographic location, viz., thigh, leg, foot, digits I–V, anterior, posterior, medial, lateral, dorsal, plantar. Descriptors based on the course or distribution of nerves, such as "sciatica" and "anterior sciatica" should not be used because they convey an unjustified implication of the involvement of the said nerve. The term "calf" can substitute for "posterior leg."

Usage: In describing a patient simultaneously suffering from spinal pain and referred pain, the distribution of both pains should be explicitly stated, e.g., "lower cervical spinal pain and referred pain to the shoulder," or "lumbosacral pain with referred pain to the gluteal region and posterior thigh," with the side to which the pain is referred being stated. This precision avoids the ambiguity of terms such as "upper cervical syndrome and headache," "typical cervical syndrome," "brachialgia," "sciatica," and "low-back syndrome."

Physiology: The anatomical basis for spinal referred pain appears to be convergence. Afferent fibers from the vertebral column synapse in the spinal cord with second-order neurons that happen also to receive afferents from other nerves. In the absence of any further localizing information, the brain is unable to determine whether the information it receives from the second-order neuron was initiated by the vertebral afferent or the other convergent fibers, and so attributes its origin to both.

Convergence is typically segmental in nature, in that referred pain is perceived as arising from those regions innervated by fibers of the anterior primary nerves of the spinal nerve that also innervates the spinal source of pain. However, convergence may also occur between consecutive spinal cord segments, resulting in more disparate patterns of referred and local pain. For example, convergence between afferents of the trigeminal nerve from the forehead and orbit with vertebral afferents in the third cervical spine nerve may result in upper cervical pain being referred to the forehead.

The essential feature of spinal referred pain that distinguishes it from neurogenic and radicular pain (see below) is that it is nociceptive in nature: the pain is initiated by stimulation of nerve endings of afferent fibers that innervate the vertebral column and its adnexa. Afferent fibers from the region of referred pain are not stimulated by the causative lesion.

RADICULAR PAIN
(see also Radicular Pain and Radiculopathy, below)

Radicular pain is distinguished from nociception by the axons being stimulated along their course; their peripheral terminals are not the site of stimulation. Ectopic activation may occur as a result of mechanical deformation of a dorsal root ganglion, mechanical stimulation of previously damaged nerve roots, inflammation of a dorsal root ganglion, and possibly by ischemic damage to dorsal root ganglia (Howe et al. 1977; Murphy 1977; Howe 1979).

Ectopic activation results in pain being perceived as arising in the territory supplied by the affected axons. Radicular pain differs from referred pain in several respects.

The disease processes that cause radicular pain are indiscriminate and inescapably also affect non-nociceptive afferents (Howe et al. 1977; Howe 1979), resulting in a sensation that is more than pure nociception. Consequently, radicular pain differs in quality from referred pain. The latter is felt deeply and is aching in quality; although its central region is recognizable and constant, its margins are hard to define (Kellgren 1938, 1939; Feinstein et al. 1954). In contrast, radicular pain is usually lancinating in quality and may be perceived along narrow bands reminiscent of but not identical to the bands of dermatomes (Norlen 1944; Smyth and Wright 1959; McCulloch and Waddell 1980). While also perceived deeply, radicular pain nevertheless has a cutaneous quality in proportion to the number of cutaneous afferent fibers being ectopically activated, i.e., it is perceived in the skin as well as deeply. Referred pain lacks any cutaneous quality.

Sciatica: This term is an anachronism and should be abandoned. It stems from an era when the mechanisms of referred pain and radicular pain were poorly understood. It was used to describe pain that appeared to travel along the course of the sciatic nerve. The unfortunate legacy of this term is that it has been applied erroneously to any or all pain of spinal origin perceived in the lower limb. Furthermore, because nerve root compression has been believed to be the cause of sciatica, many forms of referred pain in the lower limb have been erroneously ascribed to this cause.

Clinical experiments have shown that the only type of pain that is evoked by stimulating nerve roots is radicular pain as described above (Norlen 1944; Smyth and Wright 1959; McCulloch and Waddell 1980). Consequently, at the most, sciatica and radicular pain can be considered as synonymous. However, there is no justification on physiological grounds for equating sciatica and referred pain. The two are distinct in mechanism and quality.

Pain in the lower limb should be described specifically as either referred pain or radicular pain. In cases of doubt no implication should be made and the pain should be described as pain in the lower limb.

QUALITY OR DESCRIPTION OF PAIN

In this section, individual descriptions of the quality of pain have not been presented throughout the descriptions of syndromes. This is because pain in the back tends not to discriminate much among the different diagnostic groups. The following general characteristics may be noted.

Acute back pain is often cramping or knifelike, but may be merely dull or aching. It is worse with movement. Chronic back pain without a radicular component is generally aching, dull, or burning or any combination of these three features. It also tends to be made worse by movement.

Radicular pain is often stabbing or shooting with paresthesias, and tingling or lancinating elements, but may well occur against a background of more dull aching pain.

REFERENCES

Bogduk, N. and Marsland, A., On the concept of third occipital headache. J. Neurol. Neurosurg. Psychiatry, 49 (1986) 775–780.

Bogduk, N. and Marsland, A., The cervical zygapophyseal joints as a source of neck pain, Spine, 13 (1988) 610–617.

Booth, R.E., Rothman, R.H. Cervical angina, Spine, 1 (1976) 28–32.

Campbell, D.G. and Parsons, C.M., Referred head pain and its concomitants, J. Nerv. Ment. Dis., 99 (1944) 544–551.

Cloward, R.B., Cervical diskography: a contribution to the aetiology and mechanism of neck, shoulder and arm pain, Ann. Surg., 130 (1959) 1052–1064.

Dwyer, A., Aprill, C. and Bogduk, N., Cervical zygapophyseal joint pain patterns I: a study in normal volunteers, Spine, 15 (1990) 453–457.

Ehni, G. and Benner, B., Occipital neuralgia and the C1–2 arthrosis syndrome, J. Neurosurg. 61 (1984) 961–965.

Feinstein, B., Langton, J.B.K., Jameson, R.M. and Schiller, F., Experiments on referred pain from deep somatic tissues, J. Bone Joint Surg., 36A (1954) 981–997.

Hockaday, J.M. and Whitty, C.W.M., Patterns of referred pain in the normal subject, Brain, 90 (1967) 481–496.

Howe, J.F., A neurophysiological basis for the radicular pain of nerve root compression. In: J.J. Bonica, J.C. Liebeskind, and D.G. Albe-Fessard (Eds.), Proceedings of the Second World Congress on Pain. Advances in Pain Research and Therapy, Vol. 3. Raven Press, New York, 1979, pp. 647–657.

Howe, J.F., Loeser, J.D. and Calvin, W.H., Mechanosensitivity of dorsal root ganglia and chronically injured axons: a physiological basis for the radicular pain of nerve root compression, Pain, 3 (1977) 25–41.

Kellgren, J.H., Observations on referred pain arising from muscle, Clin. Sci., 3 (1938) 175–190.

Kellgren, J.H., On the distribution of referred pain arising from deep somatic structures with charts of segmental pain areas, Clin. Sci., 4 (1939) 35–46.

McCall, I.W., Park, W.M. and O'Brien, J.P., Induced pain referral from posterior lumbar elements in normal subjects, Spine 4 (1979) 441–446.

McCulloch, J.A. and Waddell, G., Variation of the lumbosacral myotomes with bony segmental anomalies J. Bone Joint Surg., 62B (1980) 475–480.

Mooney, V. and Robertson, J., The facet syndrome, Clin. Orthop., 115 (1976) 149–156.

Murphy, R.W., Nerve roots and spinal nerves in degenerative disk disease, Clin. Orthop., 129 (1977) 46–60.

Norlen, G., On the value of the neurological symptoms in sciatica for the localisation of a lumbar disk herniation. Acta Chir. Scand., Suppl., 95 (1944) 1–96.

Smyth, M.J. and Wright, V., Sciatica and the intervertebral disc: an experimental study, J. Bone Joint Surg., 40A (1959) 1401–1418.

Principles

The symptom of spinal pain should be described in terms of its location and nature using the definitions supplied on pages 11 and 12; these descriptions, however, do not establish a diagnosis.

As far as possible, the actual diagnosis of spinal pain should be expressed simultaneously along two axes: an anatomic axis specifying the structure that is the *source* of pain, including its regional or segmental location, and a pathologic axis specifying the pathological basis for the *cause* of pain, e.g., "septic arthritis of the left T5–6 zygapophysial joint."

In patients with spinal pain and referred pain or radicular pain, attention should be paid to diagnosing both parts of their pain. In some cases both forms of pain may stem from the one lesion and a single diagnosis can be formulated, e.g., "cervical spinal pain with right upper scapular referred pain due to osteomyelitis of the C6 vertebral body."

In other cases the two forms of pain may have separate but related causes; both should be enunciated, e.g., "lumbar spinal pain due to internal disruption of the L4–5 intervertebral disk and radicular pain in the right posterior thigh and calf due to stenosis of the L4–5 intervertebral foramen."

It is acknowledged that given the limitations of reliability and validity of currently available clinical techniques and special investigations, it may not always be possible to formulate a diagnosis complete in both anatomic and pathologic terms. Accordingly, this taxonomy provides for three types of diagnoses.

The schedule of classifications provides for:
1. Conditions that are associated with spinal pain whose cause can reasonably be attributed to a demonstrable lesion or otherwise recognizable diathesis;
2. Conditions that may be recognized clinically and for which there is no dispute about their definition but for which a specific diagnosis in anatomic or pathologic terms is either not available or is not justifiable; and
3. Conditions that in some circles are considered controversial or unproven, but which in other circles are staunchly endorsed.

Conditions in which the spinal pain can reasonably be attributed to a demonstrable lesion would be more appropriately coded in terms of the primary diagnosis. There is no special need to elaborate a diagnosis and classification system based on the pain they cause when these conditions are otherwise already classifiable. For example, tumors may cause spinal pain, but once the diagnosis is established, the condition should be classified as "tumor," followed by the pathologic nature of the tumor and the region of the spine that it affects. However, these entities have been included in the schedule for completeness.

For conditions that are considered still controversial or unproven, the Committee has formulated criteria that should be fully satisfied before the diagnosis is ascribed. The Committee also accepts the use of such diagnoses on a presumptive basis without the criteria being satisfied. In adopting this stance, the Committee seeks to mediate contemporary controversies by on the one hand acknowledging novel or controversial entities while on the other hand outlining criteria that if satisfied should assuage skepticism about the validity of the diagnosis. In this regard, the Committee hopes to facilitate the evolution of knowledge in this field by outlining contemporary standards of scientific thought.

In this way, the following taxonomy is designed not to be limiting or prescriptive but to provide options reflecting the diversity of current approaches and attitudes to the problem of spinal pain.

The next section below incorporates definitions of radicular pain and radiculopathy. Technically, radicular pain is not a spinal pain, for it is not perceived in any region of the vertebral column; it is perceived in the limbs or around a segment of the body wall. However, it is mentioned in the context of spinal pain for not uncommonly radicular pain is associated with spinal pain, and in some instances but not always, both forms of pain may have the same cause. It is, however, illegitimate to

diagnose or classify any form of spinal pain as radicular pain or in terms relating to radicular pain. Radicular pain in isolation is strictly a pain problem of the affected limb or body wall segment. When associated with spinal pain, the spinal pain warrants an independent classification to which the classification of the radicular pain may then be appended.

Similarly, radiculopathy may occur in conjunction with spinal pain, but radiculopathy involves loss of conduction in sensory or motor axons, or both, in a nerve root, and there is no evidence that such conduction loss can be a cause of spinal pain. Consequently, it is illegitimate to classify spinal pain in terms of any radiculopathy that may be associated with it. As with radicular pain, the spinal pain should be classified independently, supplemented if required by a classification of the radiculopathy.

In classifying spinal pain, it is immaterial whether or not the spinal pain is associated with referred pain; the extent or distribution of referred pain has no bearing on the underlying cause of the spinal pain. Both the spinal pain and the referred pain are caused by the same lesion (unless one believes the patient is suffering from two independent pain problems), and identifying the location or extent of any referred pain has little bearing on formulating a diagnosis. Consequently, in this taxonomy spinal pain problems are classified according to their location but without deference to the presence or distribution of any referred pain.

In compiling a taxonomy based on anatomical and pathological axes, the Committee has endeavored to provide a workable system of diagnostic criteria which may help to order the primary phenomena. The complete *assessment* of a patient requires attention beyond the anatomical diagnosis to consider the psychological, social, and vocational context and consequences of pain and their significance.

Radicular Pain and Radiculopathy

RADICULAR PAIN: GENERAL FEATURES

Definition: Pain perceived as arising in a limb or the trunk wall caused by ectopic activation of nociceptive afferent fibers in a spinal nerve or its roots or other neuropathic mechanisms.

Clinical Features: The pain is lancinating in quality and travels along a narrow band. It may be episodic, recurrent, or paroxysmal according to the causative lesion or any superimposed aggravating factors.

Pathology: Lesions that directly compromise the dorsal root ganglion mechanically or indirectly compromise the spinal nerve and its roots by causing ischemia or inflammation of the axons. Specific entities include:

1. Foraminal stenosis due to vertical subluxation of the intervertebral joint, osteophytes stemming from the zygapophysial joint or intervertebral disk, buckling of the ligamentum flavum, or a combination of any of the above.
2. Foraminal stenosis due to miscellaneous disorders of the zygapophysial joint such as articular factures, slipped epiphysis, ganglion, joint effusion, and synovitis.
3. Prolapsed intervertebral disk acting mechanically as a space-occupying lesion that compromises axons.
4. Prolapsed intervertebral disk material that elicits an inflammatory reaction in the vertebral canal that secondarily produces inflammation of adjacent neural elements.
5. Radiculitis caused by inflammatory exudates leaking from an intervertebral disk in the absence of frank prolapse.
6. Radiculitis caused by exudates from a zygapophysial joint.
7. Radiculitis caused by viral infection or postviral inflammation of a dorsal root ganglion, e.g., herpes zoster and postherpetic neuralgia.
8. Radiculitis due to arteritis.
9. Tabes dorsalis.

Diagnosis: The diagnosis can be ascribed on clinical grounds alone if the appropriate clinical features are present. Where possible the segmental level of the affected spinal nerve should be specified. The cause and segmental level of the affected nerve can be specified if an appropriate lesion is demonstrated by imaging techniques such as myelography, CT, or MRI. The affected nerve but not the causative lesion can be specified if in the presence of the appropriate clinical features, a selective spinal nerve block abolishes the pain.

Remarks: Radicular pain must be distinguished from referred pain (see above).

Radicular pain must, by definition, involve a region beyond the spine. There is no evidence that the mechanism underlying radicular pain can cause spinal pain alone.

Radicular pain may occur alone, in the absence of spinal pain, whereupon it should be classified as limb pain or trunk pain according to its perceived distribution. When present in conjunction with spinal pain, the two should in the first instance be defined and diagnosed separately, for there is no prima facie reason to maintain that both pains will have exactly the same cause.

RADICULOPATHY: GENERAL FEATURES

Definition: Objective loss of sensory and/or motor function as a result of conduction block in axons of a spinal nerve or its roots.

Clinical Features: Subjective sensations of numbness and weakness, confirmed objectively by neurological examination and/or by electrodiagnostic means, occurring in the distribution of a spinal nerve. Radiculopathy may occur in isolation or in association with radicular pain, referred pain, or spinal pain.

Paresthesias in a dermatomal distribution can be caused by ischemia of a spinal nerve or its roots, and may be regarded as a feature of incipient conduction block and therefore a feature of radiculopathy.

Pathology: Any lesion that causes conduction block in axons of a spinal nerve or its roots either directly by mechanical compression of the axons or indirectly by compromising their blood supply and nutrition. Specific entities include:

1. Foraminal stenosis due to vertical subluxation of the intervertebral joint, osteophytes stemming from the zygapophysial joint or intervertebral disk, buckling of the ligamentum flavum, or a combination of any of these.
2. Foraminal stenosis due to miscellaneous disorders of the zygapophysial joint such as articular factures, slipped epiphysis, ganglion, joint effusion, and synovitis.
3. Prolapsed intervertebral disk acting mechanically as a space-occupying lesion that compromises axons.
4. Chronic inflammation of the nerve root complex and its meningeal investments.

Remarks: Radiculopathy and radicular pain are not synonymous. The former relates to objective neurological signs due to conduction block. The latter is a symptom caused by ectopic impulse generation. The two conditions may nonetheless coexist and may be caused by the same lesion; or radiculopathy may follow radicular pain in the course of a disease process.

However, radiculopathy and radicular pain are both distinct from referred pain. There is no physiological or clinical evidence that referred pain can be caused by the same processes that underlie radiculopathy. Similarly, radiculopathy is not a cause of spinal pain.

Referred pain and spinal pain associated with radiculopathy consequently warrant a separate and additional diagnosis.

D. SPINAL PAIN, SECTION 2: SPINAL AND RADICULAR PAIN SYNDROMES OF THE CERVICAL AND THORACIC REGIONS

In using this section, please refer back to the remarks upon Spinal Pain and Radicular Pain, pp. 11–16.

Where spinal and radicular pain occur, the suffixes S and R are used, respectively. If both occur together, *in the same location*, e.g., in the neck, the suffix C, for combined spinal and radicular pain, should be used. If a radicular pain occurs in an area with a different location it should be coded additionally. For example, pain due to a prolapsed disk causing both local spinal and local radicular pain in the neck would be coded 133.X1kC, while concomitant radicular pain in the arm would be coded 233.X1bR as well. Codes that occur without the expectation of possible R codes, e.g., those for torticollis, do not employ the S suffix in coding.

* The asterisk is inserted in spinal and radicular codes where no letter is required in the sixth place.

IX. Cervical or Radicular Spinal Pain Syndromes

IX-1 Cervical Spinal or Radicular Pain Attributable to a Fracture		S/C codes	R only/in addition
IX-1.1(S)(R)	Fracture of a Vertebral Body	133.X1eS/C	233.X1eR
IX-1.2(S)	Fracture of a Spinous Process (Synonym: "clay-shoveler's fracture")	133.X1fS	
IX-1.3(S)(R)	Fracture of Transverse Process	133.X1gS/C	233.X1fR
IX-1.4(S)(R)	Fracture of an Articular Pillar	133.X1hS/C	233.X1gR
IX-1.5(S)(R)	Fracture of a Superior Articular Process	133.X1iS/C	233.X1hR
IX-1.6(S)(R)	Fracture of an Inferior Articular Process	133.X1jS/C	233.X1iR
IX-1.7(S)(R)	Fracture of Lamina	133.X1kS/C	233.X1uR
IX-1.8(S)(R)	Fracture of the Odontoid Process	133.X1lS/C	233.X1vR
IX-1.9(S)(R)	Fracture of the Anterior Arch of the Atlas	133.X1mS/C	233.X1pR
IX-1.10(S)(R)	Fracture of the Posterior Arch of the Atlas	133.X1nS/C	233.X1qR
IX-1.11(S)(R)	Burst Fracture of the Atlas	133.X1oS/C	233.X1wR

IX-2 Cervical Spinal or Radicular Pain Attributable to an Infection		S/C codes	R only/in addition
IX-2.1(S)(R)	Infection of a Vertebral Body (Osteomyelitis)	132.X2aS/C	232.X2iR
IX-2.2(S)(R)	Septic Arthritis of a Zygapophysial Joint	132.X2bS/C	232.X2jR
IX-2.3(S)(R)	Septic Arthritis of an Atlanto-Axial Joint	132.X2cS/C	232.X2cR
IX-2.4(S)(R)	Infection of the Paravertebral Muscles or Space	132.X2dS/C	232.X2kR
IX-2.5(S)(R)	Infection of an Intervertebral Disk (Diskitis)	132.X2eS/C	232.X2lR
IX-2.6(S)(R)	Infection of an Interbody Graft	132.XtS/C	232.X2mR
IX-2.7(S)(R)	Infection of a Posterior Fusion	132.X2gS/C	232.X2nR
IX-2.8(S)(R)	Infection of the Epidural Space (Epidural Abscess)	132.X2hS/C	232.X2oR
IX-2.9(S)(R)	Infection of the Spinal Meninges (Meningitis)	103.X2cS/C	203.X2cR
IX-2.10(S)(R)	Herpes Zoster Acute	103.X2dS/C	203.X2dR
IX-2.11(S)(R)	Post Herpetic Neuralgia	103.X2eS/C	203.X2eR
IX-2.12(S)(R)	Syphilis: Tabes Dorsalis and Hypertrophic Pachymeningitis	107.X2*S/C	207.X2*R
IX-2.13(S)(R)	Other Syphilitic Changes, Including Gumma	No Code	

IX-3 Cervical Spinal or Radicular Pain Attributable to a Neoplasm	S/C codes	R only/in addition
IX-3.1(S)(R)	Primary Tumor of a Vertebral Body	133.X4aS/C	233.X4aR
IX-3.2(S)(R)	Primary Tumor of Any Part of a Vertebra Other than Its Body	133.X4bS/C	233.X4bR
IX-3.3(S)(R)	Primary Tumor of a Zygapophysial Joint	133.X4cS/C	233.X4cR
IX-3.4(S)(R)	Primary Tumor of an Atlanto-Axial Joint	133.X4dS/C	233.X4dR
IX-3.5(S)(R)	Primary Tumor of a Paravertebral Muscle	133.X4eS/C	233.X4eR
IX-3.6(S)(R)	Primary Tumor of Epidural Fat (e.g., lipoma)	133.X4fS/C	233.X4yR
IX-3.7(S)(R)	Primary Tumor of Epidural Vessels (e.g., angioma)	133.X4gS/C	233.X4gR
IX-3.8(S)(R)	Primary Tumor of Meninges (e.g., meningioma)	103.X4aS/C	203.X4aR
IX-3.9(R)	Primary Tumor of Spinal Nerves (e.g., neurofibroma, schwannoma, neuroblastoma		203.X4bR
IX-3.10(S)(R)	Primary Tumor of Spinal Cord (e.g., glioma)	103.X4cS/C	203.X4cR
IX-3.11(S)(R)	Metastatic Tumor Affecting a Vertebra	133.X4hS/C	233.X4gR
IX-3.12(S)(R)	Metastatic Tumor Affecting the Vertebral Canal	133.X4iS/C	233.X4uR
IX-3.13(S)(R)	Other Infiltrating Neoplastic Disease of a Vertebra (e.g., lymphoma)	133.X4jS/C	233.X4qR

IX-4 Cervical Spinal or Radicular Pain Attributable to Metabolic Bone Disease	S/C codes	R only/in addition
IX-4.1(S)(R)	Osteoporosis of Age	132.X5aS/C	232.X5gR
IX-4.2(S)(R)	Osteoporosis of Unknown Cause	132.X5bS/C	232.X5hR
IX-4.3(S)(R)	Osteoporosis of Some Known Cause Other than Age	132.X5cS/C	232.X5iR
IX-4.4(S)(R)	Hyperparathyroidism	132.X5dS/C	232.X5jR
IX-4.5(S)(R)	Paget's Disease of Bone	132.X5eS/C	232.X5kR
IX-4.6(S)(R)	Metabolic Disease of Bone Not Otherwise Classified	132.X5fS/C	232.X5lR

IX-5 Cervical Spinal or Radicular Pain Attributable to Arthritis	S/C codes	R only/in addition
IX-5.1(S)(R)	Rheumatoid Arthritis	132.X3aS/C	232.X3aR
IX-5.2(S)(R)	Ankylosing Spondylitis	132.X8aS/C	232.X8aR
IX-5.3(S)(R)	Osteoarthritis	138.X6aS/C	238.X6aR
IX-5.4(S)(R)	Seronegative Spondylarthropathy Not Otherwise Classified	123.X8aS/C	223.X8aR

IX-6 Cervical Spinal or Radicular Pain Associated with a Congenital Vertebral Anomaly	S/C codes	R only/in addition
IX-6(S)(R)	Cervical Spinal or Radicular Pain Associated with a Congenital Vertebral Anomaly	123.X0*S/C	223.X0R

IX-7 Cervical Spinal Pain of Unknown or Uncertain Origin	S/C codes	R only/in addition
IX-7.1(S)(R)	Upper Cervical Spinal Pain of Unknown or Uncertain Origin	13X.X8cS/C	23X.X8cR
IX-7.2(S)(R)	Lower Cervical Spinal Pain of Unknown or Uncertain Origin	13X.X8dS/C	23X.X8dR
IX-7.3(S)(R)	Cervico-Thoracic Spinal Pain of Unknown or Uncertain Origin	13X.X8eS/C	23X.X8eR

IX-8 Acceleration-Deceleration Injury of the Neck (Cervical Sprain)			S/C codes	R only/in addition
IX-8(S)(R)	Cervical Sprain Injury		133.X1aS/C 233.X1aS/C	233.X1aR
IX-9 Torticollis (Spasmodic Torticollis)			S codes only	R only/in addition
IX-9(S)	Congenital		133.X0jS	
	Trauma		133.X1*S	
	Infection		133.X2*S	
	Unknown or Other		133.X8fS	

IX-10 Cervical Discogenic Pain			S codes only	R only/in addition
IX-10(S)(R)	Cervical Discogenic Pain	Trauma Degeneration Dysfunction	133.X1vS 133.X6bS 133.X7*S	233.X1bR 233.X6* R 233.X7* R

IX-11 Cervical Zygapophysial Joint Pain			S codes only	R only/in addition
IX-11(S)	Cervical Zygapophysial Joint Pain	Trauma Degeneration Dysfunction	133.X1pS 133.X6cS 133.X7aS	

IX-12 Cervical Muscle Sprain			S/C codes	R only/in addition
IX-12(S)(R)	Cervical Muscle Sprain		133.X1mS	233.X1kR

IX-13 Cervical Trigger Point Syndrome		S codes only	R only/in addition
IX-13.1(S)(C)	Upper Sternocleidomastoid	132.X1aS	
IX-13.2(S)(C)	Lower Sternocleidomastoid	132.X1bS	
IX-13.3(S)(C)	Upper Trapezius	132.X1cS	
IX-13.4(S)(C)	Middle Trapezius	132.X1dS	
IX-13.5(S)(C)	Lower Trapezius	132.X1eS	
IX-13.6(S)(C)	Splenius Capitis	132.X1fS	
IX-13.7(S)(C)	Upper Splenius Cervicis	132.X1gS	
IX-13.8(S)(C)	Lower Splenius Cervicis	132.X1hS	
IX-13.9(S)(C)	Semispinalis Capitis	132.X1iS	
IX-13.10(S)(C)	Levator Scapulae	132.X1jS	

IX-14 Alar Ligament Sprain		S codes only	R only/in addition
IX-14(S)	Alar Ligament Sprain	132.X1*S	

IX-15 Cervical Segmental Dysfunction		S codes only	R only/in addition
IX-15(S)(R)	Cervical Segmental Dysfunction	133.X1tS	233.X1cR

* The asterisk is inserted in spinal and radicular codes where no letter is required in the sixth place.

IX-16 Radicular Pain Attributable to a Prolapsed Cervical Disk		S/C codes	R only/in addition
IX-16(R)	Radicular Pain Attributable to a Prolapsed Cervical Disk		203.X6aR (arm)

IX-17 Traumatic Avulsion of Nerve Roots		S/C codes	R only/in addition
IX-17(S)(R)	Traumatic Avulsion of Nerve Roots	103.X1aS/C	203.X1cR

X. Thoracic Spinal or Radicular Pain Syndromes

X-1 Thoracic Spinal or Radicular Pain Attributable to a Fracture		S/C codes	R only/in addition
X-1.1(S)(R)	Fracture of a Vertebral Body	333.X1eS/C	233.X1jR
X-1.2(S)	Fracture of a Spinous Process	333.X1f (S only)	
X-1.3(S)(R)	Fracture of a Transverse Process	333.X1gS/C	233.X1kR
X-1.4(S)	Fracture of a Rib	333.X1h (S only)	
X-1.5(S)(R)	Fracture of a Superior Articular Process	333.X1tS/C	233.X1lR
X-1.6(S)(R)	Fracture of an Inferior Articular Process	333.X1jS/C	233.X1mR
X-1.7(S)(R)	Fracture of a Lamina	333.X1kS/C	233.X1nR

X-2 Thoracic Spinal or Radicular Pain Attributable to an Infection		S/C codes	R only/in addition
X-2.1(S)(R)	Infection of a Vertebral Body (osteomyelitis)	332.X2aS/C	232.X2iR
X-2.2(S)(R)	Septic Arthritis of a Zygapophysial Joint	332.X2bS/C	232.X2jR
X-2.3(S)(R)	Septic Arthritis of a Costo-Vertebral Joint	332.X2cS/C	232.X2cR
X-2.4(S)(R)	Septic Arthritis of a Costo-Transverse Joint	332.X2dS/C	232.X2kR
X-2.5(S)(R)	Infection of a Paravertebral Muscle	332.X2eS/C	232.X2lR
X-2.6(S)(R)	Infection of an Intervertebral Disk (diskitis)	332.X2fS/C	232.X2mR
X-2.7(S)(R)	Infection of a Surgical Fusion-Site	332.X2gS/C	232.X2nR
X-2.8(S)(R)	Infection of the Epidural Space (epidural abscess)	332.X2hS/C	232.X2oR
X-2.9(S)(R)	Infection of the Meninges (meningitis)	303.X2cS/C	203.X2fR
X-2.10(S)(R)	Acute Herpes Zoster (code only)	303.X2aS/C	203.X2aR
X-2.11(S)(R)	Postherpetic Neuralgia	303.X2bS/C	203.X2bR

X-3 Thoracic Spinal or Radicular Pain Attributable to a Neoplasm		S/C codes	R only/in addition
X-3.1(S)(R)	Primary Tumor of a Vertebral Body	333.X4aS/C	233.X4vR
X-3.2(S)(R)	Primary Tumor of Any Part of a Vertebra Other than Its Body	333.X4bS/C	233.X4lR
X-3.3(S)(R)	Primary Tumor of a Zygapophysial Joint	333.X4cS/C	233.X4mR
X-3.4(S)(R)	Primary Tumor of the Proximal End of a Rib	333.X4dS/C	233.X4nR
X-3.5(S)(R)	Primary Tumor of a Paravertebral Muscle	333.X4eS/C	233.X4oR
X-3.6(S)(R)	Primary Tumor of Epidural Fat (e.g., lipoma)	333.X4fS/C	233.X4pR
X-3.7(S)(R)	Primary Tumor of Epidural Vessels (e.g., angioma)	333.X4gS/C	233.X4qR
X-3.8(S)(R)	Primary Tumor of Meninges (e.g., meningioma)	303.X4aS/C	203.X4dR

* The asterisk is inserted in spinal and radicular codes where no letter is required in the sixth place.

			S/C codes	R only/in addition
X-3.9(S)(R)	Primary Tumor of Spinal Nerves (e.g., neurofibroma, schwannoma, neuroblastoma)		303.X4bS/C	203.X4eR
X-3.10(S)(R)	Primary Tumor of Spinal Cord (e.g., glioma etc.)		303.X4*S/C	203.X4fR
X-3.11(S)(R)	Metastatic Tumor Affecting a Vertebra		333.X4hS/C	233.X4hR
X-3.12(S)(R)	Metastatic Tumor Affecting a Vertebral Canal		333.X4iS/C	233.X4iR
X-3.13(S)(R)	Other Infiltrating Neoplastic Disease of a Vertebra (e.g., lymphoma)		333.X4jS/C	233.X4jR

X-4 Thoracic Spinal or Radicular Pain Attributable to Metabolic Bone Disease			S/C codes	R only/in addition
X-4.1(S)(R)	Osteoporosis of Age		332.X5aS/C	232.X5gR
X-4.2(S)(R)	Osteoporosis of Unknown Cause		332.X5bS/C	232.X5hR
X-4.3(S)(R)	Osteoporosis of Some Known Cause Other than Age		332.X5cS/C	232.X5iR
X-4.4(S)(R)	Hyperparathyroidism		332.X5dS/C	232.X5jR
X-4.5(S)(R)	Paget's Disease of Bone		332.X5eS/C	232.X5kR
X-4.6(S)(R)	Metabolic Disease of Bone Not Otherwise Classified		332.X5fS/C	232.X5lR

X-5 Thoracic Spinal or Radicular Pain Attributable to Arthritis			S/C codes	R only/in addition
X-5.1(S)(R)	Rheumatoid Arthritis		334.X3aS/C	234.X3aR
X-5.2(S)	Ankylosing Spondylitis		332.X8aS/C	
X-5.3(S)(R)	Osteoarthritis		338.X6*S/C	238.X6bR
X-5.4(S)(R)	Seronegative Spondylarthropathy Not Otherwise Classified		323.X8*S/C	223.X8*R

X-6 Thoracic Spinal or Radicular Pain Associated with a Congenital Vertebral Anomaly			S/C codes	R only/in addition
X-6(S)(R)	Thoracic Spinal Pain Associated with a Congenital Vertebral Anomaly		323.X0*S/C	223.X0aR

X-7 Pain Referred from Thoracic Viscera or Vessels and Perceived as Thoracic Spinal Pain			S/C codes	R only/in addition
X-7.1	Pericarditis	Known infection	323.X2	
		Unknown infective cause	323.X3	
		Trauma	323.X1	
		Neoplasm	323.X4	
		Toxic	323.X5	
X-7.2	Aneurysm of the Aorta		322.X6	
X-7.3	Carcinoma of the Esophagus		353.X4	

X-8 Thoracic Spinal Pain of Unknown or Uncertain Origin			S/C codes	R only/in addition
X-8.1(S)(R)	Upper Thoracic Spinal Pain of Unknown or Uncertain Origin		3XX.X8bS/C	2XX.X8fR
X-8.2(S)(R)	Midthoracic Spinal Pain of Unknown or Uncertain Origin		3XX.X8cS/C	2XX.X8gR
X-8.3(S)(R)	Lower Thoracic Spinal Pain of Unknown or Uncertain Origin		3XX.X8dS/C	2XX.X8hR
X-8.4(S)(R)	Thoracolumbar Spinal Pain of Unknown or Uncertain Origin		3XX.X8eS/C	2XX.X8iR

X-9 Thoracic Discogenic Pain			S codes only	R only/in addition
X-9(S)	Thoracic Discogenic Pain	Trauma Degeneration Dysfunctional	333.X1lS 333.X6aS 333.X7cS	

X-10 Thoracic Zygapophysial Joint Pain			S/C codes	R only/in addition
X-10(S)	Thoracic Zygapophysial Joint Pain	Trauma Degeneration Dysfunctional	333.X1mS/C 333.X6bS/C 333.X7tS/C	

X-11 Costo-Transverse Joint Pain			S codes only	R only/in addition
X-11(S)	Costo-Transverse Joint Pain	Trauma Degeneration Dysfunctional	333.X1nS 333.X6cS 333.X7eS	

X-12 Thoracic Muscle Sprain			S codes only	R only/in addition
X-12(S)	Thoracic Muscle Sprain	Trauma Dysfunctional	333.X1oS 333.X7fS	

X-13 Thoracic Trigger Point Syndrome			S codes only	R only/in addition
X-13(S)	Thoracic Trigger Point Syndrome	Trauma Degeneration Dysfunctional	332.X1aS 332.X6aS 332.X7hS	

X-14 Thoracic Muscle Spasm			S codes only	R only/in addition
X-14(S)	Thoracic Muscle Spasm	Trauma Infection Neoplasm Degenerative Dysfunctional Unknown	332.X1bS 332.X2iS 332.X4*S 332.X6bS 332.X7iS 332.X8fS	

X-15 Thoracic Segmental Dysfunction			S/C codes	R only/in addition
X-15(S)(R)	Thoracic Segmental Dysfunction	Trauma Dysfunctional	333.X1pS/C 333.X7dS/C	333.X1pR 333.X7dR

X-16 Radicular Pain Attributable to a Prolapsed Thoracic Disk			S/C codes	R only/in addition
X-16(R)	Radicular Pain Attributable to a Prolapsed Thoracic Disk	Trauma Degenerative Trauma (arm) Degenerative (arm)		303.X1aR 303.X6bR 203.X1cR 203.X6bR

* The asterisk is inserted in spinal and radicular codes where no letter is required in the sixth place.

E. LOCAL SYNDROMES OF THE UPPER LIMBS AND RELATIVELY GENERALIZED SYNDROMES OF THE UPPER AND LOWER LIMBS

XI. Local Syndromes of the Upper Limbs and Relatively Generalized Syndromes of the Upper and Lower Limbs	
1. Tumors of the Brachial Plexus	102.X4b or 202.X4b
2. Chemical Irritation of the Brachial Plexus	102.X5 or 202.X5
3. Traumatic Avulsion of the Brachial Plexus	203.X1c
4. Postradiation Pain of the Brachial Plexus (code only)	203.X5
5. Painful Arms and Moving Fingers (code only) (*see* XXXI-9 for legs)	202.X8
6. Brachial Neuritis (Brachial Neuropathy, Neuralgic Amyotrophy, Parsonage-Turner Syndrome)	202.X8a
7. Bicipital Tendinitis	231.X3
8. Subacromial Bursitis (Subdeltoid Bursitis, Supraspinatus Tendinitis)	238.X3
9. Rotator Cuff Tear—Partial or Complete	231.X1a
10. Adhesive Capsulitis and Frozen Shoulder (code only)	232.X2 (infective) 232.X3b (inflammatory) 232.X7 (dysfunctional)
11. Lateral Epicondylitis (Tennis Elbow)	235.X1a
12. Medial Epicondylitis (Golfer's Elbow)	235.X1b
13. DeQuervain's Tenosynovitis	233.X3
14. Osteoarthritis of the Hands	238.X6b
15. Cubital Tunnel Syndrome	202.X6c
16. Carpal Tunnel Syndrome	204.X6
17. Pain of Psychological Origin in the Shoulder and Arm	233.X7b (tension) 21X.X9a (delusional) 21X.X9b (conversion) 21X.X9d (with depression)
18. Crush Injury of Upper Limbs (code only)	231.X1b
19. Pain in a Limb or Limbs, Not Otherwise Specified (code only)	2XX.XXz (upper limb or limbs) 6XX.XXz (lower limb or limbs)

XII. Vascular Disease of the Limbs	
1. Raynaud's Disease	024.X7a (face) 224.X7a (arms) 624.X7b (legs)
2. Raynaud's Phenomenon	024.X7c (face) 224.X7c (arms) 624.X7c (legs)
3. Frostbite and Cold Injury	222.X1a (arms) 622.X1a (legs)
4. Erythema Pernio (Chilblains)	225.X1 (arms) 625.X1 (legs)
5. Acrocyanosis	222.X1b (arms) 622.X1b (legs)

6. Livedo Reticularis	222.68a (arms)
	622.68c (legs)
7. Volkmann's Ischemic Contracture (code only)	222.X5

XIII. Collagen Disease of the Limbs	
1. Scleroderma	226.X5 (arms)
	626.X5 (legs)
2. Ergotism	281.X6 (arms)
	681.X5 (legs)

XIV. Vasodilating Functional Disease of the Limbs	
1. Erythromelalgia	224.X8d (hands)
	624.X8d (feet)
2. Thromboangiitis Obliterans	224.X3c (arms)
	624.X3b (legs)
3. Chronic Venous Insufficiency	222.X4 (arms, neoplasm)
	222.X6 (arms)
	622.X4 (legs, neoplasm)
	622.X6 (legs)

XV. Arterial Insufficiency in the Limbs	
1. Intermittent Claudication	224.X8c (arms)
	624.X8c (legs)
2. Rest Pain	222.X8b (arms)
	622.X8b (legs)
3. Gangrene Due to Arterial Insufficiency (code only)	222.X8d (arms)
	622.X8d (legs)

XVI. Pain of Psychological Origin in the Lower Limbs	
See also I-16 and VI-1, VI-2	633.X7c (tension)
	61X.X9d (delusional)
	61X.X9e (conversion)
	61X.X9f (with depression)

F. VISCERAL AND OTHER SYNDROMES OF THE TRUNK APART FROM SPINAL AND RADICULAR PAIN

XVII. Visceral and Other Chest Pain	
1. Acute Herpes Zoster	303.X2d
2. Postherpetic Neuralgia	303.X2e
3. Other Postinfectious and Segmental Peripheral Neuralgia	306.X2 (postinfectious) 306.X8 (unknown) 306.X1 or 303.X1a (post-traumatic)
4. Angina Pectoris	324.X6 224.X6 (if mostly in the arms)
5. Myocardial Infarction	321.X6 221.X6 (if in the arms)
6. Pericarditis	323.X2 (known infection) 323.X3 (unknown infective cause) 323.X1 (trauma) 323.X4 (neoplasm) 323.X5 (toxic)
7. Aneurysm of the Aorta	322.X6 (chronic aneurysm)
8. Disease of the Diaphragm	423.X2 (infection: chest or pulmonary source) 423.X4 (neoplasm: chest or pulmonary source) 433.X2 (musculoskeletal) 453.X2 (infection: gastro-intestinal source) 453.X4a (neoplasm: gastro-intestinal source) 453.X6 (cholelithiasis)
9. Carcinoma of the Esophagus	353.X4
10. Slipping Rib Syndrome	333.X6
11. Postmastectomy Pain Syndrome: Chronic Nonmalignant	303.X9
12. Late Postmastectomy Pain or Regional Carcinoma	307.X4
13. Post-thoracotomy Pain Syndrome	303.X1d (neuroma) 333.X4a (metastasis)
14. Internal Mammary Artery Syndrome	303.X1f
15. Tietze's Syndrome—Costo-Chondritis (code only)	332.X6
16. Fractured Ribs or Sternum (code only)	335.X1
17. Xiphoidalgia Syndrome	494.X8
18. Carcinoma of the Lung or Pleura	323.X4a

XVIII. Chest Pain of Psychological Origin	
1. Muscle Tension Pain	333.X7h
2. Delusional Pain	31X.X9d
3. Conversion Pain	31X.X9e
4. With Depression	31X.X9f
See also: I-16, Pain of Psychological Origin.	

XIX. Chest Pain Referred from Abdomen or Gastrointestinal Tract	
1. Subphrenic Abscess	353.X2 (thorax)
	453.X2a (abdomen)
2. Herniated Abdominal Organs	355.X6 (thoracic pain)
	455.X6 (abdominal pain)
3. Esophageal Motility Disorders	356.X7
4. Esophagitis	355.X2 (monilial)
	355.X3a (peptic)
5. Reflux Esophagitis with Peptic Ulceration	355.X3b
6. Gastric Ulcer with Chest Pain (code only)	355.X3c
7. Duodenal Ulcer with Chest Pain (code only)	355.X3d
8. Thoracic Visceral Disease with Pain Referred to Abdomen (*See* XVII-6, Pericarditis, and XIX-2, Herniated Abdominal Organs)	

XX. Abdominal Pain of Neurological Origin	
1. Acute Herpes Zoster (code only)	403.X2d
2. Postherpetic Neuralgia (code only)	403.X2b
3. Segmental or Intercostal Neuralgia	406.X2 (postinfectious)
	406.X8 (unknown)
	406.X1 or 403.X1
	(post-traumatic)
4. Twelfth Rib Syndrome	433.X6a
5. Abdominal Cutaneous Nerve Entrapment Syndrome	433.X6b

XXI. Abdominal Pain of Visceral Origin	
1. Cardiac Failure	452.X6
2. Gallbladder Disease	456.X6
3. Post-cholecystectomy Syndrome	457.X1
4. Chronic Gastric Ulcer	455.X3a
5. Chronic Duodenal Ulcer	455.X3b
6. Carcinoma of the Stomach	453.X4c
7. Carcinoma of the Pancreas	453.X4b
8. Chronic Mesenteric Ischemia	455.X5
9. Crohn's Disease	456.X3a (colicky pain)
	452.X3a (sustained pain)
10. Chronic Constipation	453.X7a
11. Irritable Bowel Syndrome	453.X7b
12. Diverticular Disease of the Colon	454.X6
13. Carcinoma of the Colon	452.X4
14. Gastritis and Duodenitis (code only)	45X.X2c
15. Dyspepsia and Other Dysfunctional Disorders in Stomach with Pain (code only)	45X.X7c or 45X.X8
16. Radiation Enterocolitis (code only)	453.X5
17. Ulcerative Colitis and Other Chronic Colitis and Other Ulcer (code only)	453.X8a
18. Post–Gastric Surgery Syndrome, Dumping (code only)	454.X1a
19. Chronic Pancreatitis (code only)	453.XXd

20. Recurrent Abdominal Pain in Children	456.X7
21. Carcinoma of the Liver or Biliary System (code only)	453.X4
22. Carcinoma of the Kidney (Grawitz Carcinoma) (code only)	453.X4

XXII. Abdominal Pain Syndromes of Generalized Diseases	
1. Familial Mediterranean Fever (FMF)	434.X0b or 334.X0b
2. Abdominal Migraine	404.X7a
3. Intermittent Acute Porphyria	404.X5a
4. Hereditary Corproporphyria	404.X5b
5. Variegate Porphyria	404.X5c

XXIII. Abdominal Pain of Psychological Origin	
1. Muscle Tension Pain	433.X7c
2. Delusional or Hallucinatory Pain	41X.X9d
3. Conversion Pain	41X.X9e
4. Associated with Depression	41X.X9f
Abdominal Pain: Visceral Pain Referred to the Abdomen (*See* XVII-6, Pericarditis; XIX-2, Herniated Abdominal Organs; XVII-7, Aneurysm of the Aorta; and XVII-8, Diseases of the Diaphragm)	

XXIV. Diseases of the Bladder, Uterus, Ovaries, and Adnexa	
1. Mittelschmerz	765.X7a

2. Secondary Dysmenorrhea
    With Endometriosis
    With Adenomyosis or Fibrosis
    With Congenital Obstruction
    With Acquired Obstruction
    Psychological Causes
	765.X6a
	765.X4
	765.X0
	765.X6b
	765.X9a (tension)
	765.X9b (delusional)
	765.X9c (conversion)

3. Primary Dysmenorrhea	765.X7b
4. Endometriosis	764.X6
5. Posterior Parametritis	733.X2
6. Tuberculosis Salpingitis	763.X2
7. Retroversion of the Uterus	765.X7c
8. Ovarian Pain	764.X7a (cystic ovary) 764.X7b (remnant syndrome)
9. Chronic Pelvic Pain Without Obvious Pathology (CPPWOP)	763.X8
10. Pain from Urinary Tract (code only)	763.XXb or 863.XX
11. Pain of Vaginismus or Dyspareunia (code only)	864.X7
12. Carcinoma of the Bladder (code only)	763.X4

XXV. Pain in the Rectum, Perineum, and External Genitalia	
1. Neuralgia of Iliohypogastric, Ilio-Inguinal, or Genito-Femoral Nerves Testicular Pain	407.X7b 407.X1

2. Rectal, Perineal, and Genital Pain of Psychological Origin	81X.X9d (delusional) 81X.X9e (conversion) 81X.X9f (depressive)
3. Pain of Hemorrhoids (code only)	853.X5
4. Proctalgia Fugax	856.X8
5. Ulcer of Anus or Rectum (code only)	81X.XX
6. Injury of External Genitalia (code only)	832.X1
7. Carcinoma of the Prostate (code only)	862.X4

G. SPINAL PAIN, SECTION 3: SPINAL AND RADICULAR PAIN SYNDROMES OF THE LUMBAR, SACRAL, AND COCCYGEAL REGIONS

In using this section, please refer back to the remarks upon Spinal Pain and Radicular Pain, pp. 11–16.

Where spinal and radicular pain occur, the suffixes S and R are used, respectively. If both occur together, *in the same location,* e.g., in the neck, the suffix C, for combined spinal and radicular pain, should be used. If a radicular pain occurs in an area with a different location it should be coded additionally. For example, pain due to a prolapsed disk causing both local spinal and local radicular pain in the neck would be coded 133.X1kC, while concomitant radicular pain in the arm would be coded 233.X1bR as well. Codes that occur without the expectation of possible R codes, e.g., those for torticollis, do not employ the S suffix in coding.

* The asterisk is inserted in spinal and radicular codes where no letter is required in the sixth place.

XXVI. Lumbar Spinal or Radicular Pain Syndromes

XXVI-1 Lumbar Spinal or Radicular Pain Attributable to a Fracture		S/C codes	R only/in addition
XXVI-1.1(S)(R)	Fracture of a Vertebral Body	533.X1aS/C	633.X1aR
XXVI-1.2(S)	Fracture of a Spinous Process	533.X1b (S only)	
XXVI-1.3(S)(R)	Fracture of a Transverse Process	533.X1cS/C	633.X1cR
XXVI-1.4(S)(R)	Fracture of a Superior Articular Process	533.X1dS/C	633.X1dR
XXVI-1.5(S)(R)	Fracture of an Inferior Articular Process	533.X1eS/C	633.X1e
XXVI-1.6(S)(R)	Fracture of a Lamina (pars interarticularis)	533.X1fS	633.X1fR

XXVI-2 Lumbar Spinal or Radicular Pain Attributable to an Infection		S/C codes	R only/in addition
XXVI-2.1(S)(R)	Infection of a Vertebral Body (osteomyelitis)	532.X2aS/C	632.X2aR
XXVI-2.2(S)(R)	Septic Arthritis of a Zygapophysial Joint	532.X2bS/C	632.X2bR
XXVI-2.3(S)(R)	Infection of a Paravertebral Muscle (e.g., psoas abscess)	532.X2cS/C	632.X2cR
XXVI-2.4(S)(R)	Infection of an Intervertebral Disk (diskitis)	532.X2dS/C	632.X2dR
XXVI-2.5(S)(R)	Infection of a Surgical Fusion-Site	532.X2eS/C	632.X2eR
XXVI-2.6(S)(R)	Infection of a Retroperitoneal Organ or Space	532.X2fS/C	632.X2fR
XXVI-2.7(S)(R)	Infection of the Epidural Space (epidural abscess)	532.X2gS/C	632.X2gR
XXVI-2.8(S)(R)	Infection of the Meninges (meningitis)	502.X2*S/C	602.X2cR
XXVI-2.9(S)(R)	Acute Herpes zoster (code only)	503.X2dS/C (low back)	603.X2dR (leg)
XXVI-2.10(S)(R)	Postherpetic Neuralgia (code only)	503.X2bS/C (low back)	603.X2bR (leg)

XXVI-3 Lumbar Spinal or Radicular Pain Attributable to a Neoplasm		S/C codes	R only/in addition
XXVI-3.1(S)(R)	Primary Tumor of a Vertebral Body	533.X4aS/C	633.X4aR
XXVI-3.2(S)(R)	Primary Tumor of Any Part of a Vertebra Other than Its Body	533.X4bS/C	633.X4bR
XXVI-3.3(S)(R)	Primary Tumor of a Zygapophysial Joint	533.X4cS/C	633.X4cR
XXVI-3.4(S)(R)	Primary Tumor of a Paravertebral Muscle	533.X4dS/C	633.X4dR
XXVI-3.5(S)(R)	Primary Tumor of Epidural Fat (e.g., lipoma)	533.X4eS/C	633.X4eR
XXVI-3.6(S)(R)	Primary Tumor of Epidural Vessels (e.g., angioma)	533.X4fS/C	633.X4fR

XXVI-3.7(S)(R)	Primary Tumor of Meninges (e.g., meningioma)	503.X4aS/C	603.X4aR
XXVI-3.8(S)(R)	Primary Tumor of a Spinal Nerve (e.g., neurofibroma, schwannoma, neuroblastoma)	503.X4bS/C 503.X4cS/C	603.X4bR 603.X4cR
XXVI-3.9(S)(R)	Primary Tumor of Spinal Cord (e.g., glioma, etc.)	533.X4gS/C	633.X4gR
XXVI-3.10(S)(R)	Metastatic Tumor Affecting a Vertebra	533.X4hS/C	633.X4hR
XXVI-3.11(S)(R)	Metastatic Tumor Affecting the Vertebral Canal	533.X4iS/C	633.X4iR
XXVI-3.12(S)(R)	Other Infiltrating Neoplastic Disease of a Vertebra (e.g., lymphoma)	533.X4jS/C	633.X4jR

XXVI-4 Lumbar Spinal or Radicular Pain Attributable to Metabolic Bone Disease		S/C codes	R only/in addition
XXVI-4.1(S)(R)	Osteoporosis of Age	532.X5aS/C	632.X5aR
XXVI-4.2(S)(R)	Osteoporosis of Unknown Cause	532.X5bS/C	632.X5bR
XXVI-4.3(S)(R)	Osteoporosis of Some Known Cause Other than Age	532.X5cS/C	632.X5cR
XXVI-4.4(S)(R)	Hyperparathyroidism	532.X5dS/C	632.X5dR
XXVI-4.5(S)(R)	Paget's Disease of Bone	532.X5eS/C	632.X5eR
XXVI-4.6(S)(R)	Metabolic Disease of Bone Not Otherwise Classified	532.X5fS/C	632.X5fR

XXVI-5 Lumbar Spinal or Radicular Pain Attributable to Arthritis		S/C codes	R only/in addition
XXVI-5.1(S)(R)	Rheumatoid Arthritis	534.X3aS/C	634.X3aR
XXVI-5.2(S)(R)	Ankylosing Spondylitis	532.X8*S/C	632.X8*R
XXVI-5.3(S)(R)	Osteoarthritis	538.X6aS/C	638.X6aR
XXVI-5.4(S)(R)	Seronegative Spondylarthropathy Not Otherwise Classified	532.X8bS/C	632.X8bR

XXVI-6 Lumbar Spinal or Radicular Pain Associated with a Congenital Vertebral Anomaly		S/C codes	R only/in addition
XXVI-6(S)(R)	Lumbar Spinal or Radicular Pain Associated with a Congenital Vertebral Anomaly	523.X0aS/C	623.X0aR

XXVI-7 Pseudoarthrosis of a Transitional Vertebra		S/C codes	R only/in addition
XXVI-7(S)(R)	Pseudoarthrosis of a Transitional Vertebra	523.X0bS/C	623.X0bR

XXVI-8 Pain Referred from Abdominal Viscera or Vessels and Perceived as Lumbar Spinal Pain		S/C codes	R only/in addition
XXVI-8.1(S)	Aortic Aneurysm (*see also* XVII-7)	522.X6S	
XXVI-8.2(S)	Gastric Ulcer (*see also* XXI-4)	555.X3aS	
XXVI-8.3(S)	Duodenal Ulcer (*see also* XXI-5)	555.X3bS	
XXVI-8.4(S)	Mesenteric Ischemia (*see also* XXI-8)	555.X5S	
XXVI-8.5(S)	Pancreatitis (*see also* XXI-19)	553.XXfS	
XXVI-8.6(S)	Perforation of a Retroperitoneal Organ	552.X3S	

XXVI-9 Lumbar Spinal Pain of Unknown Uncertain Origin		S codes only	R only/in addition
XXVI-9.1(S)	Upper Lumbar Spinal Pain of Unknown or Uncertain Origin	5XX.X8cS	

XXVI-9.2(S)	Lower Lumbar Spinal Pain of Unknown or Uncertain Origin		5XX.X8dS	
XXVI-9.3(S)	Lumbosacral Spinal Pain of Unknown or Uncertain Origin		5XX.X8eS	

XXVI-10 Lumbar Spinal or Radicular Pain after Failed Spinal Surgery			S/C codes	R only/in addition
XXVI-10(S)(R)	Lumbar Spinal or Radicular Pain after Failed Spinal Surgery		533.X1gS/C	632.X1hR

XXVI-11 Lumbar Discogenic Pain			S codes only	R only/in addition
XXVI-11(S)	Lumbar Discogenic Pain	Trauma	533.X1i S	
		Degenerative	533.X6aS	
		Dysfunctional	533.X7cS	

XXVI-12 Internal Disk Disruption			S codes only	R only/in addition
XXVI-12(S)	Internal Disk Disruption	Trauma	533.X1tS	
		Degenerative	533.X6bS	
		Dysfunctional	533.X7*S	

XXVI-13 Lumbar Zygapophysial Joint Pain			S/C codes	R only/in addition
XXVI-13(S)(R)	Lumbar Zygapophysial Joint or Radicular Pain	Trauma	533.X1kS/C	633.X1*R
		Degenerative	533.X6oS/C	633.X6aR

XXVI-14 Lumbar Muscle Sprain			S codes only	R only/in addition
XXVI-14(S)	Lumbar Muscle Sprain		533.X1lS	

XXVI-15 Lumbar Trigger Point Syndrome			S codes only	R only/in addition
XXVI-15.1(S)	Multifidus		532.X1aS	
XXVI-15.2(S)	Longissimus Thoracis		532.X1bS	
XXVI-15.3(S)	Iliocostalis Lumborum		532.X1cS	
XXVI-15.4(S)	Lumbar Trigger Point Syndrome Not Otherwise Specified		532.X1*S	

XXVI-16 Lumbar Muscle Spasm			S codes only	R only/in addition
XXVI-16(S)	Lumbar Muscle Spasm	Trauma	532.X1tS	
		Infection	532.X2hS	
		Neoplasm	532.X4aS	
		Degenerative	532.X6aS	
		Dysfunctional	532.X7dS	
		Unknown	532.X8fS	

* The asterisk is inserted in spinal and radicular codes where no letter is required in the sixth place.

XXVI-17 Lumbar Segmental Dysfunction		S codes only	R only/in addition
XXVI-17(S)	Lumbar Segmental Dysfunction	533.X1hS 533.X7eS	

XXVI-18 Lumbar Ligament Sprain		S codes only	R only/in addition
XXVI-18(S)	Lumbar Ligament Sprain	533.X1mS	

XXVI-19 Sprain of the Anulus Fibrosus		S codes only	R only/in addition
XXVI-19(S)	Sprain of the Anulus Fibrosus	533.X1nS	

XXVI-20 Interspinous Pseudoarthrosis (Kissing Spines, Baastrup's Disease)		S codes only	R only/in addition
XXVI-20(S)	Interspinous Pseudoarthrosis (Kissing Spines, Baastrup's Disease)	533.X1oS	

XXVI-21 Lumbar Instability		S codes only	R only/in addition
XXVI-21(S)	Lumbar Instability	533.X7jS	

XXVI-22 Spondylolysis		S codes only	R only/in addition
XXVI-22(S)	Spondylolysis	53X.X0*S	

XXVI-23 Prolapsed Intervertebral Disk		S/C codes	R only/in addition
XXVI-23(S)(R)	Prolapsed Intervertebral Disk (code only)	502.X1cS/C	602.X1aR

XXVII. Sacral Spinal or Radicular Pain Syndromes

* Note: S codes include R codes unless specified as "S only."

XXVII-1 Sacral Spinal or Radicular Pain Attributable to a Fracture		S/C codes	R only/in addition
XXVII-1.1(S)(R)	Sacral Spinal Pain Attributable to a Fracture	533.X2l S/C	

XXVII-2 Sacral Spinal or Radicular Pain Attributable to an Infection		S/C codes	R only/in addition
XXVII-2.1(S)(R)	Infection of the Sacrum (osteomyelitis)	533.X2aS/C	633.X2aR
XXVII-2.2(S)	Septic Arthritis of the Sacroiliac Joint	533.X2bS (S only)	
XXVII-2.3(S)	Infection of a Paravertebral Muscle (psoas abscess)	533.X2cS (S only)	
XXVII-2.4(S)	Infection of a Surgical Fusion-Site	533.X2dS (S only)	
XXVII-2.5(S)	Infection of a Retroperitoneal Organ or Space	533.X2eS (S only)	
XXVII-2.6(S)(R)	Infection of the Epidural Space (epidural abscess)	533.X2fS/C	633.X2bR
XXVII-2.7(S)(R)	Infection of the Meninges (meningitis)	502.X2dS/C	602.X2dR

XXVII-3 Sacral Spinal or Radicular Pain Attributable to a Neoplasm		S/C codes	R only/in addition
XXVII-3.1(S)(R)	Primary Tumor of the Sacrum	533.X4tS/C	633.X4kR
XXVII-3.2(S)	Primary Tumor of the Sacroiliac Joint	533.X4k S (S only)	
XXVII-3.3(S)	Primary Tumor of a Parasacral Muscle	533.X4mS (S only)	
XXVII-3.4(S)(R)	Primary Tumor of Epidural Fat (e.g., lipoma)	533.X4nS/C	633.X4lR
XXVII-3.5(S)(R)	Primary Tumor of Epidural Vessels (e.g., angioma)	533.X4oS/C	633.X4mR
XXVII-3.6(S)(R)	Primary Tumor of Meninges (e.g., meningioma)	503.X4dS/C	603.X4dR
XXVII-3.7(S)(R)	Primary Tumor of a Spinal Nerve (e.g., neurofibroma, schwannoma, neuroblastoma)	503.X4eS/C	603.X4eR
XXVII-3.8(S)(R)	Metastatic Tumor Affecting the Sacrum	533.X4pS/C	633.X4nR
XXVII-3.9(S)(R)	Metastatic Tumor Affecting the Sacral Canal	533.X4qS/C	633.X4oR
XXVII-3.10 (S)(R)	Other Infiltrating Neoplastic Disease Affecting the Sacrum (e.g., lymphoma)	533.X4rS/C	633.X4pR

XXVII-4 Sacral Spinal or Radicular Pain Attributable to Metabolic Bone Disease		S/C codes	R only/in addition
XXVII-4.1(S)(R)	Osteoporosis of Age	532.X5gS/C	632.X5gR
XXVII-4.2(S)(R)	Osteoporosis of Unknown Cause	532.X5hS/C	632.X5hR
XXVII-4.3(S)(R)	Osteoporosis of Some Unknown Cause Other than Age	532.X5iS/C	632.X5iR
XXVII-4.4(S)(R)	Hyperparathyroidism	532.X5jS/C	632.X5jR
XXVII-4.5(S)(R)	Paget's Disease of Bone	532.X5kS/C	632.X5kR
XXVII-4.6(S)(R)	Metabolic Disease of Bone Otherwise Not Classified	532.X5lS/C	632.X5lR

XXVII-5 Sacral Spinal or Radicular Pain Attributable to Arthritis		S/C codes	R only/in addition
XXVII-5.1(S)	Rheumatoid Arthritis of the Sacroiliac Joint	534.X3bS (S only)	
XXVII-5.2(S)	Ankylosing Spondylitis	532.X8aS (S only)	
XXVII-5.3(S)(R)	Seronegative Spondylarthropathy Not Otherwise Classified	523.X8aS/C	623.X8aR
XXVII-5.4(S)	Sacroiliitis (evident on bone scan)	532.X8gS (S only)	
XXVII-5.5(S)	Osteitis Condensans Ilii	532.X8uS (S only)	

XXVII-6 Spinal Stenosis: Cauda Equina Lesion		S/C codes	R only/in addition
XXVII-6(S)(R)	Spinal Stenosis: Cauda Equina Lesion	533.X6*S/C (back)	633.X6*R (legs)

XXVII-7 Sacral Spinal or Radicular Pain Associated with a Congenital Vertebral Anomaly		S/C codes	R only/in addition
XXVII-7(S)(R)	Sacral Spinal or Radicular Pain Associated with a Congenital Vertebral Anomaly	533.X0*S/C	533.X0*R 633.X0*R

* The asterisk is inserted in spinal and radicular codes where no letter is required in the sixth place.

XXVII-8 Pain Referred from Abdominal or Pelvic Viscera or Vessels Perceived as Sacral Spinal Pain		S/C codes	R only/in addition
XXVII-8.0	Dysmenorrhea (*see* XXIV-2 and XXIV-3) Endometriosis (*see* XXIV-4) Posterior Parametritis (*see* XXIV-5) Retroversion of the Uterus (*see* XXIV-7) Carcinoma of the Rectum (*see* XXIX-5.1)		
XXVII-8.1(S)	Irritation of Presacral Tissues by Blood	533.X6aS/C	
XXVII-8.2(S)	Irritation of Presacral Tissues by Contents of Ruptured Viscera	533.X6bS/C	

XXVII-9 Sacral Spinal Pain of Unknown or Uncertain Origin		S codes only	R only/in addition
XXVII-9(S)	Sacral Spinal Pain of Unknown or Uncertain Origin	5XX.X8*S	

XXVII-10 Sacroiliac Joint Pain		S codes only	R only/in addition
XXVII-10(S)	Sacroiliac Joint Pain	533.X6dS	

XXVIII. Coccygeal Pain Syndromes

XXVIII-1 Coccygeal Pain of Unknown or Uncertain Origin		S codes only	R only/in addition
XXVIII-1(S)	Coccygeal Pain of Unknown or Uncertain Origin	5XX.X8hS	

XXVIII-2 Posterior Sacrococcygeal Joint Pain			S codes only	R only/in addition
XXVIII-2(S)	Posterior Sacrococcygeal Joint Pain	Trauma Degenerative	533.X1pS 533.X6eS	

XXIX. Diffuse or Generalized Spinal Pain

XXIX-1 Generalized Spinal Pain Attributable to Multiple Fractures		S/C codes	R only/in addition
XXIX-1(S)	Generalized Spinal Pain Attributable to Multiple Fractures	933.X1*S/C	933.X1*R

XXIX-2 Generalized Spinal Pain Attributable to Disseminated Neoplastic Disease		S/C codes	R only/in addition
XXIX-2.1(S)	Disseminated Primary Tumors Affecting the Vertebral Column or Its Adnexa (e.g., multiple myeloma)	933.X4aS/C	933.X4aR
XXIX-2.2(S)	Disseminated Metastatic Tumors Affecting the Vertebral Column or Its Adnexa	933.X4bS/C	933.X4bR
XXIX-2.3(S)	Infiltrating Neoplastic Disease of the Vertebral Column or Its Adnexa, Other than Primary or Metastatic Tumors (e.g., lymphoma)	933.X4cS/C	933.X4cR

XXIX-3 Generalized Spinal Pain Attributable to Metabolic Bone Disease		S/C codes	R only/in addition
XXIX-3.1(S)	Osteoporosis of Age	933.X5aS/C	933.X5aR
XXIX-3.2(S)	Osteoporosis of Unknown Cause	933.X5bS/C	933.X5bR
XXIX-3.3(S)	Osteoporosis of Some Known Cause Other than Age	933.X5cS/C	933.X5cR

XXIX-3.4(S)	Hyperparathyroidism	933.X5dS/C	933.X5dR
XXIX-3.5(S)	Paget's Disease of Bone	933.X5eS/C	933.X5eR
XXIX-3.6(S)	Metabolic Disease of Bone Not Otherwise Classified	933.X5fS/C	933.X5fR

XXIX-4 Generalized Spinal Pain Attributable to Arthritis		S/C codes	R only/in addition
XXIX-4.1(S)	Rheumatoid Arthritis	932.X3aS/C	932.X3aR
XXIX-4.2(S)	Ankylosing Spondylitis	932.X3bS/C	932.X3bR
XXIX-4.3(S)	Osteoarthritis	932.X8*S/C	932.X8*R
XXIX-4.4(S)	Seronegative Spondylarthropathy Not Otherwise Classified	932.X8bS/C	932.X8bR

XXIX-5 Back Pain of Other Visceral or Neurological Origin Involving the Spine		S/C codes	R only/in addition
XXIX-5.1(S)	Carcinoma of the Rectum (code only) Pelvic pain Perineal pain	753.X4*S/C 853.X4*S/C	753.X4*R 853.X4*R
XXIX-5.2(S)	Tumor Infiltration of the Lumbosacral Plexus	502.X4dS/C	502.X4dR
XXIX-5.3(S)	Tumor Infiltration of the Sacrum and Sacral Nerves Nerve infiltration Musculoskeletal deposits (*See also* XXIX-5.1 and XXIX-5.2)	702.X4*S/C 732.X4*S/C	792.X4*R 732.X4*R

XXX. Low Back Pain of Psychological Origin with Spinal Referral		S codes only	R only/in addition
XXX-1(S)	Low Back Pain of Psychological Origin with Spinal Referral Tension Delusional Conversion Depression (*See also* I-16)	533.X7bS 51X.X9aS 51X.X9bS 51X.X9fS	

* The asterisk is inserted in spinal and radicular codes where no letter is required in the sixth place.

H. LOCAL SYNDROMES OF THE LOWER LIMBS

XXXI. Local Syndromes in the Leg or Foot: Pain of Neurological Origin	
1. Lateral Femoral Cutaneous Neuropathy (Meralgia Paresthetica)	602.X1a
2. Obturator Neuralgia	602.X6a (obturator hernia) 602.X1b (surgery) 602.X2a (inflammation) 602.X4a (neoplasm)
3. Femoral Neuralgia	602.X2b (inflammation) 602.X4b (neoplasm) 602.X6b (arthropathy)
4. Sciatica Neuralgia	602.X1c
5. Interdigital Neuralgia of the Foot (Morton's Metatarsalgia)	603.X1d
6. Injection Neuropathy (code only)	602.X5
7. Gluteal Syndromes	632.X1e
8. Piriformis Syndrome	632.X1f
9. Painful Legs and Moving Toes (*see* XI-5 for arms)	602.X8
10. Metastatic Disease	633.X4

11. Peroneal Muscular Atrophy (Charcot-Marie-Tooth Disease)
                Pain affecting joints only
 	
                Pain affecting the belly of the muscle
	
	203.X0 and 603.X0 (most often
	     203.60 and 603.60)
	205.X0 and 605.X0 (most often
	     205.60 and 605.60)

XXXII. Pain Syndromes of Hip and Thigh of Musculoskeletal Origin	
1. Ischial Bursitis	533.X3
2. Trochanteric Bursitis	634.X3d
3. Osteoarthritis of the Hip	638.X6b

XXXIII. Musculoskeletal Syndromes of the Lower Limbs	
1. Spinal Stenosis (*see* XXVII-6)	633.X6
2. Osteoarthritis of the Knee	638.X6c
3. Night Cramps	634.X8
4. Plantar Fasciitis	633.X3

PART II

DETAILED DESCRIPTIONS OF PAIN SYNDROMES

ITEMS USUALLY PROVIDED IN DESCRIPTIONS
OF PAIN SYNDROMES

Definition

Site

System(s)

Main Features   — prevalence, sex ratio if known, age of onset, pain quality, time pattern, occurrence in bouts or continuously, intensity, usual duration

Associated Symptoms   — aggravating and relieving agents

Signs

Laboratory Findings

Usual Course   — including treatment, if treatment contributes to diagnosis

Complications

Social and Physical Disability

Pathology   — or other contributing factors

Summary of Essential Features and Diagnostic Criteria

Criteria   — when available

Differential Diagnosis

Code(s)

References   — optional

A. RELATIVELY GENERALIZED SYNDROMES

GROUP I: RELATIVELY GENERALIZED SYNDROMES

Peripheral Neuropathy (I-1)

Definition
Constant or intermittent burning, aching, or lancinating limb pains due to generalized or focal diseases of peripheral nerves.

Site
Usually distal (especially the feet) with burning pain, but often more proximal and deep with aching. Focal with mononeuropathies, in the territory of the affected nerve (e.g., meralgia paresthetica).

System
Peripheral nervous system.

Main Features
Prevalence: common in neuropathies of diabetes, amyloid, alcoholism, polyarteritis, Guillain-Barré Syndrome (for which see I-36), neuralgic amyotrophy, Fabry's disease. *Age of Onset:* variable, usually after second decade. *Pain Quality:* (a) burning, superficial, distal pain often with dysesthesia, constant. May be in the territory of a single affected nerve; (b) deep aching, especially nocturnal, constant; and (c) sharp lancinating "tabetic" pains, especially in legs, intermittent.

Associated Symptoms
Sensory loss, especially to pinprick and temperature; sometimes weakness and muscle atrophy (especially in neuralgic amyotrophy); sometimes reflex loss; sometimes signs of loss of sympathetic function; smooth, fine skin; hair loss.

Laboratory Findings
(a) Features of the primary disease, e.g., diabetes; and (b) features of neuropathy: reduced or absent sensory potentials, slowing of motor and sensory conduction velocities, EMG evidence of muscle denervation.

Usual Course
Distal burning and deep aching pains are often longlasting, and the disease processes are relatively unresponsive to therapy. Pain resolves spontaneously in weeks or months in self-limited conditions such as Guillain-Barré syndrome or neuralgic amyotrophy.

Complications
Drug abuse, depression.

Social and Physical Disabilities
Decreased mobility.

Pathology
Nerve fiber damage, usually axonal degeneration. Pain especially occurs with small fiber damage (sensory fibers). Nerve biopsy may reveal the above, plus features of the specific disease process, e.g., amyloid.

Summary of Essential Features and Diagnostic Criteria
Chronic distal burning or deep aching pain with signs of sensory loss with or without muscle weakness, atrophy, and reflex loss.

Differential Diagnosis
Spinal cord disease, muscle disease.

Code
203.X2a	Arms: infective
203.X3a	Arms: inflammatory or immune reactions
203.X5a	Arms: toxic, metabolic, etc.
203.X8a	Arms: unknown or other
603.X2a	Legs: infective
603.X3a	Legs: inflammatory or immune reactions
603.X5a	Legs: toxic, metabolic, etc
603.X8a	Legs: unknown or other
X03.X4d	Von Recklinghausen's disease

References
Thomas, P.K., Pain in peripheral neuropathy: clinical and morphological aspects. In: J. Ochoa and W. Culp (Eds.), Abnormal Nerves and Muscles as Impulse Generators, Oxford University Press, New York, 1982.

Asburn, A.K. and Fields, H.L., Pain due to peripheral nerve damage: an hypothesis, Neurology, 34 (1984) 1587–1590.

Stump Pain (I-2)

Definition
Pain at the site of an extremity amputation.

Site
Upper or lower extremity at the region of amputation. Pain is not referred to the absent body part but is perceived in the stump itself, usually in region of transected nerve(s).

System
Peripheral nervous system; perhaps central nervous system.

Main Features
Sharp, often jabbing pain in stump, usually aggravated by pressure on, or infection in, the stump. Pain often

elicited by tapping over neuroma in transected nerve or nerves.

Associated Symptoms
Refusal to utilize prosthesis.

Signs
Pain elicited by percussion over stump neuromata.

Laboratory Findings
None.

Usual Course
Develops several weeks to months after amputation; persists indefinitely if untreated.

Relief
(a) Alter prosthesis to avoid pressure on neuromata; (b) resect neuromata so that they no longer lie in pressure areas; and (c) utilize neurosurgical procedures such as rhizotomy and ganglionectomy or spinal cord or peripheral nerve stimulation in properly selected patients.

Complications
Refusal to use prosthesis.

Social and Physical Disabilities
Severe pain can preclude normal daily activities; failure to utilize prosthesis can add to functional limitations.

Pathology
Neuroma at site of nerve transection.

Essential Features
Pain in stump.

Differential Diagnosis
Phantom limb pain, radiculopathy.

Code
203.X1a   Arms
603.X1a   Legs

Phantom Pain (I-3)

Definition
Pain referred to a surgically removed limb or portion thereof.

Site
In the absent body part.

System
Central nervous system.

Main Features
Follows amputation, may commence at time of amputation or months to years later. Varies greatly in severity

from person to person. Reports of prevalence vary from < 1% to > 50% of amputees. Believed to be more common if loss of limb occurs later in life, in limbs than in breast amputation, in the breast before the menopause rather than after it, and particularly if pain was present before the part was lost. Pain may be continuous, often with intermittent exacerbations. Usually cramping, aching, burning; may have superimposed shocklike components. Seems to be less likely if the initial amputation is treated actively and a prosthesis is promptly utilized. Phantom limb pain is almost always associated with distorted image of lost part.

Associated Symptoms
Aggravated by stress, systemic disease, poor stump health.

Signs
Loss of body part.

Usual Course
Complaints persist indefinitely; frequently with gradual amelioration over years.

Relief
No therapeutic regimen has more than a 30% long-term efficacy. TENS, anticonvulsants, antidepressants, or phenothiazines may be helpful. Sympathectomy or surgical procedures upon spinal cord and brain, including stimulation, are sometimes helpful.

Social and Physical Disabilities
May preclude gainful employment or normal daily activities.

Pathology
Related to deafferentation of neurons and their spontaneous and evoked hyperexcitability.

Essential Features
Pain in an absent body part.

Differential Diagnosis
Stump pain.

Code
203.X7a   Arms
603.X7a   Legs

Complex Regional Pain Syndromes (CRPS)

This title is being introduced to cover the painful syndromes which formerly were described under the headings of "Reflex Sympathetic Dystrophy" and "Causalgia." There has been dissatisfaction with the term "reflex sympathetic dystrophy" because not all the cases seem to have sympathetically maintained pain, and not all were dystrophic. The conditions usually follow injury which appears regionally and have a distal predominance of abnormal findings, exceeding the expected clinical course of the inciting event in both magnitude and duration and often resulting in significant impairment of motor function. The syndrome broadly corresponding to what was formerly described as reflex sympathetic dystrophy is now termed CRPS Type I (Reflex Sympathetic Dystrophy), and causalgia is described as CRPS Type II (Causalgia).

In the previous edition of this classification, causalgia was presented before reflex sympathetic dystrophy. However, because the present descriptions recognize that causalgia begins with a nerve injury but develops the signs of CRPS Type I as well, it has been felt better to give the description of CRPS Type I before that of causalgia. This means that the initial identifying numbers in the classification have been changed, CRPS Type I becoming syndrome I-4; CRPS Type II becoming syndrome I-5.

Sympathetically maintained pain (SMP) may be found in association with these syndromes. It is taken to be pain that is maintained by sympathetic efferent innervation or by circulating catecholamines. This is a feature of several types of painful conditions and is not an essential requirement of any one condition. It is understood that pain relieved by a specific sympatholytic procedure may be considered SMP. This does not imply a mechanism for the pain but simply follows the common clinical observation that in certain cases sympatholytic interventions will lead to a reduction of pain. It is also notable that a patient may have SMP and *sympathetically independent pain* (SIP) at the same time. SMP may occur in some patients with CRPS, but certainly does not occur in all.

Complex Regional Pain Syndrome, Type I (Reflex Sympathetic Dystrophy) (I-4)

Definition
CRPS Type I is a syndrome that usually develops after an initiating noxious event, is not limited to the distribution of a single peripheral nerve, and is apparently disproportionate to the inciting event. It is associated at some point with evidence of edema, changes in skin blood flow, abnormal sudomotor activity in the region of the pain, or allodynia or hyperalgesia.

Site
Usually the distal aspect of an affected extremity or with a distal to proximal gradient.

System
Peripheral nervous system; possibly the central nervous system.

Main Features
Pain often follows trauma, which is usually mild and is not associated with significant nerve injury. It may follow a fracture, a soft tissue lesion, or immobilization related to visceral disease, e.g., angina or stroke. The onset of symptoms usually occurs within one month of the inciting event. The pain is frequently described as burning and continuous and exacerbated by movement, continuous stimulation, or stress. The intensity of pain fluctuates over time, and allodynia or hyperalgesia may be found which are not limited to the territory of a single peripheral nerve. Abnormalities of blood flow occur including changes in skin temperature and color. Edema is usually present and may be soft or firm. Increased or decreased sweating may appear. The symptoms and signs may spread proximally or involve other extremities. Impairment of motor function is frequently seen.

Associated Symptoms and Signs
Atrophy of the skin, nails, and other soft tissues, alterations in hair growth, and loss of joint mobility may develop. Impairment of motor function can include weakness, tremor, and, in rare instances, dystonia. Symptoms and signs fluctuate at times. Sympathetically maintained pain may be present and may be demonstrated with pharmacological blocking or provocation techniques. Affective symptoms or disorders occur secondary to the pain and disability. Guarding of the affected part is usually observed.

Laboratory Findings
Noncontact skin temperature measurement indicates a side-to-side asymmetry of greater than 1°C. Due to the unstable nature of the temperature changes in this disorder, measurements at different times are recommended. Measurements of skin blood flow may show an increase or a reduction. Testing of sudomotor function, both at rest and evoked, indicates side-to-side asymmetry. The bone uptake phase of a three-phase bone scan may reveal a characteristic pattern of subcutaneous blood pool changes. Radiographic examination may demonstrate patchy bone demineralization.

Usual Course
Variable.

Relief
In cases with sympathetically maintained pain, sympatholytic interventions may provide temporary or permanent pain relief.

Complications
Phlebitis, inappropriate drug use, and suicide.

Social and Physical Impairment
Inability to perform activities of daily living and occupational and recreational activities.

Pathology
Unknown.

Diagnostic Criteria
1. The presence of an initiating noxious event, or a cause of immobilization.
2. Continuing pain, allodynia, or hyperalgesia with which the pain is disproportionate to any inciting event.
3. Evidence at some time of edema, changes in skin blood flow, or abnormal sudomotor activity in the region of the pain.
4. This diagnosis is excluded by the existence of conditions that would otherwise account for the degree of pain and dysfunction.

Note: Criteria 2–4 must be satisfied.

Differential Diagnosis
CRPS Type II (causalgia) unrecognized local pathology (e.g., fracture, strain, sprain), traumatic vasospasm, cellulitis, Raynaud's disease, thromboangiitis obliterans, thrombosis.

Code
203.X1h   Arms
603.X1h   Legs

Complex Regional Pain Syndrome, Type II (Causalgia) (I-5)

Definition
Burning pain, allodynia, and hyperpathia usually in the hand or foot after partial injury of a nerve or one of its major branches.

Site
In the region of the limb innervated by the damaged nerve.

Main Features
The onset usually occurs immediately after partial nerve injury but may be delayed for months. The nerves most commonly involved are the median, the sciatic, the tibial, and the ulnar. Causalgia of the radial nerve is very rare. Spontaneous pain occurs which is described as constant and burning, and is exacerbated by light touch, stress, temperature change or movement of the involved limb, visual and auditory stimuli (e.g., sudden sound or bright light), and emotional disturbances. The intensity of the pain may fluctuate over time, and allodynia/hyperalgesia occur but are not limited to the territory of a single peripheral nerve. Abnormalities in skin blood flow may develop including changes in skin temperature and skin color. Edema is usually present and may be soft or hard, and either hyperhidrosis or hypohidrosis may be present. The symptoms and signs may spread proximally, and infrequently may involve other extremities. Impairment of motor function is frequently seen.

Associated Symptoms and Signs
Atrophy of the skin, nails, and other soft tissues, alterations in hair growth, and loss of joint mobility may occur. Impairment of motor function may include weakness, tremor, and in rare instances dystonia. The symptoms and signs may fluctuate. Sympathetically maintained pain may be present. Affective disorders appear. Guarding of the affected part is usually found.

Laboratory Findings
Noncontact measurement of skin temperature indicates a side-to-side asymmetry of greater than 1.1°C. Because of the unstable nature of the temperature changes in this disorder, measurements at different times are recommended. Testing of sudomotor function both at rest and evoked indicates side-to-side asymmetry. The bone uptake phase with three-phase bone scan reveals a characteristic pattern of periarticular uptake. Radiographic examination may demonstrate patchy bone demineralization.

Usual Course
Variable.

Relief
In cases with sympathetically maintained pain, sympatholytic interventions may provide temporary or permanent pain relief.

Complications
Phlebitis, inappropriate drug use, and suicide.

Social and Physical Impairment
Inability to perform activities of daily living and occupational and recreational activities.

Pathology
Unknown.

Diagnostic Criteria
1. The presence of continuing pain, allodynia, or hyperalgesia after a nerve injury, not necessarily limited to the distribution of the injured nerve.
2. Evidence at some time of edema, changes in skin blood flow, or abnormal sudomotor activity in the region of the pain.
3. This diagnosis is excluded by the existence of conditions that would otherwise account for the degree of pain and dysfunction.

Note: All three criteria must be satisfied.

Differential Diagnosis

CRPS Type I (Reflex Sympathetic Dystrophy), unrecognized local pathology (e.g., fracture, strain, sprain), traumatic vasospasm, cellulitis, Raynaud's disease, thromboangiitis obliterans, thrombosis.

Code

207.X1h   Arms
607.X1h   Legs

Central Pain (I-6)

Definition

Regional pain caused by a primary lesion or dysfunction in the central nervous system, usually associated with abnormal sensibility to temperature and to noxious stimulation.

Site

The regional distribution of the pain correlates neuroanatomically with the location of the lesion in the brain and spinal cord. It may include all or most of one side, all parts of the body caudal to a level (like the lower half of the body), or both extremities on one side. It may also be restricted simply to the face or part of one extremity.

System

Central nervous system.

Main Features

Age of Onset: all ages may be affected. The onset may be instantaneous but usually occurs after a delay of weeks or months, rarely a few years, and the pain increases gradually. *Pain Quality:* many different qualities of pain occur, the most common being burning, aching, pricking, and lancinating. Often the patient experiences more than one kind of pain. Dysesthesias are common. The pain is usually spontaneous and continuous, and exacerbated or evoked by somatic stimuli such as light touch, heat, cold, or movement. Some patients have no pain at rest but suffer from evoked pain, paresthesias, and dysesthesias. The pain can be augmented by startle stimuli (e.g., sudden sound or light), by visceral activity (e.g., micturition), or by anxiety and emotional arousal. The pain may be superficial or deep. *Intensity:* varies from mild but irritating to intolerable.

Associated Symptoms and Signs

There may be various neurological symptoms and signs such as monoparesis, hemiparesis, or paraparesis, together with somatosensory abnormalities in the affected areas. Impaired sensibility for temperature and noxious stimulation are leading signs. Increased threshold for at least one modality is most common, and this is frequently accompanied by dysesthetic or painful reactions to somatic stimuli, particularly touch and cold. Such reactions commonly meet the criteria for allodynia, hyperalgesia, and hyperpathia. In some patients it is difficult to show the altered sensibility with standard clinical tests. The threshold for tactile, vibration, and kinesthetic sensibility may be increased or normal.

Laboratory Findings

MRI or CT may show a relevant lesion.

Usual Course

In some cases improvement occurs with time, but in most patients the pain persists.

Relief

TENS may give relief in a few patients but can also transiently exacerbate the pain. Anticonvulsant drugs help in some instances, especially carbamazepine and particularly for paroxysmal elements of the pain. Certain antidepressants (e.g., amitriptyline) seem to give the best relief, and some think that phenothiazines (e.g., chlorpromazine, fluphenazine) may be helpful.

Social and Physical Disabilities

This pain is a great physical and psychological burden to most patients. In consequence their social life and work are often much impaired. Allodynia in response to external stimuli and movements may hamper rehabilitation and prevent activities, thus making the patient physically handicapped.

Pathology

Cerebrovascular lesions (infarcts, hemorrhages), multiple sclerosis, and spinal cord injuries are the most common causes. Central pain is also common in syringomyelia, syringobulbia, and spinal vascular malformation, and may occur after operations like cordotomy. Increasing evidence indicates that central pain only occurs in patients who have lesions affecting the spino-thalamo-cortical pathways, which are important for temperature and pain sensibility. The lesion can be located at any level along the neuraxis, from the dorsal horn of the spinal cord to the cerebral cortex. The lesion sometimes may involve the medial lemniscal pathways.

Diagnostic Criteria

Regional pain attributable to a lesion or disease in the central nervous system and accompanied by abnormal sensibility for temperature and pain, most often hyperpathia.

Differential Diagnosis

Nociceptive, peripheral neurogenic, and psychiatric causes of pain should be excluded as far as possible. Sensory abnormalities will in most cases allow a diagnosis for positive reasons.

Code

If three or more major sites are involved, code first digit as 9:

903.X5c	Vascular
903.X1c	Trauma
903.X2c	Infection
903.X3c	Inflammatory
903.X4c	Neoplasm
903.X8c	Unknown

If only one or two sites are involved, code first digit according to specific site or sites; for example, for head or face, code 003.X5c.

Syndrome of Syringomyelia (I-7)

Definition

Aching or burning pain usually in a limb, commonly with muscle wasting due to tubular cavitation gradually developing in the spinal cord.

Site

Pain in shoulder, arm, chest, or leg, rarely in the face, occasionally bilateral.

System

Central nervous system.

Main Features

Pain is usually unilateral and continuous in an area that corresponds to the site of cavitation of spinal cord or brainstem, most frequently in the shoulder-girdle and arm. It may be a periodic diffuse dull ache but sometimes, and particularly when the pain is situated in forearm and hand, may have an intense burning quality. The pain may be severe and referred to deep structures in the limb, not responding to rest or minor sedation.

Associated Symptoms

Muscular weakness in affected region.

Signs

There is commonly muscle wasting beginning in small muscles of the hand and ascending to the forearm and shoulder-girdle with fasciculation and an early loss of tendon reflexes. Scoliosis kyphosis may occur. Characteristically, pain and temperature sensations are impaired but other sensations are intact. The area of sensory impairment typically has a shawl distribution over the front and back of the upper thorax. A Horner's syndrome may appear.

Usual Course

The disease usually begins in the second or third decade and slowly progresses.

Social and Physical Disability

The disease may be present for 15 to 20 years, progressing slowly, but still compatible with an active, self-supporting life. After 15 or 20 years the problems of pain, weakness, and general infirmity usually result in increasing invalidism, eventually leading to total dependency.

Pathology

A tubular cavitation develops slowly in the spinal cord, extending over many segments. The most common location is in the lower cervical cord near the central canal. There is loss of anterior horn cells and interruption of spinothalamic fibers. The cavity may be lined by a thick layer of glial tissue. Cavities may be bilateral and asymmetric and may communicate with an enlarged central canal. Ascent of the cavity into the brain stem produces syringobulbia. The canal may extend the entire length of the cord. Associated findings may be ectopic cerebellar tonsils, hydrocephalus, cerebellar hypoplasia, and astrocytoma or ependymoma of the spinal cord.

Essential Features

Pain in the relevant distribution of slowly progressing muscle weakness and wasting and impairment of sensation to pinprick and temperature, while other sensory modalities remain intact.

Differential Diagnosis

Other conditions which have to be considered are: (1) amyotrophic lateral sclerosis, (2) multiple sclerosis, (3) tumor of the spinal cord, (4) skeletal anomalies of the cervical spine, (5) platybasia, and (6) cervical spondylosis.

Code

007.X0	Face
207.X0	Arm
607.X0	Leg

Polymyalgia Rheumatica (I-8)

Definition

Diffuse aching, and usually stiffness, in neck, hip girdle, or shoulder girdle, usually associated with a markedly raised sedimentation rate, sometimes associated with giant cell vasculitis, and promptly responsive to steroids.

System

Musculoskeletal system.

Main Features

Incidence about 54 per 100,000 in those over 30 years of age. Deep muscular aching pain usually begins in the neck, shoulder girdle, and upper arms, but may only involve the pelvis and proximal parts of the thighs. Morning stiffness and stiffness after inactivity are prominent features.

Associated Symptoms
Malaise, fatigue, depression, low grade fever, weight loss, and giant cell arteritis.

Aggravating Factors
Movement.

Signs
No muscle tenderness or weakness.

Laboratory Findings
Anemia of chronic disease, raised sedimentation rate (usually greater than 50 mm/hour Westergren).

Relief
Dramatic response to oral corticosteroids, usually in low doses, e.g., 5–20 mg prednisone daily.

Complications
Blindness from giant cell arteritis.

Pathology
Giant cell vasculitis.

Essential Features
Diffuse pain with malaise, elevated sedimentation rate, response to steroids.

Diagnostic Criteria
1. Symmetrical proximal limb myalgia and severe stiffness.
2. Symptoms lasting longer than two weeks.
3. Age of onset: 50 years or older.
4. Erythrocyte sedimentation rate (Westergren) 40 mm or higher.
5. Morning stiffness exceeding one hour.

The diagnosis is to be made if three or more of the above criteria are present, or if one of the above criteria and pathologic evidence of giant cell arteritis is present.

Differential Diagnosis
Polymyositis, fibrositis, hyperthyroidism.

Code
X32.X3a

References
Bird H.A., Esselinkcz, W., Dixon, A.St.J., Mowat, A.G. and Wood, P.H.N., An evaluation of criteria for polymyalgia rheumatica, Ann. Rheum. Dis., 38 (1979) 434.

Ayoub, W.T., Franklin, C.M. and Torretti, D., Polymyalgia rheumatica: duration of therapy and long-term outcome, Am. J. Med., 37 (1985) 309.

Fibromyalgia (or Fibrositis) (I-9)

N.B.: We consider Myofascial Pain Syndrome (diffuse or not) to have a somewhat different meaning and think it adds confusion to use the term when discussing fibromyalgia.

Definition
Diffuse musculoskeletal aching and pain with multiple predictable tender points.

Site
Multiple anatomic areas.

System
Musculoskeletal system (muscles, ligaments, tendons, joints).

Main Features
Primary fibromyalgia, without important associated disease, is uncommon compared to concomitant fibromyalgia. It may occur in childhood but is most common in the fourth and fifth decades. The sex ratio is 6:1 female to male. Concomitant fibromyalgia occurs with any other musculoskeletal condition, where it may act to intensify the pain of the associated condition. The syndrome is chronic, and remissions are uncommon. *Pain:* Widespread aching of more than three months' duration, often poorly circumscribed and perceived as deep, usually referred to muscle or bony prominences. Most common areas are cervical, thoracic, and lumbar. Although pain in the trunk and proximal girdle is aching, distal limb pain is often perceived as associated with swelling, numbness, or stiff feeling. Day-to-day fluctuation in pain intensity and shifting from one area to another are characteristic, although the pain is usually continuous. Stiffness is present in 80% and is perceived as an increased resistance to joint movement, particularly toward the end of the range of movement. Both pain and stiffness are maximal within the broad sclerotomic and myotomic areas of reference of the lower segments of the cervical and lumbar spine. *Fatigue* is present in 80%, and is often severe enough to interfere with daily activities. Sleep disturbance is present in 75%, and waking is unrefreshed or tired. *Multiple tender points:* Discrete local areas of deep tenderness widely dispersed throughout the body and involving a variety of otherwise normal tissues are a pathognomonic feature provided about 60% of examined sites are tender. Tender points are found within muscle and over tendons, muscle insertions, and bony prominences. Tender point sites are "tender" in many normal individuals but are reported as "painful," often with grimace or withdrawal when palpated, in those with fibromyalgia. The predictable location of these tender points and their multiplicity are essential features of the syndrome.

Associated Symptoms and Signs

Paresthesias: Most often involving the upper extremities, are found in 60%.

Headaches: Noted in 53%.

Irritable Bowel Syndrome: Noted in 30%.

Anxiety: Noted in 48%.

Skinfold Tenderness: The rolling of the skin and subcutaneous tissues of the upper scapula region between the examiner's thumb and index finger elicits tenderness in 60%.

Reactive Hyperemia: Redness of the skin developing after palpation of tender points over the trapezius and contiguous regions is found in half the patients.

Autonomic Phenomena: Reactive hyperemia is the most commonly recognized feature, but temperature changes and mild soft tissue swelling involving the distal upper extremities are also frequently reported.

Aggravating and Relieving Features

Cold, poor sleep, anxiety, humidity, weather change, fatigue, and mental stress intensify symptoms in 60–70%. Symptoms are typically made worse or brought on by prolonged or vigorous work activity. Warmth (78%) temporarily improves symptoms.

Signs

Tender points, widely and symmetrically distributed, are the characteristic sign of the syndrome. They are not found in other musculoskeletal syndromes.

Relief

Relief may be provided by reassurance and explanation about the nature of the syndrome and possible mechanisms of pain: anxiety may thus be reduced, expensive and hazardous investigations and treatments limited, and use of medication reduced. Low dose amitriptyline, cyclobenzaprine, and aerobic exercise have been shown, in placebo controlled double blind studies, to improve symptoms.

Pathology

Nonspecific muscle changes have been found in some biopsy studies. Blood flow during exercise is reduced, and decreased oxygen uptake in muscles has been noted. Two studies have found increased levels of substance P in the cerebrospinal fluid of patients. In general, these findings, some of which may be secondary phenomena, have been insufficient to explain the major signs and symptoms of the syndrome.

Etiology

Unknown. The syndrome may begin in childhood or early life without obvious association. It also is noted frequently following trauma, and has been known to develop after apparent viral illness. Finally, it may appear insidiously in later life. Thus the syndrome may be the final common pathway, perhaps as hyperalgesia, for a number of causative factors. Trauma or degenerative changes in the cervical or lumbar regions might precipitate the syndrome. Intrinsic changes in levels of neurotransmitters might play a factor. A syndrome similar to fibromyalgia can be induced temporarily with experimental reduction in non-REM sleep. Low grade symptoms may be increased by mental stress or fatigue. An association with *previous* major depression in patients and families has suggested a genetic factor.

Classification Criteria for Primary and Concomitant Fibromyalgia (from Wolfe et al. 1990)

1. History of Widespread Pain

Definition

Pain is considered widespread when all of the following are present: pain in the left side of the body, pain in the right side of the body, pain above the waist and below the waist. In addition, axial skeletal pain (cervical spine or anterior chest or thoracic spine or low back) must be present. In this definition, shoulder and buttock pain is considered as pain for each involved side. "Low back" pain is considered lower segment pain.

2. Pain in 11 of 18 Tender Point Sites on Digital Palpation

Definition

Pain, on digital palpation, must be present in at least 11 of the following 18 tender point sites:

Occiput: bilateral, at the suboccipital muscle insertions.
Low Cervical: bilateral, at the anterior aspects of the intertransverse spaces at C5–C7.
Trapezius: bilateral, at the midpoint of the upper border.
Supraspinatus: bilateral, at origins above the scapula spine near the medial border.
Second Rib: bilateral, at the second costochondral junctions, just lateral to the junctions on upper surfaces.
Lateral Epicondyle: bilateral, 2 cm distal to the epicondyles.
Gluteal: bilateral, in upper outer quadrants of buttocks in anterior fold of muscle.
Greater Trochanter: bilateral, posterior to the trochanteric prominence.
Knees: bilateral, at the medial fat pad proximal to the joint line.

Digital palpation should be performed with an approximate force of 4 kg.

For a tender point to be considered "positive," the subject must state that the palpation was painful. "Tender" is not to be considered painful.

For classification purposes, patients will be said to have fibromyalgia if both criteria are satisfied. Widespread pain must have been present for at least three months. The presence of a second clinical disorder does not exclude the diagnosis of fibromyalgia.

Code
X33.X8a

References
Wolfe, F., Smythe, H.A., Yunus, M.B., et al., The American College of Rheumatology 1990 criteria for the classification of fibromyalgia: report of the Multicenter Criteria Committee, Arthritis Rheum., 33 (1990) 160 172.

Bennett, R.M. and Goldenberg, D.L. (Eds.), The fibromyalgia syndrome, Rheumatic Disease Clinics of North America, vol. 15, no. 1, WB Saunders, Philadelphia, 1989.

Note: Specific Myofascial Pain Syndromes

Synonyms: fibrositis (syndrome), myalgia, muscular rheumatism, nonarticular rheumatism.

Specific myofascial syndromes may occur in any voluntary muscle with referred pain, local and referred tenderness, and a tense shortened muscle. The pain has the same qualities as that of the diffuse syndromes. Passive stretch or strong voluntary contraction in the shortened position of the muscle is painful. Satellite tender points may develop within the area of pain reference of the initial trigger point. Other phenomena resemble those of the diffuse syndromes. Diagnosis depends upon the demonstration of a trigger point (tender point) and reproduction of the pain by maneuvers which place stress upon proximal structures or nerve roots. This suggests that the syndrome is an epiphenomenon secondary to proximal pathology such as nerve root irritation. Relief may be obtained by stretch and spray techniques, tender point compression, or tender point injection including the use of "dry" needling.

Some individual syndromes are described here, e.g., sternocleidomastoid and trapezius. Others may be coded as required according to individual muscles that are identified as being a site of trouble.

Rheumatoid Arthritis (I-10)

Definition
Aching, burning joint pain due to systemic inflammatory disease affecting all synovial joints, muscle, ligaments, and tendons in accordance with diagnostic criteria below.

Site
Symmetrical involvement of small and large joints.

System
Musculoskeletal system and connective tissue.

Main Features
Diffuse aching, burning pain in joints, usually moderately severe; usually intermittent with exacerbations and remissions. The condition affects about 1% of the population and is more common in women. Diagnostic criteria of the American Rheumatism Association describe and further define the illness. They are as follows: (1) morning stiffness, (2) pain on motion or tenderness at one joint or more, (3) swelling of one joint, (4) swelling of at least one other joint, and (5) symmetrical joint swelling.

All of the above have to be of at least six weeks' duration. Further criteria include: (6) subcutaneous nodules, (7) typical radiographic changes, (8) positive test for rheumatoid factor in the serum, (9) a poor response in the mucin clot test in the synovial fluid, (10) synovial histopathology consistent with rheumatoid arthritis, and (11) characteristic nodule pathology.

Classical rheumatoid arthritis requires seven criteria to be diagnosed. Definite rheumatoid arthritis may be diagnosed on five criteria, and probable rheumatoid arthritis on three criteria.

Associated Symptoms
Morning stiffness usually greater than half an hour's duration; chronic fatigue. Inflammation may affect eyes, heart, lungs.

Signs
Tenderness, swelling, loss of range of motion of joints, ligaments, tendons. Chronic destruction and joint deformity are common.

Laboratory Findings
Anemia, raised ESR (erythrocyte sedimentation rate), rheumatoid factor in the serum in the majority of cases.

Relief
Usually good relief of pain and stiffness can be obtained with nonsteroidal anti-inflammatory drugs, but some patients require therapy with gold or other agents.

Pathology
Chronic inflammatory process of synovium, ligaments, or tendons. There may be systemic vasculitis.

Essential Features
Aching, burning joint pain with characteristic pathology.

Diagnostic Criteria
1. Morning stiffness in and around joints lasting at least one hour before maximal improvement.

2. Simultaneous soft tissue swelling or fluid in at least three joint areas observed by a physician. The 14 possible areas are right or left proximal interphalangeal joints (PIP), metacarpal phalangeal (MCP), wrist, elbow, knee, ankle, and metatarsal phalangeal joints (MTP).

3. At least one area of soft tissue swelling or effusion in a wrist, MCP, or PIP joint.

4. Symmetrical arthritis. Simultaneous involvement of the same joint areas as defined in 2 above in both sides of the body (bilateral involvement of PIP, MCP, or MTP is acceptable without absolute symmetry).

5. Rheumatoid nodules.

6. Positive serum rheumatoid factor, demonstrable by any method for which any result has been positive in less than 5% of normal control subjects.

7. Radiographic changes typical of rheumatoid arthritis on posterior-anterior hand and wrist radiographs; this must include erosions or unequivocal bony decalcification which is periarticular.

A patient fulfilling four of these seven criteria can be said to have rheumatoid arthritis. Criteria 1–4 must have been present for at least six weeks.

Differential Diagnosis
Systemic lupus erythematosus, palindromic rheumatism, mixed connective tissue disease, psoriatic arthropathy, calcium pyrophosphate deposition disease, seronegative spondyloarthropathies, hemochromatosis (rarely).

Code
X34.X3a

Reference
Arnett, F.C., Edworthy, S.M., Bloch, D.A., et al., The American Rheumatism Association 1987 revised criteria for the classification of rheumatoid arthritis, Arthritis Rheum., 31 (1988) 315–324.

Osteoarthritis (I-11)

Definition
Deep, aching pain due to a "degenerative" process in a single joint or multiple joints, either as a primary phenomenon or secondary to other disease.

Site
Joints most commonly involved are distal and proximal interphalangeal joints of the hands, the carpo-metacarpal thumb joint, the knees, the hips, and cervical and lumbar spines. Many joints or only a few joints may be affected, e.g., at C5 or L5, the hip or knee; proximal joints may be involved alone or only distal interphalangeal joints.

System
Musculoskeletal system.

Main Features
There is deep, aching pain which may be severe as the disease progresses. The pain is felt at the joint or joints involved but may be referred to adjacent muscle groups. Usually the pain increases in proportion to the amount of use of the joint. As the disease progresses there is pain at rest and later nocturnal pain. The pain tends to become more continuous as the severity of the process increases. Stiffness occurs after protracted periods of inactivity and in the morning but lasts less than half an hour as a rule.

There is a discrepancy between radiological prevalence and clinical complaints. Radiological evidence of osteoarthritis occurs in 80% of individuals over 55 years of age. Only about 25% of those with radiographic changes report symptoms. The incidence increases with age. There is a greater prevalence relatively in men under the age of 45 compared with women, and in women over the age of 45 compared with men.

Aggravating Features
Use, fatigue.

Signs
Clinically, joint line tenderness may be found and crepitus on active or passive joint motion; noninflammatory effusions are common. Later stage disease is accompanied by gross deformity, bony-hypertrophy, contracture. X-ray evidence of joint space narrowing, sclerosis, cysts, and osteophytes may occur.

Laboratory Findings
None specific.

Usual Course
Initially there is pain with use and minimal X-ray and clinical findings. Later pain becomes more prolonged as the disease progresses and nocturnal pain occurs. The course is one of gradually progressive pain and deformity.

Relief
Some have relief with nonsteroidal anti-inflammatory agents or with non-narcotic analgesics. Joint rest in the early stages relieves the pain. Occasional relief in the early phases may appear from intra-articular steroids.

Physical Disability
Progressive limitation of ambulation occurs in large weight-bearing joints.

Pathology
This is loosely described as a "degenerative" disease of articular cartilage.

Essential Features
Deep, aching pain associated with the characteristic "degenerative" changes in joints.

Diagnostic Criteria

No official diagnostic criteria exist for osteoarthritis, although criteria have been proposed for osteoarthritis of the knee joint.

Noninflammatory arthritis of one or several diarthrodial joints, occurring in the absence of any known predisposing cause, with loss of cartilage and/or bony sclerosis (or osteophyte formation) demonstrable by X-rays.

Differential Diagnosis

Calcium pyrophosphate deposition disease; presence of congenital traumatic, inflammatory, endocrinological, or metabolic disease to which the osteoarthritis may be secondary.

Code

X38.X6a

Calcium Pyrophosphate Dihydrate Deposition Disease (CPPD) (I-12)

Definition

Attacks of aching, sharp, and throbbing pain with acute or chronic recurrent inflammation of a joint caused by calcium pyrophosphate crystals.

Site

Usually one joint, sometimes more, often alternating. Knees, wrists, and metacarpo-phalangeal joints are most frequent sites.

System

Musculoskeletal system.

Main Features

The disorder occurs clinically in about 1 in 1000 adults, more often in the elderly, but radiology shows the presence of the disease in 5% of adults at the time of death. There are four major clinical presentations: (1) *pseudogout:* acute redness, heat, swelling, and severe pain which is aching, sharp, or throbbing in one or a few joints; the attacks last from 2 days to several weeks, with freedom from pain between attacks; (2) *pseudorheumatoid arthritis:* marked by deep aching and swelling in multiple joints, with attacks lasting weeks to months; (3) *pseudo-osteoarthritis*: see the description of osteoarthritic features; and (4) *pseudarthritis with acute attacks*: the pain being the same as in osteoarthritis but with superimposed acute painful swollen joints.

Signs

Aspiration of calcium pyrophosphate crystals from the joint is diagnostic. X-rays show calcification in the cartilage of the wrists, knees, and symphysis pubis.

Relief

Acute attacks respond well to nonsteroidal anti-inflammatory drugs, with or without local corticosteroid injections.

Complications

Chronic disabling arthritis.

Associated Disorders

Hyperparathyroidism, hemochromatosis. There may be hereditary, sporadic, or metabolic causes.

Pathology

Acute and chronic inflammation or degeneration.

Diagnostic Criteria

1. Demonstration of CPPD crystals in tissues or synovial fluid by definitive means such as X-ray diffraction.
2. Crystals compatible with CPPD demonstrable by compensated polarized light microscopy.
3. Typical calcifications seen on roentgenograms.

A definite diagnosis can be made if 1 above is present, or if 2 and 3 are present. A probable diagnosis can be made if 2 or 3 is present.

Differential Diagnosis

Gout, infection, palindromic rheumatism, osteoarthritis.

Code

X38.X0 or X38.X5a

Reference

Ryan, L.M. and McCarty, D.J., Calcium pyrophosphate crystal deposition disease: pseudogout articular chondrocalcinosis. In: D.J. McCarty (Ed.), Arthritis and Allied Conditions, 10th ed., Lea & Febiger, Philadelphia, 1985, pp. 1515–1546.

Gout (I-13)

Definition

Paroxysmal attacks of aching, sharp, or throbbing pain, usually severe and due to inflammation of a joint caused by monosodium urate crystals.

Site

First metatarso-phalangeal joints, midtarsal joints, ankles, knees, wrists, fingers, or elbows.

Main Features

More common in men in the fourth to sixth decades of life and in postmenopausal women. Acute severe paroxysmal attacks of pain occur with redness, heat, swelling, and tenderness, usually in one joint. The pain is aching, sharp, and throbbing. The patient is often unable to accept the weight of bedclothes on the joint and unable to bear weight on the affected joint. Attacks last two days to several weeks in duration.

Associated Symptoms
In the acute phase, patients may be febrile and have leukocytosis.

Aggravating Factors
Trauma, alcohol ingestion, surgery, starvation.

Signs
Redness, heat, and tender swelling of the joint, which may be extremely painful to move. Intracellular urate crystals aspirated from the joint are diagnostic.

Laboratory Findings
Serum urate may vary during the acute attack. Leukocytosis and raised sedimentation rate are seen during the attack.

Usual Course
Initially the disorder is monoarticular; in 50% of patients the first metatarso-phalangeal joint is involved in the great toe. Acute attacks are separated by variable symptom-free intervals. Attacks may become polyarticular and recur at shorter intervals and may eventually resolve incompletely leaving chronic, progressive crippling arthritis.

Relief
Responds well to nonsteroidal anti-inflammatory agents, intravenous colchine, and local steroid injections.

Complications
Renal calculi, tophaceous deposits, and chronic arthritis with joint damage.

Pathology
Acute inflammatory response induced by uric acid crystals.

Essential Features
Paroxysmal joint pains with sodium monourate deposition.

Diagnostic Criteria
1. Demonstration of intracellular sodium urate monohydrate crystals in synovial fluid leukocytes by polarizing microscopy or other acceptable methods of identifying crystals.
2. Demonstration of sodium urate monohydrate crystals in an aspirate or biopsy of a tophus by methods similar to those in 1.
3. In the absence of specific crystal identification, a history of monoarticular arthritis followed by an asymptomatic intercritical period, rapid resolution of synovitis following Colchicine administration, and the presence of hyperuricemia.

Any one of the three above is sufficient to make the diagnosis.

Differential Diagnosis
Calcium pyrophosphate deposition disease, infection, palindromic rheumatism.

Code
X38.X5b

Reference
Holmes, E.W., Clinical gout and the pathogenesis of hyperuricemia. In: D.J. McCarty (Ed.), Arthritis and Allied Conditions, 10th ed., Lea & Febiger, Philadelphia, 1985, pp. 1445–1480.

Hemophilic Arthropathy (I-14)

Definition
Bouts of acute, constant, nagging, burning, bursting, and incapacitating pain or chronic, aching, nagging, gnawing, and grating pain occurring in patients with congenital blood coagulation factor deficiencies and secondary to hemarthrosis.

Site
The most common joints affected initially are the knees, ankles, and elbows. Shoulders, hips, and wrist joints are affected next most often. As the first joints become progressively affected, other remaining articular and muscle areas are involved with changes of disuse atrophy or progressive hemorrhagic episodes.

System
Musculoskeletal system.

Main Features
Prevalence: hemophilic joint hemorrhages occur in severely and moderately affected male hemophiliacs. They only rarely occur in female Factor VIII and Factor IX carriers and in homozygous severely affected patients with von Willebrand's disease. Acute hemarthrosis occurs most commonly in the juvenile in association with minor trauma. In the adult, spontaneous hemorrhages and pain occur in association also with minor or severe trauma. Characteristically the acute pain is associated with such hemarthrosis, which is relieved by replacement therapy and rest of the affected limb. A reactive synovitis results from repeated hemarthroses, which may be simply spontaneous small recurrent hemorrhages. The pain associated with them is extremely difficult to treat because of the underlying inflammatory reaction.

Time Course: The acute pain is marked by fullness and stiffness and constant nagging, burning, or bursting qualities. It is incapacitating and will cause severe pain for at least a week depending upon the degree of intracapsular swelling and pressure. It will recur episodically from the causes indicated. Chronic pain is often a dull ache, worse with movement, but can be debilitating, gnawing, and grating. At the stage of destructive joint changes the chronic pain is unremitting and relieved mainly by rest and analgesics. These syndromes are exacerbated by accompanying joint and muscle degeneration due to lack of mobility rather than repeated hemorrhages.

Associated Symptoms
Depressive or passive/aggressive symptoms often accompany hemorrhages and are secondary to the extent of pain or to the realization of vulnerability to hemorrhage, which is beyond the control of the hemophiliac. If bleeding occurs into a muscle or potential space, e.g., retroperitoneal and iliopsoas muscle, this can mimic joint hemorrhage and can cause severe nerve compression syndromes, e.g., of the femoral nerve. Numerous psychosomatic complaints are associated with the chronic and acute pain of chronic synovitis, arthritis, and hemarthrosis.

Signs
Reactive Synovitis: There is a chronic swelling of the joint with a "boggy" consistency to the swelling, which is tender to palpation. Marked limitation of joint movement often with signs of adjacent involvement of muscle groups due to disuse atrophy. *Chronic Joint Degeneration:* Severe bony remodeling with decrease in joint movement, adjacent muscular atrophy with subsequent fixation of the joint and loss of effective use.

Laboratory Findings
X-rays with the large hemarthrosis show little except for soft tissue swelling. In reactive synovitis there is often evidence of osteoporosis accompanied by overgrowth of the epiphyses but not evidence of joint destruction. In chronic arthropathy there is cartilage destruction and narrowing of the joint space. Gross misalignment of the joint surfaces progresses. Cysts, rarefactions, subcondylar cysts, and an overgrowth of the epiphysis are noted. This progresses through to fibrous joint contracture, loss of joint space, extensive enlargement of the epiphysis, and substantial disorganization of the joint structures. The articular cartilage shows extensive degeneration with fibrillation and eburnated bone ends.

Usual Course
Until the availability of therapy with blood clotting factor concentrate, there was an inexorable deterioration of the affected joints following the initial repeated spontaneous hemarthroses in the severely affected individual. This joint deterioration was associated with pain as described in the section regarding time course. The introduction of concentrated clotting factor transfusions has avoided the consequence of repeated acute severe hemarthroses. However, it is by no means certain whether the pain pattern of chronic synovitis and arthritis can be avoided or merely delayed using such therapy. Therapy

with blood clotting factor concentrate is available on a regular basis only in North America and Europe at this time.

Relief
Acute Hemarthrosis: Adequate intravenous replacement with appropriate coagulation factors with subsequent graded exercise and physiotherapy will provide good relief. Aspiration of the joint will be necessary under coagulation factor cover if there is excessive intracapsular pressure. Analgesics are required for acute pain management. *Reactive and Chronic Hemarthrosis:* Prophylactic factor replacement is required in association with analgesics and carefully selected anti-inflammatory agents, e.g., steroids or ibuprofen. Pain control using analgesics and transcutaneous nerve stimulation is also useful, and physiotherapy is of considerable assistance in managing both symptoms and signs. Synovectomy may be of use for the control of pain secondary to the recurrent bleeding. *Chronic Destructive Arthropathy:* Replacement therapy is of little assistance in relieving pain and disability. Carefully selected anti-inflammatory agents and rest are the major therapies of use. Physiotherapy after control of acute symptoms is useful. Joint replacement is a final choice for chronic pain management.

Complications
Analgesic abuse is a common problem in hemophilia due to the acute and chronic pain syndromes associated with hemophilic arthropathy. This problem can be avoided in the younger age group by not using narcotic analgesics for chronic pain management and relying upon principles of comprehensive hemophilia care. These include regular physiotherapy, exercise, and making full use of available social and professional opportunities.

Social and Physical Disability
Severe crippling and physical disability, with prolonged school and work absences, have traditionally been associated with this form of arthropathy. Consequently, affected individuals have not been able to achieve satisfactory school and job schedules. It is considered that the higher suicide rate is related not only to the family and psychosocial aspects of the disease but also to the chronic pain syndromes that these individuals experience.

Pathology
This depends upon the phase of the disorder. Generally two pathologic phases are associated with the hemophilic joint. Phase one involves an early synovial soft tissue reaction caused by intraarticular bleeding. Synovial hypertrophy with hemosiderin deposition and mild perivascular inflammation are present. Cartilage degeneration and joint degeneration similar to that seen in osteoarthritis and rheumatoid arthritis is seen in the

second-phase joint. Associated with this type of phase two change is synovial thickening and hyperplasia which falls into numerous folds and clusters of villi. The amount of hemosiderin deposited is increased compared to phase one.

Summary of Essential Features and Diagnostic Criteria

Acute and chronic pain as the result of acute hemarthrosis with chronic synovial cartilaginous and bony degeneration is exacerbated by spontaneous and trauma-related hemorrhage.

Diagnostic Criteria

Pain associated with hemophiliac arthropathy must satisfy both 1 and 2.

1. Spontaneous intracapsular hemorrhages in an individual with an inherited hemostatic defect.
2. Demonstrable synovial bleeding with or without bony joint contour abnormalities.

Differential Diagnosis

In the presence of a severe (less than 0.01 units/ml) hemophilic factor deficiency, no other diagnosis is possible. In the mildly affected individual (greater than 0.05 units/ml), all other causes of degenerative arthritis, particularly in the older affected individual, must be considered.

Code

X34.X0a

References

Arnold, W.D. and Hilgartner, M.W., Haemophilia arthropathy: current concepts of pathogenesis and management, J. Bone Joint Surg., 59A (1977) 287–305.

Duthie, R.B., Matthews, J.M., Rizza, C.R. and Steele, W.M., The Management of Musculoskeletal Problems in the Hemophiliac, 1st ed., Blackwell, Oxford, 1972.

Hilgartner, M.W., Hemophiliac arthropathy. Adv. Paediatr., 21 (1975) 139–165.

Hoskinson, J. and Duthie, R.B., Management of musculoskeletal problems in the hemophiliac. Orthop. Clinics North Amer., WB Saunders, Philadelphia, 1978, pp. 455–480.

Burns (I-15)

Definition

Acute and severe pain at first, following burns, later continuous with exacerbations, gradually declining.

Site

Anywhere on the body surface and deep to it.

System

Usually only epidermis and/or dermis, but any system may be involved.

Main Features

Prevalence: is approximately 3 per 1000 of population. Ten percent of these will require hospital admission. Any age can be affected, but the highest incidence (18%) is between 20 and 29 years. Children are the next largest group, with 30% of these being in the 1–2 year age group. *Sex Ratio:* approximately 1:1, but 3:2 males to females in children.

Pain Quality: initially the pain is acute and intense. It is frequently described as throbbing, smarting, and stinging, and marked exacerbations of stabbing pain occur with any movement or procedure. Thus, it is particularly intense where there are skin creases or flexures or where pressure is applied, such as palms, soles, genitalia, ears, or resting surfaces. This applies especially to partial thickness burns. Despite the destruction of all cutaneous nerve endings, full thickness burns are often painful with a quality described as deep, dull, or aching.

Intensity and Duration: the pain tends to diminish in intensity as healing takes place. In addition, the quality of the pain changes, and at one to two weeks after the burn is usually described as sore, aching, tender, tiring, and tight. After three or four weeks it is described as itchy or tingling. These descriptions also apply to pain at donor sites. Pain is exacerbated by procedures such as "tanking" for the removal of eschar, and physiotherapy. In addition, frequent surgery is often necessary, with an accompanying increase in pain. Relief may be promoted by the use of opioid premedication prior to procedures, time-contingent analgesics, inhalational analgesia during procedures, ensuring that the burnt areas never dry out, protecting the burn with creams, and achieving skin cover by some means as soon as possible.

Associated Symptoms

Dyspnea may occur as a result of smoke inhalation. Disuse may lead to causalgia-like symptoms.

Usual Course

Tends to settle with skin healing. Burnt areas may be tender and sore for up to a year. Itch and irritation may continue for two or three weeks.

Complications

If healing occurs, it is unusual to have persistent pain unless deep structures (muscle, bones, major nerves) are involved. Cellulitis in burnt areas or donor sites may lead to a marked increase in the severity of pain.

Social and Physical Disability

This is most frequent where the burn is extensive, and such cases often require sustained treatment and prolonged hospitalization. Psychological treatment is also needed where scars affect the patient's ability to function socially or physically, for example, as a result of scars of the hands, face, or genitalia.

Pathology

Loss of skin integrity with consequent loss of fluid and thermoregulation and an increased likelihood of infection. Burns are classified in three degrees of severity based on burn depth. A superficial burn involves the epidermis only. A partial thickness burn involves epidermis and dermis at varying depths, and a full thickness burn involves epidermis, dermis, and at times deeper tissues. Electrical burns may cause considerable damage to deeper tissues by direct effect and by occlusion of blood vessels. The severity of damage is related to the temperature to which the area was exposed, the duration of exposure, and the thickness of the skin involved. The agents responsible may be thermal, electrical, or chemical.

Summary of Essential Features and Diagnostic Criteria

Pain with the appropriate time course following burns.

Differential Diagnosis

Possibly hysterical conversion pain or pain of psychological origin may prolong or exacerbate the original effects of the injury. This may be more important in work-related injuries or where there is litigation.

Code

X42.X1 or X82.X1

Pain of Psychological Origin: Muscle Tension Pain (I-16.1)

Definition

Virtually continuous pain in any part of the body due to sustained muscle contraction and provoked by emotional causes or by persistent overuse of particular muscles.

Site

Any region with pain reference from voluntary muscle.

System

Central nervous system (psychological and social).

Main Features

Prevalence: often diagnosed. Even approximate prevalence is unknown. *Sex Ratio:* females more than males, 4:1 in those who consult doctors. *Age of Onset:* from age 8 onward, usually before age 30. *Start:* gradual emergence intermittent at first, as mild diffuse ache or unpleasant feeling, increasing to a definite pain part of the time. Fluctuation during the day is typical. These exacerbations seem to emerge after several years of lesser headache. *Pain Quality:* dull ache, usually does not throb; severe during exacerbations, often or almost always with throbbing. Some describe tight bands or gripping headache. They may be a minority. Others describe pressure sensations. *Occurrence and Duration:* most days per week, usually every day for most of the day. Occasionally in long-standing severe cases pain may wake the patient from sleep. *Precipitants and Exacerbating Factors:* emotional stress, anxiety and depression, physical exercise, alcohol.

Associated Symptoms

Many patients have anxiety, depression, irritability, or more than one of these combined.

Signs

Muscle tenderness occurs but may also be found in other conditions and in normal individuals.

Relief

Resolution or treatment of emotional problems, anxiety, or depression often diminishes symptoms. Relaxation treatment helps. Anxiolytics may help but should be avoided since some patients become depressed and others develop dependence. Tricyclic antidepressants are frequently very useful. Analgesics help only a little.

Complications

Analgesics, narcotic, and other drug abuse.

Social and Physical Disability

Reduction of activities and of work.

Pathology

Unsettled.

Differential Diagnosis

From delusional and conversion pains; from muscle spasm provoked by local disease; and from other causes of dysfunction in particular regions, e.g., migraine, post-traumatic headache, cervical spine disorders, depression, hallucinatory headache, and conversion hysteria.

Code

X33.X7b

Note: "b" coding used to allow the "a" coding to be employed if an acute syndrome needs to be specified.

Pain of Psychological Origin: Delusional or Hallucinatory (I-16.2)

Definition

Pain of psychological origin and attributed by the patient to a specific delusional cause.

Site

Any part of the body. May be symmetrical, e.g., in a fronto-temporal-occipital ring distribution, or in one place, e.g., at vertex, precordial, genital.

Main Features

Prevalence: rare; estimated to be present in less than 2% of patients with chronic pain without lesions. *Age of Onset:* not apparently reported in children; onset in late adolescence or at any time in adult life. *Pain Quality:* may be sensory or affective or both, not necessarily bizarre; essential characteristic is attribution of the pain by the patient to a specific delusional cause, e.g., to a crown of thorns in a patient who had messianic delusions. *Time Pattern:* in accordance with the delusion. *Intensity:* from mild to severe. *Usual Duration:* in accordance with the causal psychological illness.

Associated Symptoms and Modifying Factors

May be exacerbated by psychological stress, relieved by treatment causing remission of illness. No physical signs or laboratory findings.

Complications

In accordance with causal condition; usually lasts for a few weeks in manic-depressive or schizo-affective psychoses, may be sustained for months or years in established schizophrenia if resistant to treatment. Occasionally chronic pain without any formal delusions remits to be succeeded by a paranoid or schizophrenic psychosis.

Social and Physical Disabilities

In accordance with the mental state and its consequences. Drug addiction not reported.

Etiology

Manic-depressive, schizophrenic, or possibly other psychoses.

Essential Features

Those required for diagnosis are pain, without a lesion or overt physical mechanism and founded upon a delusional or hallucinatory state.

Differential Diagnosis

From undisclosed or missed lesions in psychotic patients, or migraine, giving rise to delusional misinterpretations; from tension headaches; from hysterical, hypochondriacal, or conversion states.

Code

X1X.X9a

Note: X = to be completed individually according to circumstances in each case.

Pain of Psychological Origin: Hysterical, Conversion, or Hypochondriacal (I-16.3)

Definition

Pain specifically attributable to the thought process, emotional state, or personality of the patient in the absence of an organic or delusional cause or tension mechanism.

Site

May be symmetrical; if lateralized, possibly more often on the left precordium, genitals; may be at any single point over the cranium or face, can involve tongue or oral cavity or any other body region. Usually diffuse in fronto-temporo-occipital region or in maxillary area.

Main Features

Prevalence: true population prevalence unknown. Frequency increases from general practice populations to specialized headache or pain clinics or psychiatric departments. Estimates of 11% and 43% have been found in psychiatric departments, depending on the sample. *Sex Ratio:* estimated female to male ratio 2:1 or greater—particularly if multiple complaints occur. *Onset:* may be at any time from childhood onward but most often in late adolescence. *Pain Quality:* described mostly in simple sensory terms, but complex or affective descriptions occur in some cases. *Time Pattern:* Pain is usually continuous throughout most of the waking hours but fluctuates somewhat in intensity, does not wake the patient from sleep. *Duration:* usually lasts for more than six months.

Associated Symptoms

Loss of function without a physical basis (anesthesia, paralyses, etc.) may be present. Pain is often present in other areas. There may be frequent visits to physicians to obtain relief despite medical reassurance, or excessive use of analgesics as well as other psychotropic drugs for complaints of depression, neither type of remedy proving effective. The pain may have a symbolic significance, e.g., identifying the patient with someone who died of brain tumor. Psychological interpretations are frequently not acceptable to the patient, although emotional conflict may have provoked the condition. These patients tend to marry but have poor marital relationships.

La belle indifference can occur but is not common. Depressive complaints and resentment are more frequent. The personality is often of a dependent-histrionic-labile type ("hysterical personality" or "passive dependent personality"). A history of past conversion symptoms is helpful in diagnosis.

There are three overlapping types in this category. The first is largely *monosymptomatic,* is relatively rare, and consists of patients who have pain in one or two regions only, who have only recently developed pain, and who have clear evidence of emotional conflicts, perhaps with an associated paralysis or anesthesia, and a relatively good prognosis. Some patients who primarily have a depressive illness also present with pain as the main somatic symptom. Their pain may be interpreted delusionally or may be based on a tension pain, etc., or may be hysterical.

The second type is of patients with more numerous or *multiple complaints,* often of many and varied types without a physical basis. In the history these often number more than 10, including classical conversion or pseudoneurological symptoms (paralyses, weakness, impairment of special senses, difficulty in swallowing, etc.), gastrointestinal, cardiovascular (palpitations, shortness of breath), disturbances in sexual function (impaired libido, reduced potency), etc., as well as pains in different parts.

In the third, or *hypochondriacal,* subtype, the patient presents excessive concern or fear of the symptoms and a conviction that disease is present despite thorough physical examination, appropriate investigation, and careful reassurance. There may also be other signs of preoccupation with somatic health, e.g., great anxiety over constipation, the color of the urine, etc.

As emphasized, the subtypes overlap. The most common pattern in pain clinics is the second one described. A hypochondriacal pattern may be observed either alone or with the first or the second subtype, more often with the second. In all types, physical treatments (manipulation, physiotherapy, surgery) tend to produce brief improvements which are not maintained. In the second and third types, a disorder of emotional development is often present.

Note: Depressive pain has been distributed among the above three types and also into the delusional and tension pain groups. This is done because there does not seem to be a single mechanism for pain associated with depression, even though such pain is frequent. The words "depressive pain" as indicating a particular type or mechanism should be avoided.

Aggravating Factors
Emotional stress may be a predisposing factor and is almost always important in the monosymptomatic type. Experience of physical illness or pain due to emotional stress in person or in a family member or close associate may be a predisposing factor.

Usual Course
Usually chronic in the first subtype. In relatively acute monosymptomatic conditions, environmental change

and sometimes individual psychotherapy may promote recovery.

Complications
Dependence on minor tranquilizers; salicylate addiction; narcotic addiction; drug-induced confusional states; excessive investigations; unsuccessful surgery, sometimes repeatedly.

Social and Physical Disability
Often associated with marital disharmony, inability to sustain regular employment, sometimes loss of function or limbs due to surgery.

Essential Features
Pain without adequate organic or pathophysiological explanation. Separate evidence other than the prime complaint to support the view that psychiatric illness is present. Proof of the presence of psychological factors in addition by virtue of both of the following: (1) an appropriate and important relationship in time exists between the onset or exacerbation of the pain and an emotional conflict or need, and (2) the pain enables the individual to avoid some activity that is unwelcome to him or her or to obtain support from the environment that otherwise might not be forthcoming.

The condition must not be attributable to any psychiatric disorder other than the following, and it should conform to the requirements for the diagnoses of Dissociative [conversion] Disorders (F44) or Somatoform Disorder (F45) in the International Classification of Diseases, 10th edition, or to those for somatization disorder (300.81) or conversion disorder (300.11), somatoform pain disorder (307.80), or hypochondriasis (300.70) in the American Psychiatric Association Diagnostic and Statistical Manual, 3rd edition revised (DSM-III-R).

Differential Diagnosis
(1) From physical causes of pain, e.g., tumor, acromegaly, Paget's disease of bone, etc.; (2) from physical illnesses that may present with multiple, often diffuse symptoms, e.g., hypothyroidism, hyperparathyroid-ism, disseminated lupus erythematosis, multiple sclerosis, porphyria; (3) from schizophrenia, endogenous depression, reactive depression, or major depressive disorder according to DSM-III-R, from pain of psychological origin associated with depression; and (4) from tension pain, particularly headache. The differential diagnosis from tension headache usually will be based on one or more of the following: (a) the level of observed anxiety is not sufficient to account for tension which might produce the symptom; (b) the personality conforms to the hysterical or hypochondriacal pattern and the complaint to an acute conflict situation or to a pattern of multiple symptoms; and (c) relaxation exercises and sedation do not provide relief.

Code
X1X.X9b

References
International Classification of Diseases, 10th ed., World Health Organization, Geneva, 1992

Diagnostic and Statistical Manual, 3rd ed., Revised, American Psychiatric Association, Washington, D.C., 1987.

Pain of Psychological Origin: Associated with Depression (I-16.4)

Definition
Pain occurring in the course of a depressive illness, usually not preceding the depression and not attributable to any other cause.

Site
Any part of the body; may be symmetrical, e.g., in a fronto-temporal occipital ring distribution, or in one place, e.g., at vertex, precordial, low back, genital.

Main Features
Prevalence: probably common. Likely to appear in the majority of patients with an independent depressive illness, more often in nonendogenous depression, and less often in illness with an endogenous pattern. *Sex Ratio:* more common in females. *Pain Quality:* may be sensory or affective, or both, not necessarily bizarre; worse with intercurrent stress, increased anxiety. The pain may occur at the site of previous trauma (accidental or surgical) and may therefore be confused with a recurrence of the original condition. Usually aching or throbbing, may be described as sharp. May have both sensory and affective components. *Intensity:* varies from mild to severe. *Duration* and intensity often in accordance with the length and severity of the depression.

Associated Symptoms
Anxiety and irritability are common.

Signs
Tenderness may occur, but may also be found in other conditions and in normal individuals.

Relief
Improvement in the pain occurs with the improvement of the depression. The response to psychological treatments or antidepressants is better than to analgesics.

Social and Physical Disability
Reduction of activities and work.

Etiology
A link with reductions in cerebral monoamines or monoamine receptors has been suggested.

Differential Diagnosis
Muscle tension pain with depression, delusional, or hallucinatory pain; in depression or with schizophrenia, muscle spasm provoked by local disease; and other causes of dysfunction in particular regions, e.g., migraine, post-traumatic headache, cervical spine disorders, hysterical or hypochondriacal pain.

It is important not to confuse the situation of depression causing pain as a secondary phenomenon with depression which commonly occurs when chronic pain arising for physical reasons is troublesome.

Code
X1X.X9d

Note: Unlike muscle contraction pain, hysterical pain, or delusional pain, no clear mechanism is recognized for this category. If the patient has a depressive illness with delusions, the pain should be classified under Pain of Psychological Origin: Delusional or Hallucinatory. If muscle contraction predominates and can be demonstrated as a cause for the pain, that diagnosis may be preferred. Patients with anxiety and depression who do not have evident muscle contraction may have pain in this category. Previously, depressive pain was distributed between other types of pain of psychological origin, including delusional and tension pain groups and hysterical and hypochondriacal pains. The reason for this was the lack of a definite mechanism with good supporting evidence for a separate category of depressive pain. While the evidence that there is a specific mechanism is still poor, the occurrence of pain in consequence of depression is common, and was not adequately covered by the alternative categories mentioned.

Reference
Magni, G., On the relationship between chronic pain and depression when there is no organic lesion, Pain, 31 (1987) 1–21.

A Note on Factitious Illness and Malingering (I-17)

Factitious illness is of concern to psychiatrists because both it and malingering are frequently associated with personality disorder. Physicians in any discipline may encounter the problem in differential diagnosis. No coding is given for pain in these circumstances because it will be either induced by physical change or counterfeit. In the first instance it can be coded under the appropriate physical heading. In the second case, the complaint of pain does not represent the presence of pain. ICD-10 does not appear to provide a code for malingering, which suggests that the final application of the label of malingering is a judicial (legal) process and not a medical one. The role of the doctor in this task may be limited to drawing attention to discrepancies and inconsistencies in the history and clinical findings.

Regional Sprains or Strains (I-18)

Code
X33.X1d

Sickle Cell Arthropathy (I-19)

Code
X34.X0c

Purpuric Arthropathy (I-20)

Code
X34.X0d

Stiff Man Syndrome (I-21)

Code
934.X8

Paralysis Agitans (I-22)

Code
902.X7

Epilepsy (I-23)

Code
X04.X7

Polyarteritis Nodosa (I-24)

Code
X5X.X3

Psoriatic Arthropathy and Other Secondary Arthropathies (I-25)

Code
X34.X8c

Painful Scar (I-26)

Code
X4X.X1b

Systemic Lupus Erythematosis, Systemic Sclerosis and Fibrosclerosis, Polymyositis, and Dermatomyositis (I-27)

Code
X33.X3b

Infective Arthropathies (I-28)

Code
X33.X3c

Traumatic Arthropathy (I-29)

Code
X33.X1a

Osteomyelitis (I-30)

Code
X32.X2f

Osteitis Deformans (I-31)

Code
X32.X5b

Osteochondritis (I-32)

Code
X32.X5c

Osteoporosis (I-33)

Code
X32.X5d

Muscle Spasm (I-34)

Code
X37.X7

Local Pain, No Cause Specified (I-35)

Code
X7X.XXa or X3X.X8e

Guillain-Barré Syndrome (I-36)

Definition
Pain arising from an acute demyelinating neuropathy.

Site
Back, extremities, abdomen.

System
Peripheral nervous system, musculoskeletal system.

Main Features
Deep aching pain involving the low back region, buttocks, thighs, and calves is common (> 50%) in the first week or two of the illness. Pain may also occur in the shoulder girdle and upper extremity but is less frequent. Beyond the first month, burning tingling extremity pain occurs in about 25% of patients.

Note: While in the Guillain-Barré syndrome weakness typically occurs first in the feet and the legs and then later in the arms, the worst pain is in the low back, buttocks, thighs, and calves.

Associated Symptoms
During the acute phase there may be muscle pain and pains of cramps in the extremities associated with muscle tenderness. Constipation can produce lower abdominal and pelvic pain.

Signs
Extremity weakness and areflexia are essential features of the neuropathy. Back and leg pain are commonly exacerbated by nerve root traction maneuvers such as straight-leg raising.

Laboratory Findings
EMG evidence of demyelination (conduction block) and secondary axonal degeneration. Cerebrospinal fluid shows elevated protein with relatively normal cell count.

Usual Course
Aching back and extremity pain, sometimes of a severe nature, usually resolves over the first four weeks. Dysesthetic extremity pain persists indefinitely in 5–10% of patients.

Relief
Acetaminophen or nonsteroidal anti-inflammatory drugs for mild to moderate pain. Opioid analgesics for severe pain—continuous parenteral infusion or epidural administration may be required. Active and passive exercise program. Bowel stimulants to prevent constipation. Padding to prevent pressure palsies.

Complications
Persistent weakness and contractures from incomplete recovery. Ulnar and peroneal pressure palsies from immobilization.

Pathology
Peripheral nerve demyelination with secondary axonal degeneration.

Differential Diagnosis
Pain secondary to neuropathies stimulating Guillain-Barré syndrome: porphyria, diphtheritic infection, toxic neuropathies (e.g., lead, solvent abuse such as glue sniffing).

Code
901.X3

B. RELATIVELY LOCALIZED SYNDROMES OF THE HEAD AND NECK

GROUP II: NEURALGIAS OF THE HEAD AND FACE

Trigeminal Neuralgia (Tic Douloureux) (II-1)

Definition
Sudden, usually unilateral, severe brief stabbing recurrent pains in the distribution of one or more branches of the Vth cranial nerve.

Site
Strictly limited to the distribution of the Vth nerve; unilateral in about 95% of the cases. Usually involves one branch; may involve two or, rarely, even all three branches. The second, third, and first branches of the Vth cranial nerve are involved in the foregoing order of frequency. The pain is more frequent on the right side.

System
Nervous system.

Main Features
Prevalence: relatively rare. *Incidence:* men 2.7, women 5.0 per 100,000 per annum in USA. Most patients have a lesion compressing the nerve where it leaves the brain stem. In patients with multiple sclerosis, there is also an increased incidence of tic douloureux. *Sex Ratio:* women affected perhaps more commonly than men. *Age of Onset:* after fourth decade, with peak onset in fifth to seventh decades; earlier onset does occur, but onset before age 30 is uncommon. *Pain Quality:* sharp, agonizing electric shock–like stabs or pain felt superficially in the skin or buccal mucosa, triggered by light mechanical contact from a more or less restricted site (trigger point or trigger zone), usually of brief duration—a few seconds (but reportedly occasionally up to 1–2 minutes)—followed by a refractory period of up to a few minutes. *Time Pattern:* paroxysms may occur at intervals or many times daily or, in rare instances, succeed one another almost continuously. Periodicity is characteristic, with episodes occurring for a few weeks to a month or two, followed by a pain-free interval of months or years and then recurrence of another bout. *Intensity:* extremely severe, probably one of the most intense of all acute pains.

Precipitation
Pain paroxysms can be triggered by trivial sensations from various trigger zones, that is, areas with increased sensitivity, which are located within the area of trigeminal innervation. The trigger phenomenon can be elicited by light touch, shaving, washing, chewing, etc.

Associated Symptoms and Signs
Occasionally, a mild flush may be noted during paroxysms. In true trigeminal neuralgia, apart from the trigger point, gross neurological examination is usually negative; in many patients, however, careful sensory testing to light touch will show a subtle sensory loss. No particular aggravating factors.

Relief
From carbamazepine, diphenyl hydantoin, and baclofen. If medical measures fail, radio-frequency treatment of the ganglion or microsurgical decompression of the trigeminal root are appropriate.

Usual Course
Recurrent bouts over months to years, interspersed with more or less prolonged asymptomatic phases.

Complications
Usually none. During exacerbations, nourishment may be a (transitory) problem.

Social and Physical Disability
Only as related to the recurrent pain episodes.

Pathology
When present, always involves the peripheral trigeminal (primary afferent) neuron. Impingement on the root by vascular loops, etc., appears to be the most common cause. Demyelination and hypermyelination on electron microscopy.

Essential Features
Unilateral, sudden, transient, intense paroxysms of superficially located pain, strictly confined to the distribution of one or more branches of the trigeminal nerve, usually precipitated by light mechanical activation of a trigger point. No sensory or reflex deficit detectable by routine neurologic testing.

Differential Diagnosis
Must be differentiated from symptomatic trigeminal neuralgia due to a small tumor such as an epidermoid or small meningioma involving either the root or the ganglion. Sensory and reflex deficits in the face may be detected in a significant proportion of such cases. Differential diagnosis between trigeminal neuralgia of mandibular division and glossopharyngeal neuralgia may, in rare instances, be difficult. Jabs and Jolts syndrome ("multiple jabs," "ice-pick pain"). SUNCT syndrome.

Code
006.X8a

References
Fromm, G.H. (Ed.), The Medical and Surgical Management of Trigeminal Neuralgia, Future Publishing Company, Mount Kisco, N.Y., 1987.

Loeser, J.D., Tic douloureux and atypical face pain. In: P.D. Wall and R. Melzack (Eds.), Textbook of Pain, 3rd ed., Churchill Livingstone, Edinburgh, 1994, pp. 699–710.

Rovit, R.L., Murali, R. and Jannetta, P.J., Trigeminal Neuralgia, Williams & Wilkins, Baltimore, 1990.

Secondary Neuralgia (Trigeminal) from Central Nervous System Lesions (II-2)

Definition
Sudden, severe, brief, stabbing recurrent pains in the distribution of one or more branches of the Vth cranial nerve, attributable to a recognized lesion such as tumor or aneurysm.

Site
Usually limited to distribution of trigeminal nerve.

System
Nervous system.

Main Features
Prevalence: rare; probably less than 2% of cases of tic douloureux. *Sex Ratio:* not remarkable. *Age of Onset:* corresponds to that of appearance of tumors. *Pain Quality:* paroxysmal pain may be indistinguishable from "true" tic douloureux. Nonparoxysmal pain of dull or more constant type may occur. *Time Pattern:* may mimic tic douloureux. Attack pattern may be less typical with longer-lasting paroxysms or nonparoxysmal pain. *Intensity:* may be as severe as in tic douloureux. *Usual Duration:* indeterminate.

Associated Symptoms and Signs and Laboratory Findings
Sensory changes (hypoesthesia in trigeminal area) or loss of corneal reflex. Motor deficit is difficult to detect until late phase. X-ray, CAT scan, or MRI may reveal mass lesion in Meckel's cave or in pontine cistern.

Relief
Surgical intervention directed to the underlying cause. Occasionally, partial relief from drugs for "essential" trigeminal neuralgia.

Usual Course
Progression, usually very gradual.

Complications
Related to location of tumor.

Social and Physical Disability
Related to painful episodes and neurologic deficit when present.

Pathology
Meningioma of Meckel's cave, epidermoid cyst, and less frequently vascular malformation (arterio-venous aneurysm or tortuous basilar artery) of cerebello-pontine angle are among the most frequent causes of this rare condition.

Essential Features
Paroxysmal neuralgia in the trigeminal innervation zone, with one or more atypical features such as hyperesthesia or depression of corneal reflex, or longer-lasting paroxysms.

Differential Diagnosis
"Essential" trigeminal neuralgia.

Code
006.X4	Tumor
006.X0	Aneurysm
002.X2b	Arnold-Chiari syndrome: congenital; code only

References
Rovit, R.L., Murali, R. and Jannetta, P.G., Trigeminal Neuralgia, Williams & Wilkins, Baltimore, 1990.

Secondary Trigeminal Neuralgia from Facial Trauma (II-3)

Definition
Chronic throbbing or burning pain with paroxysmal exacerbations in the distribution of a peripheral trigeminal nerve subsequent to injury.

Site
Maxillofacial region.

System
Nervous system.

Main Features
Prevalence: 5–10% following facial fractures; common after reconstructive orthognathic surgery; 1–5% after removal of impacted teeth. *Pain Quality:* biphasic with sharp, triggered paroxysms and dull throbbing or burning background pain. *Occurrence:* constant with triggered episodes. *Intensity:* moderate. *Duration:* constant.

Signs
Tender palpable nodules over peripheral nerves; neurotrophic effects.

Usual Course
Progressive for six months, then stable until treated with microsurgery, graft-repair reanastomosis; transcutaneous stimulation and anticonvulsant pharmacotherapy.

Social and Physical Disabilities
Impaired mastication and speech.

Pathology
Neuromata; deafferentation, hypersensitivity.

Differential Diagnosis
Idiopathic trigeminal neuralgia, secondary trigeminal neuralgia from intracranial lesions, postherpetic neuralgia, odontalgia, musculoskeletal pain.

Code
006.X1

Acute Herpes Zoster (Trigeminal) (II-4)

Definition
Pain associated with acute herpetic lesions in the distribution of a branch or branches of the Vth cranial nerve.

Site
Face. Pain limited to distribution of trigeminal nerve (usually first division).

System
Trigeminal nerve.

Main Features
Prevalence: infrequent. *Sex Ratio:* not remarkable. *Age of Onset:* adults, more common in middle and old age. *Pain Quality:* burning, tingling pain with occasional lancinating components felt in the skin. *Time Pattern:* pain usually precedes the onset of herpetic eruption by one or two days (preherpetic neuralgia); may develop coincident with or after eruption. *Intensity:* severe. *Usual Duration:* one to several weeks.

Associated Symptoms
May be general malaise, low fever, headaches.

Signs and Laboratory Findings
Clusters of small cutaneous vesicles, almost invariably in the distribution of the ophthalmic distribution of the trigeminal. Frequently associated with lymphoma in treatment. Elevated protein and pleocytosis in spinal fluid.

Usual Course
Spontaneous and permanent remission. In the older age group, progression to chronic (postherpetic) neuralgia is not uncommon.

Complications
Acute glaucoma and corneal ulceration due to vesicles have been reported.

Social and Physical Disability
Related to cosmetic aspects and to pain.

Pathology
Small cell infiltrates in affected skin and bullous cutaneous changes. Similar infiltrates in ganglion and root entry zone.

Summary of Essential Features and Diagnostic Criteria
Herpetic vesicular eruption in distribution of first division of trigeminal nerve. History of burning pain in the perieruptive period.

Differential Diagnosis
Syndrome is usually unmistakable. Often related to impaired resistance, e.g., in the elderly or in the presence of carcinomatous metastases.

Code
002.x2a

Postherpetic Neuralgia (Trigeminal) (II-5)

Definition
Chronic pain with skin changes in the distribution of one or more roots of the Vth cranial nerve subsequent to acute herpes zoster.

Site
Face. Usually distribution of first (ophthalmic) division.

System
Trigeminal nerve.

Main Features
Prevalence: relatively infrequent. *Age of Onset:* sixth and later decades. *Sex Ratio:* more common in males. *Quality:* burning, tearing, itching dysesthesias and crawling dysesthesias in skin of affected area. Exacerbated by mechanical contact. *Time Pattern:* Constantly present with exacerbations. May last for years but spontaneous subsidence is not uncommon. *Intensity:* usually moderate, but constancy and intractability in many instances, contribute to intolerable nature of complaint. *Usual Duration:* months to years.

Associated Symptoms
Depression, irritability.

Signs and Laboratory Findings
Cutaneous scarring, loss of normal pigmentation in area of earlier herpetic eruption. Hypoesthesia to touch, hypoalgesia, hyperesthesia to touch, and hyperpathia may occur.

Usual Course
Chronic, intractable, may last for years. Some cases "burn out" spontaneously.

Complications
None.

Social and Physical Disability
Severe impairment of most or all social activities due to constant pain. Suicide occasionally.

Pathology
Loss of many large fibers in affected sensory nerve. Chronic inflammatory changes in trigeminal ganglion and demyelination in root entry zone.

Summary of Essential Features and Diagnostic Criteria
Chronic burning, dysesthesias, paresthesias, and intractable cutaneous pain in distribution of the ophthalmic division of the trigeminal associated with cutaneous scarring and history of herpetic eruption in an elderly patient.

Differential Diagnosis
The syndrome is usually characteristic. Other conditions, e.g., metastatic carcinoma under treatment, may promote its occurrence.

Code
003.X2b

Geniculate Neuralgia (VIIth Cranial Nerve): Ramsay Hunt Syndrome (II-6)

Definition
Severe lancinating pains felt deeply in external auditory canal subsequent to an attack of acute herpes zoster.

Site
External auditory meatus with retroauricular radiation.

System
The sensory fibers of the facial nerve.

Main Features
Prevalence: rare; few cases in world literature. *Sex ratio:* no data. *Pain Quality:* sharp, lancinating, shocklike pains felt deeply in external auditory canal. *Intensity:* severe.

Signs and Laboratory Findings
Usually follows an eruption of herpetic vesicles which appear in the concha and over the mastoid.

Complications
None.

Social and Physical Disability
Only as related to the pain episodes.

Pathology
No reported case with pathological examination.

Summary of Essential Features and Diagnostic Criteria
Onset of lancinating pain in external meatus several days to a week or so after herpetic eruption on concha.

Differential Diagnosis
Differentiate from otic variety of glossopharyngeal neuralgia, which does not have herpetic prodromata.

Code
006.X2

Neuralgia of the Nervus Intermedius (II-7)

Note: This condition is admittedly very rare and is presented as a tentative category about which there is still some controversy.

Definition
Sudden, unilateral, severe, brief, stabbing, recurrent pain in the distribution of the nervus intermedius.

Site
In ear canal, deep in ear, and in posterior pharynx.

System
Nervous system.

Main Features
Prevalence: very rare. Probably .03 per 100,000 per annum in USA. *Sex Ratio:* women equal to men. *Age of Onset:* fifth to seventh decade most common. *Pain Quality:* sharp agonizing electric shock–like stabs of pain felt in the ear canal, middle ear, or posterior pharynx, usually of brief duration, often with a refractory period after multiple jabs of pain. *Time Pattern:* paroxysms may occur at intervals or may occur in a brief

flurry. Periodicity is characteristic, with episodes occurring for weeks or months, and then months or years without any pain. *Intensity:* extremely severe; probably one of the most intense of all acute pains.

Precipitation
Pain paroxysms can be triggered by non-noxious stimulation from the posterior pharynx or ear canal.

Associated Signs and Symptoms
None.

Relief
From carbamazepine and baclofen. Or from surgical procedures: microsurgical decompression of the nervus intermedius or section of the nerve.

Usual Course
Recurrent bouts over months to years, interspersed with asymptomatic phases.

Complications
Usually none.

Social and Physical Disability
Related to recurrent pain episodes.

Pathology
Most patients have impingement on the nervus intermedius at its root entry zone.

Essential Features
Unilateral, sudden, transient, intense paroxysms of electric shock–like pain in the ear or posterior pharynx. No sensory or motor deficit is detectable by routine neurologic testing.

Differential Diagnosis
Must be differentiated from tic douloureux involving the Vth nerve, glossopharyngeal neuralgia, and geniculate neuralgia of the VIIth nerve due to herpes zoster.

Code
006.X8c

Reference
Furlow, L.P., Tic douloureux of the nervus intermedius, JAMA, 119 (1942) 255

Glossopharyngeal Neuralgia (IXth Cranial Nerve) (II-8)

Definition
Sudden severe brief stabbing recurrent pains in the distribution of the glossopharyngeal nerve.

Site
Tonsillar fossa and adjacent area of fauces. Radiation to external auditory canal (otic variety) or to neck (cervical variety).

System
Peripheral and central mechanisms involving glossopharyngeal nerve fibers.

Main Features
Prevalence: very rare. *Incidence:* 0.5 per 100,000 per annum in USA. Sharp, stabbing bouts of severe pain, often triggered by mechanical contact with faucial area on one side, also by swallowing and by ingestion of cold or acid fluids. *Pain Quality:* sharp, stabbing bursts of high-intensity pain, felt deep in throat or ear. *Time Pattern:* episodic bouts occurring spontaneously several times daily or triggered by any of above mentioned stimuli. *Intensity:* very severe, interferes with eating. *Usual Duration:* episodes last for weeks to a month or two and subside spontaneously. Tendency to recurrence is common.

Associated Symptoms
Cardiac arrhythmia and syncope may occur during paroxysms in some cases.

Signs and Laboratory Findings
The important and only sign is the presence of a trigger point, usually on fauces or tonsil; sometimes it may be absent.

Usual Course
Fluctuating; bouts of pain interspersed by prolonged asymptomatic periods.

Complications
Transitory cardiac arrhythmias, as noted.

Social and Physical Disability
Only as related to pain episodes.

Pathology
Unknown. Vascular loops impinging on roots may be a cause.

Summary of Essential Features and Diagnostic Criteria
Paroxysmal bursts of sharp, lancinating pain, spontaneous or evoked by mechanical stimulation of tonsillar area, often with radiation to external ear or to angle of jaw and adjacent neck. Application of local anesthetic to tonsil (or trigger point) relieves pain.

Differential Diagnosis
Usually characteristic syndrome. May be confused with trigeminal neuralgia limited to mandibular division.

Code
006.X8b

Neuralgia of the Superior Laryngeal Nerve (Vagus Nerve Neuralgia) (II-9)

Definition
Paroxysms of unilateral lancinating pain radiating from the side of the thyroid cartilage or pyriform sinus to the angle of the jaw and occasionally to the ear.

Site
Unilateral, possibly more on the left in the neck from the side of the thyroid cartilage or pyriform sinus to the angle of the jaw and occasionally to the ear.

System
Nervous system.

Main Features
Prevalence: rare. May be a variant of glossopharyngeal neuralgia, which has also been called vago-glossopharyngeal neuralgia. Combined ratio of vago-glossopharyngeal neuralgia to trigeminal neuralgia is about 1:80. *Sex Ratio:* about equal. *Pain Quality:* usually severe, lancinating pain often precipitated by talking, swallowing, coughing, yawning, or stimulation of the nerve at its point of entrance into the larynx. Mild forms do occur.

Associated Symptoms
Local tenderness. Possibly autonomic phenomena, e.g., salivation, flushing; possibly tinnitus and vertigo.

Signs
Presence of a trigger zone.

Laboratory Findings
None.

Relief
Relief from analgesic nerve block, alcohol nerve block, or nerve section.

Complications
Loss of weight.

Social and Physical Disability
As related to pain episodes.

Pathology
There may be a history of local infection. A large styloid process or calcified stylohyoid ligament may be contributory (cf. Eagle's syndrome).

Essential Features
Sudden attacks of unilateral lancinating pain in the area of the thyroid cartilage radiating to the angle of the jaw and occasionally to the ear.

Differential Diagnosis
Glossopharyngeal neuralgia, carotidynia, local lesions, e.g., carcinoma.

Code
006.X8e

Occipital Neuralgia (II-10)

Definition
Pain, usually deep and aching, in the distribution of the second cervical dorsal root.

Site
Suboccipital area, unilateral in the second cervical root distribution from occiput to vertex. May radiate still farther forward, see below.

System
Nervous system.

Main Features
Prevalence: quite common; no epidemiological data; most often follows acceleration-deceleration injuries. *Sex Ratio:* women more frequently affected, but statistical data lacking. *Age of Onset:* from second decade to old age; more common in third to fifth decades. *Pain Quality:* deep, aching, pressure pain in suboccipital area, sometimes stabbing also. Unilateral usually; may radiate toward vertex or to fronto-orbital area and/or face. *Time Pattern:* irregular, usually worse later in day. *Intensity:* from moderate to severe.

Associated Symptoms
Hyperesthesia of scalp. A variety of symptoms such as vertigo, tinnitus, tears, etc., have been described in some cases, but these are probably transitional forms to cluster headache. Nerve block may give effective relief.

Signs and Laboratory Findings
Diminished sensation to pinprick in area of C2 and tenderness of great occipital nerve may be found.

Usual Course
Chronic, recurrent episodes. May cease spontaneously on occasion.

Complications
None.

Social and Physical Disability
Only as related to pain episodes.

Pathology
Unknown. Perhaps related to increased muscle activity in cervical muscles. May be secondary to trauma, including flexion-extension (whiplash) injury.

Summary of Essential Features and Diagnostic Criteria

Intermittent episodes of deep, aching, and sometimes stabbing pain in suboccipital area on one side. Marked tendency to chronicity. Often associated with tender posterior cervical muscles. Can be bilateral.

Differential Diagnosis

Cluster headaches, posterior fossa and high cervical tumor, herniated cervical disk, uncomplicated flexion-extension injury, metastatic neoplasm at the base of the skull.

Code

004.X8 or
004.X1 (if subsequent to trauma)

References

Behrman, S., Traumatic neuropathy of second cervical spinal nerves, Br. Med. J., 286 (1983) 1312–1313.

Hypoglossal Neuralgia (II-11)

Code
006.X8

Glossopharyngeal Pain from Trauma (II-12)

Code
003.X1a

Hypoglossal Pain from Trauma (II-13)

Code
003.X1b

Tolosa-Hunt Syndrome (Painful Ophthalmoplegia) (II-14)

Definition

Episodes of unilateral pain in the ocular and periocular area combined with ipsilateral paresis of oculomotor nerves (ophthalmoplegia) and of the first branch of the Vth cranial nerve. The episodes are most often circumscribed in time, but may be repetitive.

Site
Unilateral; ocular and periocular area.

System Involved
Peripheral nervous and autonomic nervous systems.

Main Features

Prevalence: rare. *Sex Ratio:* no sex preponderance. *Age of Onset:* generally in adults; mean age of onset, around 40. *Pain Quality:* pain usually precedes the ophthalmoplegia. Continuous moderate to severe ache in the ocular and periocular area or *behind* the eye, no triggering. *Time Pattern:* episodes last weeks or months with a continuous or intermittent pattern. Recurrences with several such episodes may occur. *Intensity:* moderate to severe. *Usual Duration:* untreated 8.4 ± 7.4 weeks (mean ± SD), according to Bruyn and Hoes (1986).

Precipitating Factors
Not known.

Associated Symptoms and Signs

Frequently strabismus. Affection of various cranial nerves, i.e., numbers III, IV, V, and VI, either alone or in various combinations. The pupil is usually spared. Nausea and vomiting are rare.

Laboratory Findings

Orbital phlebography renders positive findings in approximately 60–65% of cases. Such findings are: thin caliber, segmental narrowing, and even occlusion and opening of new vessels. Such changes are particularly present in the so-called third segment of the ophthalmic vein and in the cavernous sinus. The pathology of these findings has not been adequately demonstrated. Oculomotor nerve palsy can be ophthalmologically verified.

Relief
From corticosteroids.

Usual Course

Self-limiting, but at times rather protracted. There may be a solitary episode or a tendency to recurrence. Milder forms apparently exist; during recurrences in particular, the pattern may be less characteristic. Occasionally, residual symptoms are found.

Social and Physical Disability
As related to pain episodes.

Pathology
Fibrous tissue formation in cavernous sinus area, involving various structures, vein wall, etc.

Essential Features
Coexistence of orbital and periorbital pain and ophthalmoplegia on the same side.

Differential Diagnosis
Raeder's paratrigeminal syndrome, ophthalmoplegic migraine, other rare cavernous sinus syndromes, sympto-

matic forms (e.g., tumors of the orbit or base of the brain).

Code
002.X3a

References

Tolosa, E., Periarteritic lesions of the carotid siphon with the clinical features of a carotid infraclinoidal aneurysm, J. Neurol. Neurosurg. Psychiatry, 17 (1965) 300–302.

Hunt, W.E., Meagher, J.N., LeFever, H.E., et al., Painful ophthalmoplegia: its relation to indolent inflammation of the cavernous sinus, Neurology (Minneap.), 11 (1961) 56–62.

Hannerz, J., Ericson, K. and Bergstrand, G., Orbital phlebography in patients with Tolosa-Hunt syndrome in comparison with normal subject, Acta Radiol. (Diagn.), 1125 (1984) 457–463.

Bruyn, G.W. and Hoes, M.J., The Tolosa-Hunt syndrome. In: P.G. Vinken, G.W. Bruyn, H.L. Klawans and F.C. Rose (Eds.), Handbook of Clinical Neurology 48 (rev. ser. 4), Elsevier, Amsterdam, 1986, pp. 291–307.

SUNCT Syndrome (Shortlasting, Unilateral Neuralgiform Pain with Conjunctival Injection and Tearing) (II-15)

Definition
Repetitive paroxysms of unilateral shortlasting pain usually 15–120 seconds duration, mainly in the ocular and periocular area, of a neuralgiform nature and moderate to severe intensity, usually appearing only during daytime and accompanied by ipsilateral marked conjunctival injection, lacrimation, a low to moderate degree of rhinorrhea, and (subclinical) forehead sweating. SUNCT is not responsive to indomethacin or carbamazepine, and has, so far, mostly been observed in males.

Site
The ocular and periocular area, occasionally with spread to the fronto-temporal area, upper jaw, or roof of the mouth. The headache is generally strictly unilateral without change of sides, but cases with an accompanying late stage and moderate involvement of the opposite side have been observed.

System
Not firmly identified. The pain appears neurogenic, but there is also involvement of vascular factors.

Main Features
Prevalence: probably rare. *Sex Ratio:* so far, mostly males. *Age of Onset:* middle to old age. *Pain Quality:* the onset is abrupt, the discontinuation of the attack may be a little more gradual. Occasionally, some slight interparoxysmal discomfort occurs. The pain is steady and nonpulsating. Attacks may be *triggered* by various types of minor stimuli within the innervation zone of the Vth cranial nerve but also by neck movements. *Time Pattern:* the attack frequency varies much. In circumscribed periods lasting weeks to months, there may be many attacks per hour, at other times only a few per day or even less. Attacks are shortlasting, i.e., 15–120 seconds duration. Remissions last from months to years. In the early stages, attacks appear in bouts; eventually, a chronic course develops. No neurological deficits. *Intensity:* Moderate to severe pain.

Precipitating Factors
Attacks may be triggered by minor stimuli within the distribution of the Vth cranial nerve, but also partly by neck movements.

Associated Symptoms and Signs
Conjunctival injection, lacrimation, nasal stuffiness, and to a lesser extent, rhinorrhea and forehead sweating (which is apparently always subclinical) occur on the pain side. The onset of the conjunctival injection and lacrimation may have an almost explosive character during severe attacks.

Relief
No benefit from indomethacin or carbamazepine. No really effective treatment is yet available. Cortisone may possibly be of some avail.

Usual Course
At an early stage, an intermittent pattern which may or may not be permanent.

Social and Physical Disability
During the worst periods, some patients cannot do their ordinary work.

Pathology
Unknown.

Essential Features
Shortlasting, unilateral paroxysms of ocular pain, associated with ipsilateral autonomic phenomena like conjunctival injection, lacrimation, etc. In some cases, attacks may be triggered mechanically. Male preponderance.

Differential Diagnosis
Trigeminal neuralgia, Syndrome of "Jabs and Jolts" ("multiple jabs"), chronic paroxysmal hemicrania, cluster headache, "symptomatic SUNCT," Newton-Hoyt-Taniguchi syndrome.

Code
006.X8j

References

Bussone, G., Leone, M., Dalla Volta, G., Strada, L., Gasparotti, R. and Di Mona, V., Shortlasting, unilateral neuralgiform headache attacks with tearing and conjunctival injection: the first "symptomatic" case? Cephalalgia, 11 (1991) 123–127.

Sjaastad, O., Saunte, C., Salvesen, R., Fredriksen, T.A., Seim, A., Roe, O.D., Fostad, K., Lobben, O.-P. and Zhao, J.-M., Shortlasting, unilateral neuralgiform headache attacks with conjunctival injection, tearing, sweating, and rhinorrhea, Cephalalgia, 9 (1989) 147–156.

Taniguchi, R.M., Goree, J.A. and Odom, G.L., Spontaneous carotid-cavernous shunts presenting diagnostic problems, J. Neurosurg., 35 (1971) 384–391.

Raeder's Syndrome (Raeder's Paratrigeminal Syndrome) (II-16)

Definition

Horner's syndrome of the IIIrd cranial nerve type combined with aching steady pain in the ocular and periocular area, with or without parasellar cranial nerve involvement; the Vth nerve is most often involved, but also the IInd, IIIrd, IVth, and VIth cranial nerves may be affected, all on one side. The cases with and without parasellar cranial nerve involvement have been placed in two groups, I and II, respectively (Boniuk and Schlezinger 1962). Sweating is reduced on the symptomatic side in IIIrd nerve disorders, including Raeder's syndrome, but apparently only in the medial part of the forehead (corresponding to the sympathetic fibers that follow the internal carotid and ultimately perhaps the supraorbital arteries).

Site

Unilateral pain in the ocular and periocular area, temporal and aural areas, forehead, and occasionally also the anterior vertex.

System

Autonomic nervous system. Cranial nerves.

Main Features

Prevalence: rare. *Clinical Patterns:* two forms have been described: (I) the original form (described by the Norwegian ophthalmologist Raeder [1924]) with parasellar cranial nerve involvement and (II) a form without parasellar nerve involvement (Boniuk and Schlezinger 1962). If parasellar cranial nerve involvement is no longer an obligatory diagnostic requirement, then the localization of the underlying disorder no longer has to be the "paratrigeminal" space: It can be anywhere from the superior cervical ganglion and its rostral connections and toward the periphery. Many of the Boniuk and Schlezinger type cases, nevertheless, probably originate in or close to the area of pathology of type I cases. *Sex Ratio:* almost only males. A few acceptable female cases have been reported. *Age of Onset:* usually middle–old age. *Pain Quality:* the pain is not excruciating, nor is it continuously severe. It rather fluctuates between the moderate and severe stages. At times, it attains the character of an attack, frequently in the early and late stages; the pain is generally aching and nonpulsatile. *Time Pattern:* there is a relatively longlasting period of moderate to severe pain with a crescendo, a plateau, and a declining phase, and this period may or may not have been preceded by a longlasting phase or rare and/or mild headaches. The period of severe pain usually lasts for weeks to months, after which time there may be a period of lingering pain. There is only a little tendency to recurrence. *Intensity:* moderate to severe; fluctuating.

Precipitating Factors

Possibly cardiovascular factors may predispose.

Associated Symptoms and Signs

Ptosis (of a mild degree), miosis, and hypohidrosis in the medial part of the forehead (but no enophthalmus) on the symptomatic side. There are no further findings in Boniuk and Schlezinger type II. In type I cases, involvement of the IInd, IIIrd, IVth, Vth, and VIth cranial nerves appears in various combinations; most frequently the Vth nerve is affected. Cases with only a *discrete* affection (hypoesthesia, dysesthesia) of the Vth nerve (first branch) seem to be the most common type.

Relief

Group I cases may need surgery for the causal condition. Group II cases benefit from analgesics. No specific therapy is known at present and no special benefit occurs with indomethacin. Whether cortisone acts beneficially (as in the Tolosa-Hunt syndrome) is not adequately documented.

Duration and Usual Course

In most cases there is a circumscribed, self-limiting headache, lasting some weeks to months. In the occasional case, such periods may be repeated one or more times. Group II cases have a good prognosis and may not need extensive investigation. Group I cases differ from Group II cases from a diagnostic and prognostic point of view because the underlying pathology may be a tumor, skull fracture, etc. Such cases are in need of thorough investigation.

Complications

Type I: from the paratrigeminal tumor (or other pathology).

Social and Physical Disability

During the acute stage the incapacity may be considerable.

Pathology
Type I: tumor or other (serious) pathology paratrigeminally until proven otherwise. Type II: not known.

Essential Features
Painful, type III Horner's syndrome—unilaterally, with or without parasellar II–VI cranial nerve affection; the involvement of the Vth cranial nerve is usually *discrete*.

Differential Diagnosis
The Tolosa-Hunt syndrome. Other cavernous sinus syndromes, cluster headache. Hemicrania continua is also a diagnostic possibility; hypothetically, orbital space-occupying disorders (but they hardly give rise to Horner's syndrome).

Code
Type I: 002.X4   Tumor
002.X1a   Trauma
002.X3b   Inflammatory, etc.
Type II: 002.X8   Unknown

References
Boniuk, M. and Schlezinger, N.S., Raeder's paratrigeminal syndrome, Am. J. Ophthalmol., 54 (1962) 1074–1084.

Raeder, J.G., Paratrigeminal paralysis of oculo-pupillary sympathetic, Brain, 47 (1924) 149–158.

Salvesen, R., de Souza Carvalho, D. and Sjaastad, O., Horner's syndrome: sweat gland and pupillary responsiveness in two cases with a probable 3rd nerve dysfunction, Cephalalgia, 9 (1989) 63–70.

GROUP III: CRANIOFACIAL PAIN OF MUSCULOSKELETAL ORIGIN

Acute Tension Headache (III-1)

Definition
Acute, relatively shortlasting, diffuse (or more localized) dull head pain related to anxiety, depression, or emotional tension.

Main Features
As for presumed chronic tension headache except as follows: Very frequent. Affects the majority of the population. Sex ratio probably equal. The pain is dull—sometimes somewhat more marked—bilateral, and nonthrobbing, with gradual onset, steady rise, plateau, and then a decline in intensity. No nausea, vomiting, or photophobia. Does not usually need any therapy, unless the pattern is repetitive.

Acute, self-limiting, relatively shortlasting (for a few hours or less); repeated separate attacks with very varying frequency. Eases with the elimination of the (acute) cause.

Pathology
In spite of the fact that it shares the appellation with the chronic variety, it may well be that the two forms differ in more than just temporal and intensity respects. They may be different types of headache.

Code
034.X7a

References
Kudrow, L., Muscle contraction headaches. In: P.J. Vinken, G.W. Bruyn, H.L. Klawans and F.C. Rose (Eds.), Handbook of Clinical Neurology 48 (rev. ser. 4), Elsevier, Amsterdam, 1986, pp. 343–352.

Tension Headache: Chronic Form (Scalp Muscle Contraction Headache) (III-2)

Definition
Virtually continuous, dull aching head pain, usually symmetrical and frequently global. This headache is frequently, but not in all cases, associated with muscle "tension." The term *tension* is, nevertheless, retained; tension may also be taken to indicate stress, strain, anxiety, and emotional tension. There is a frequent association between these factors and also depressive states and this headache. In the later stages, exacerbations with a tinge of pounding headache and with nausea (and, less typically, vomiting) may occasionally occur, although less typically and with less intensity than in common migraine.

Site
Frontal, orbital, fronto-occipital, occipital, nuchal, or whole scalp area. Diffuse or bandlike, usually bilateral, sometimes more on one side during exacerbations.

System
Not known. Possibly musculoskeletal, possibly central nervous system, or vessels.

Main Features
Prevalence: Often diagnosed; even approximate prevalence is unknown, mainly because of lack of precise diagnostic criteria. *Sex Ratio:* Females more than males; ratio approximately 4:1 in those who consult their physician. *Onset:* From age 8 onward, usually before age 30.

Start: Gradual emergence as mild, diffuse ache or unpleasant feeling, intermittent at first, increasing with time to a more definite pain that gradually will become more and more chronic. Fluctuation during the day is typical. In a proportion of cases, exacerbations with additional symptoms seem to emerge after several years of lesser headache. *Occurrence and Duration:* Every day or most days, for most of the day. Occasionally, in longstanding severe cases, pain may wake the patient from sleep. *Pain Quality:* Dull ache, usually does not throb, more severe during exacerbations, and then occasionally with throbbing. Some describe tight band feeling or gripping headache.

Precipitants and Exacerbating Factors
Emotional stress, anxiety and depression, physical exercise, alcohol (which may also have the opposite effect).

Associated Symptoms
Many patients are hypersensitive and have anxiety, depression, or both. Irritability, nausea, vomiting, photophobia, phonophobia, and pulsatile pain may occur during exacerbations in the later stages of this headache. Vomiting is, however, most unusual.

Signs
Muscle tenderness of the pericranial and/or nuchal muscles occurs but may also be found in other conditions and in healthy individuals. Tension headache with and without muscle tenderness may differ both from a pathogenetic and from a therapeutic point of view (e.g., with regard to response to tricyclic antidepressants).

Relief
Treatment of emotional problems, anxiety, or depression may diminish symptoms. Relaxation and biofeedback treatment help. Anxiolytics may help but should generally be avoided since some patients become depressed and others develop dependence. Tricyclic antidepressants are frequently very useful, but their effect may possibly differ in patients with and without muscular tenderness. Some of them, e.g., amitriptyline, have independent analgesic properties which may account for some of their usefulness. Analgesics help only a little, and discontinuation of some chronically used drugs may be of some avail.

Usual Course
Chronic course. Hard to treat in most cases.

Complications
Analgesics, narcotics, and other drug abuse. Detoxification is often mandatory in order to improve the situation and end a vicious circle of withdrawal headaches and medication.

Social and Physical Disability
Reduction of activities and of work.

Pathology
Unsettled. Evidence of chronic muscle tenderness in many cases. Apparently, there is increased muscle activity, sometimes demonstrable on EMG. Both phenomena may, however, also be present in patients with migraine. There is a lack of adequate, long-term studies comparing controls with patients, in particular after appropriate exposures.

Essential Features
Bilateral, usually low-grade to mild, more or less chronic headache, with fewer accompanying features than in common migraine, starting early in life, and occurring much more frequently in the female.

Differential Diagnosis
Mainly from other *bilateral* headaches. Multiple attacks of acute tension headache, which *may* be an altogether different headache, may masquerade as chronic tension headache. Common migraine, "mixed vascular-tension headache," chronic abuse of analgesics, refractive errors, heterophoria ("eye strain"), post-traumatic headache (bilateral cases, which probably exist), cervicogenic headache (in the bilateral cases, that sooner or later may be recognized as being characteristic of this disorder), cervical spine disorders, depression, conversion hysteria, and hallucinatory headache.

The differential diagnosis vs. common migraine is particularly challenging. The occurrence of migraine or migraine-like headache in the close family, the frequently occurring unilaterality (with *change of side*), the "anterior" onset of attacks (or exacerbations), the more marked degree of nausea, vomiting, photophobia, and phonophobia, and pulsating headache, all in common migraine, are factors of crucial importance in distinguishing the two headaches. The ergotamine effect (and probably also the sumatriptan effect) is also clearly more marked in common migraine.

Code
033.X7c

References
Friedman, A.P., von Storch, T. and Merritt, H.H., Migraine and tension headaches: a clinical study of two thousand cases, Neurology 4 (1954) 773–774.

Kudrow, L., Paradoxical effects of frequent analgesic use. In: M. Critchley, A.K. Friedman, S. Gorini and F. Sicuteri (Eds.), Advances in Neurology, Raven Press, New York, 33 (1982) 335–341.

Pfaffenrath, V., Wermuth, A. and Pöllmann, W., Der Spannungskopfschmerz: eine Übersicht, Fortschr. Neurol. Psychiat., 56 (1988) 403–418.

Ziegler, D.K. and Hassanein, R.S., Migraine muscle-contraction dichotomy studied by statistical analysis of headache symptoms. In: F.C. Rose (Ed.), Advances in Migraine Research and Therapy, Raven Press, New York, 1982.

Temporomandibular Pain and Dysfunction Syndrome (III-3)
(also called Temporomandibular Joint Disorder)

Definition
Aching in the muscles of mastication, sometimes with an occasional brief severe pain on chewing, often associated with restricted jaw movement and clicking or popping sounds.

Site
Temporomandibular, intra-auricular, temporal, occipital, masseteric, neck, and shoulder regions.

System
Musculoskeletal system.

Main Features
Prevalence: unknown. Epidemiological studies have shown that up to 10% of people between the ages of 15 and 35 experience clicking of the jaw with dysfunction at some point in time. *Sex Ratio:* most patients are female. *Age of Onset:* patients presenting with temporomandibular pain and dysfunction have an age range of 5–60 years. *Pain Quality:* the pain is usually described as intermittent, unilateral, dull, and aching, but can be constant. The pain is often exacerbated by jaw movement, e.g., chewing hard food or yawning. Combinations of aching and severe exacerbations may also occur. *Time Pattern:* the pain may be continuous by day or brief. It is often worse on waking. *Duration:* symptoms can persist for years with fluctuations.

Clicking of the joint or popping noises in the ears are frequently present. Limitations of opening, deviation of the jaw on opening, and a feeling that the teeth do not meet together properly are common.

Signs
Restricted mandibular opening with or without deviation of the jaw to the affected side on opening; tenderness to palpation of the muscles of mastication; clicking or popping at the joint on auscultation or palpation; changes in the ability to occlude the teeth fully.

Imaging
Normal temporomandibular joint radiographic structure, variable disk displacement seen on arthrography, occasional osteoarthritic changes. Magnetic resonance imaging may show disk displacement with or without reducibility. The clinical significance of disk displacement and its relationship to the syndrome are not established.

Usual Course
Variable. Because of its fluctuating course, the response to treatment is difficult to evaluate. Psychosocial factors account for a significant portion of the outcome. The effectiveness of common treatments, e.g., occlusal splints and psychotherapy, has not been shown to be superior to placebo. A high potential for morbidity makes TM joint surgery problematic.

With conservative treatment, many patients are kept reasonably comfortable and productive. Long-term outcome studies are unavailable. However, small sample studies indicate that many experience symptoms indefinitely.

Complications
Possible degenerative joint disease, depression and anxiety, drug dependence. In some intractable cases widespread diffuse aching facial pain develops.

Social and Physical Disability
Interference with mastication and social and vocational activity, development of secondary psychological changes.

Pathology and Etiology
Muscle spasm appears in most cases. Disk displacement with or without reducibility appears in some cases. The etiology is unknown. Psychological stress and bruxism are widely believed to be contributory factors, although evidence for this is lacking. Trauma is known to be related to a minority of cases.

Summary of Essential Features and Diagnostic Criteria
Muscle tenderness; temporomandibular joint clicking; difficulty in opening the jaw and sometimes deviation on opening; a dull ache or severe episodes associated with jaw opening, or both.

Differential Diagnosis
Degenerative joint disease, rheumatoid arthritis, traumatic arthralgia, temporal arteritis, otitis media, parotitis, mandibular osteomyelitis, stylohyoid process syndrome, deafferentation pains, pain of psychological origin.

Code
034.X8a

References
Griffiths, R.H., Report of the president's conference on the examination, diagnosis and management of temporomandibular disorders. D. Laskin, W. Greenfield, E. Gale, J. Rugh, P. Neff, C. Alling and W.A. Ayer (Eds.), J. Am. Dent. Assoc., 166 (1983) 75–77.

Rudy, T.E., Turk, D..C, Zaki, H.S. and Curtin, H.B., An empirical taxometric alternative to traditional classification of temporomandibular disorders, Pain, 36 (1989) 311–320.

Schnurr, R.F., Brooke, R.I. and Rollman, G.B., Psychosocial correlates of temporomandibular joint pain and dysfunction, Pain, 42 (1990) 153.

Marbach, J.J., Lennon, M.C. and Dohrenwend, B.P., Candidate risk factors for temporomandibular pain and dysfunction syndrome: psychosocial, health behavior, physical illness and injury, Pain, 34 (1988) 139–147.

Osteoarthritis of the Temporomandibular Joint (III-4)

Code
033.X6

Rheumatoid Arthritis of the Temporomandibular Joint (III-5)

Definition
Part of the systemic disorder of rheumatoid arthritis with granulation tissue proliferating onto the articular surface.

Site
Temporomandibular joint, external acoustic meatus.

System
Musculoskeletal system.

Main Features
Prevalence: Caucasian, approximately 50% occurrence with general rheumatoid arthritis. *Sex Ratio:* female predilection. *Age of Onset:* juvenile or pubertal; adult onset 40–60 years. *Start:* spontaneous onset. *Pain Quality:* boring, penetrating, aching. *Occurrence:* constant with diurnal variation. *Intensity:* moderate A.M., mild P.M. *Duration:* minutes to hours.

Signs
Preauricular erythema, crepitus, tenderness of external acoustic meatus, restriction and deformation of other joints, open bite eventually.

Laboratory and Radiological Findings
Positive latex fixation, radiographic joint space narrowing.

Usual Course
Five to nine months acute painful course followed by joint restriction and ankylosis; responsive to condyloplasty without recurrence.

Relief
Heat, joint physiotherapy, anti-inflammatory agents.

Complication
Fibrous or bony ankylosis.

Social and Physical Disability
Mastication impairment, associated orthopedic restrictions.

Pathology
Synovitis, foam cell degeneration ("Pannus Cell" formation), secondary resorption of the articular surfaces, adhesions to the articular disk, fibrous adhesions, narrowing and loss of joint space.

Diagnostic Criteria
Multiple joint involvement, radiographic joint space loss and condylar deformation, positive lab findings.

Differential Diagnosis
Includes degenerative joint disease, traumatic arthritis, inflammatory arthritis, myofascial pain dysfunction.

Code
032.X3b

Dystonic Disorders, Facial Dyskinesia (III-6)

Code
003.X8

Crushing Injury of Head or Face (III-7)

Code
032.X1

GROUP IV: LESIONS OF THE EAR, NOSE, AND ORAL CAVITY

Maxillary Sinusitis (IV-1)

Definition
Constant burning pain with zygomatic and dental tenderness from inflammation of the maxillary sinus.

Site
Upper cheek and sometimes teeth.

System
Respiratory system.

Main Features
Prevalence: common. *Sex Ratio:* no difference. *Age of Onset:* usually adults. *Onset:* spontaneous. *Pain Quality:* dull ache, unilaterally or bilaterally, sense of fullness and tenderness in the overlying cheek. *Occurrence:* usually associated with nasal cold. Other nasal disease or dental disease causes 20% of cases. *Intensity:* mild to severe. *Duration:* days.

The illness develops when swelling of the nasal mucosa blocks the ostium so that drainage can no longer occur into the nose. When the cause is a common cold, the other nasal sinuses may become involved. Dental cases arise from infection associated with the apex of one of the molar or premolar teeth. They may also be associated with operative procedures including a tooth root being pushed accidentally into the sinus during extraction, or endodontic instruments and materials being pushed too far.

In chronic cases there may be no pain or only mild, diffuse discomfort from time to time.

Signs
Zygomatic area of face may be slightly flushed and slightly swollen ("puffy"). Pain exacerbated by bending. Tenderness of upper molar and premolar teeth and over cheek.

Laboratory Findings
Radiography may show fluid level or a tooth root. In chronic cases radiographic examination reveals a sinus more opaque than normal.

Usual Course
Subsides in several days to a week.

Relief
Analgesics, sometimes with drainage by lying down on the opposite side.

Pathology
Inflammation of the lining of the maxillary sinus.

Diagnostic Criteria
Pain or discomfort over the maxillary antrum coupled with evidence of infection such as local inflammation, radiographic signs of thickening or a fluid level, and relief by antibiotics or drainage.

Differential Diagnosis
Periapical disease of the associated teeth, malignant disease.

Code
031.X2a.

Odontalgia: Toothache 1. Due to Dentino-Enamel Defects (IV-2)

Definition
Shortlasting diffuse orofacial pain due to dentino-enamel defects and evoked by local stimuli.

Site
Orofacial pain.

System
Musculoskeletal system.

Main Features
Prevalence: extremely common. *Sex Ratio:* no difference. *Age of Onset:* 2 years of age to any age. *Start:* stimulus evoked, not spontaneous, heat, cold, mechanical, osmotic. *Pain Quality:* bright to dull. *Occurrence:* intermittent. *Intensity:* mild to moderate. *Duration:* less than a second to minutes.

Signs
Dental caries, fracture, crack, or lost restoration.

Laboratory and Radiological Findings
Radiographic evidence of caries.

Usual Course
If neglected, there may be mineralization within the dentine, resulting in less frequent pain or no pain; or pulpal involvement.

Relief
By protecting defective area with a dressing or restoration.

Complications
Laceration of soft tissues by sharp edge of tooth.

Pathology
Dental caries, trauma, operative procedures.

Diagnostic Criteria
Visually observed defects, or defects palpated with a probe, plus radiographic examination.

Differential Diagnosis
Pulp disease, periapical disease.

Code
034.X2b

Odontalgia: Toothache 2. Pulpitis (IV-3)

Definition
Orofacial pain due to pulpal inflammation, often evoked by local stimuli.

Site
Face, jaw, mouth.

System
Musculoskeletal system.

Main Features
Prevalence: very common. *Sex Ratio:* no difference. *Age of Onset:* after eruption of teeth. *Start:* milder cases may be started by hot or cold stimuli. In severe cases may be spontaneous (no external stimulus needed) but is exacerbated by heat and cold stimuli. *Pain Quality:* sharp or dull ache, may throb. *Occurrence:* with food intake in milder cases. Daily until treated in severe cases. *Intensity:* can be moderate, usually severe. *Duration:* bouts lasting minutes or hours; may continue for days.

Signs
Deep dental caries, seen both directly and on radiography.

Laboratory and Radiological Findings
Radiologic evidence of caries usually extending to pulp chamber.

Usual Course
If untreated, the pulp dies and infection spreads to the periapical tissues, producing acute or chronic periapical periodontitis which is likely to be acute but might be chronic. Death of the pulp ends pain from this source, but by then pain may already have started from the acute periapical periodontitis.

Relief
By analgesics, sometimes by cold fluids, extirpation of the dental pulp; extraction of the tooth.

Complication
Spread of infection to the periodontal tissues, jaws, lymph glands.

Pathology
Histopathological examination of the pulp reveals acute inflammation.

Diagnostic Criteria
Spontaneous pain confirms. Tooth not tender to percussion unless periodontitis has supervened.

Differential Diagnosis
Other forms of dental disease, rarely can mimic trigeminal neuralgia, sinusitis, vascular facial pain syndromes.

Code
031.X2c

Odontalgia: Toothache 3. Periapical Periodontitis and Abscess (IV-4)

Definition
Severe throbbing pain in the tooth without major pathology.

Site
Teeth and gingivae.

System
Musculoskeletal system.

Main Features
Sex Ratio: female preponderance. *Age of Onset:* adults. *Pain Quality:* teeth hypersensitive to stimuli. Severe throbbing pain in teeth and gingivae usually continuous, may vary from aching mild pain to intense pain, especially with hot or cold stimuli to the teeth. May be widespread or well localized, frequently precipitated by a dental procedure. May move from tooth to tooth. *Duration:* may be from a few minutes to several hours.

Associated Symptoms
Emotional problems. May be associated with hypotensive therapy. Also complaints of temporomandibular pain and dysfunction syndrome, oral dysesthesia, and pains of psychological origin. May be a symptom of depressive or monosymptomatic hypochondriacal psychosis. Often excessive concern with oral hygiene.

Signs and Laboratory Findings
Teeth hypersensitive to heat and cold.

Relief
Antidepressants. Small doses of phenothiazines. Counseling; avoidance of unnecessary pulp extirpations and extractions.

Pathology
Possibly hyperalgesia of pulp and periodontal pain receptors due to persistent vasodilation.

Summary of Essential Features and Diagnostic Criteria

Continuous throbbing pain in the tooth, hypersensitive to temperature and pressure. No organic pathology.

Diagnostic Criteria

Patient with history of tooth pain associated with endodontic therapy and/or extractions. Remaining teeth while clinically sound and vital are tender to thermal stimuli and to percussion.

Code

031.X2d

References

Rees, R.T. and Harris, M., Atypical odontalgia, Brit. J. Oral Surg., 16 (1979) 212–218.

Brooke, R.I., Atypical odontalgia, Oral Surg., 49 (1980) 196–199.

Marbach, J.J., Phantom tooth pain, J. Endodontics, 4 (1978) 362–372.

Odontalgia: Toothache 4. Tooth Pain Not Associated with Lesions (Atypical Odontalgia) (IV-5)

Definition

Severe throbbing pain in the tooth without major pathology.

Site

Teeth and gingivae.

System

Musculoskeletal system.

Main Features

Sex Ratio: female preponderance. *Age of Onset:* adults. *Pain Quality:* teeth hypersensitive to stimuli. Severe throbbing pain in teeth and gingivae usually continuous, may vary from aching mild pain to intense pain, especially with hot or cold stimuli to the teeth. May be widespread or well localized, frequently precipitated by a dental procedure. May move from tooth to tooth. *Duration:* may be from a few minutes to several hours.

Associated Symptoms

Emotional problems. May be associated with hypotensive therapy. Also complaints of temporomandibular pain and dysfunction syndrome, oral dysesthesia, and pains of psychological origin. May be a symptom of depressive or monosymptomatic hypochondriacal psychosis. Often excessive concern with oral hygiene.

Signs and Laboratory Findings

Teeth hypersensitive to heat and cold.

Relief

Antidepressants. Small doses of phenothiazines. Counseling; avoidance of unnecessary pulp extirpations and extractions.

Pathology

Possibly hyperalgesia of pulp and periodontal pain receptors due to persistent vasodilation.

Summary of Essential Features and Diagnostic Criteria

Continuous throbbing pain in the tooth, hypersensitive to temperature and pressure. No organic pathology.

Diagnostic Criteria

Patient with history of tooth pain associated with endodontic therapy and/or extractions. Remaining teeth while clinically sound and vital are tender to thermal stimuli and to percussion.

Code

034.X8b

References

Brooke, R.I., Atypical odontalgia, Oral Surg., 49 (1980) 196–199.

Marbach, J.J., Phantom tooth pain, J. Endodontics, 4 (1978) 362–372.

Rees, R.T. and Harris, M., Atypical odontalgia, Brit. J. Oral Surg., 16 (1979) 212–218.

Glossodynia and Sore Mouth (IV-6)
(also known as Burning Tongue or Oral Dysesthesia)

Definition

Burning pain in the tongue or other oral mucous membranes.

Site

Most often tip and lateral borders of tongue. Anterior hard palate, lips, and alveolar mucosa are often involved, but any mucosal area can be affected. Most often bilateral.

Main Features

Prevalence: common in postmenopausal women: 10–40% of women attending postmenopausal clinics, 15% of women aged 40–49 in general dental practices, 1.5–2.5% of random samples of general or dental populations. *Sex Ratio:* women predominate. *Age of Onset:* mainly over 50 years of age. *Quality:* burning, tender, annoying, tiring, nagging pain; discomforting (McGill Pain Questionnaire). *Time Pattern:* usually constant once it begins, but may be variable; increases in intensity from midmorning to late evening. *Intensity:* on 150 mm VAS (visual analog scale): least, in A.M., 22 ± 25 mm;

usual in afternoon, 63 ± 27 mm; and most by late evening, 105 ± 29 mm.

Associated Symptoms
Dry mouth (63% of subjects), persistent dysgeusic taste (63%), altered taste perception (35%), thirst (37%). Burning increased with tension (78%), fatigue (54%), speaking (44%), and hot foods (38%), and decreased with sleeping (69%), eating (58%), cold (52%), distraction (48%), and alcohol (27%). Many patients anxious and depressed. Topical anesthetic applied to painful sites decreases pain. Temporary relief by food or drink is almost pathognomonic. Denture intolerance can occur.

Signs and Laboratory Findings
Usually normal but there has been experimental evidence of altered taste perception, lowered heat pain tolerance of the tongue and alterations in salivary composition, although not quantity. Occasionally, there may be evidence of connective tissue disease (e.g., positive rheumatoid factor, antinuclear factor, increased sedimentation rate, decreased complement levels). Sometimes low iron, B_{12}, folate or other vitamin B or zinc levels, but correction of nutritional factors infrequently alleviates symptoms.

Usual Course
Fifty percent spontaneous remission within 6–7 years of onset; sometimes intractable. Often responds well to tricyclic antidepressant drugs in low doses (30–60 mg). Treatment frequently more difficult in patients who have burning only when dentures in place.

Complications
Secondary emotional changes.

Pathology
Unknown, but frequently occurs around the time of menopause.

Summary of Essential Features and Diagnostic Criteria
Burning tongue or other parts of oral mucosa, usually bilateral, dysgeusic taste, altered taste perception, dry mouth, denture intolerance.

Differential Diagnosis
Atypical facial pain; atypical odontalgia; atypical trigeminal neuralgia; oral candidiasis; erosive lichen planus; geographic tongue; vitamin, iron, or zinc deficiency.

Code
051.X5   If known
051.X8   Alternative

References
Basker, R.M., Sturdee, D.W. and Davenport, J.C., Patients with burning mouths: a clinical investigation of causative factors, including the climacteric and diabetes, Brit. Dent. J., 145 (1978) 9–16.

Grushka, M. and Sessle, B.J., Burning mouth syndrome, Dent. Clin. N.A., 35 (1991) 171–184.

Van der Waal, I., The Burning Syndrome, Munksgaard, Copenhagen, 1990.

Cracked Tooth Syndrome (IV-7)

Definition
Brief, sharp pain in a tooth, often not understood until a piece fractures off the tooth.

Site
Mouth.

System
Musculoskeletal system.

Main Features
Prevalence: fairly common. *Sex Ratio:* no difference. *Age of Onset:* third decade onward. *Start:* brief pain on biting or chewing. *Pain Quality:* sharp. *Intensity:* moderate. *Duration:* few seconds.

Signs
It may be a visible crack. Percussion of this cusp provokes the pain. The cusp might move away from the tooth when manipulated.

Usual Course
The pain recurs with biting and chewing until the cusp finally separates completely.

Relief
It is relieved when the cracked portion of the tooth finally fractures off, or if the crack is detected by the dentist and the defective portion is restored.

Complications
None.

Social and Physical Disability
Eating is more difficult.

Pathology
A crack in the tooth allows chemicals and microorganisms to enter and make the dentine at the pulpal side of the crack hypersensitive, possibly by a mild underlying pulpitis.

Diagnostic Criteria
A sharp brief pain on biting or chewing. There is pain on percussing the affected cusp but not the other cusps. The piece finally fractures off.

Differential Diagnosis
Other forms of toothache mainly from the dentine and the pulp.

Code
034.X1

Dry Socket (IV-8)

Definition
Unilateral pain in the jaw, usually lower, usually associated with additional tenderness due to submandibular lymphadenitis following dental extraction and due to a localized osteitis.

Site
Face, jaw, mouth, upper neck.

System
Musculoskeletal system.

Main Features
Prevalence: fairly common. *Sex Ratio:* no difference. *Age of Onset:* any age from when the teeth can be extracted. *Start:* two days after a dental extraction, the pain starts without stimulation. The submandibular lymph glands soon become involved with added tenderness. *Pain Quality:* constant, dull ache, may throb, associated with severe halitosis. *Intensity:* moderate, exacerbated by mechanical stimulation. *Duration:* hours to days.

After tooth extraction, blood normally fills the socket and clots, the clot gradually becoming organized with new bone formation. Dry socket occurs when this fails to happen either because there is no bleeding due to too much adrenaline in the local anesthetic solution, or because the blood is diluted by washing the mouth out, or because the clot is broken down by infection. In such circumstances the bone in the socket is no longer protected, and there is severe pain made worse by physical interference. Food gathers in the socket and decomposes, producing a foul taste and severe halitosis.

Signs
A recent extraction socket with no clot (and therefore dry), with food debris.

Laboratory and Radiological Findings
Recent empty tooth socket.

Usual Course
Continuous unless treated. Gingiva tends to grow over the socket.

Relief
It is relieved by washing out the socket and packing it with ribbon gauze covered with Whitehead's varnish (an iodoform resinous material).

Complication
Submandibular lymphadenitis.

Social and Physical Disability
Severe halitosis.

Diagnostic Criteria
Continuous ache which starts two days after tooth extraction. Socket not closed by blood clot. Food debris within. Halitosis. Pain from mechanical stimuli. Submandibular lymphadenitis.

Differential Diagnosis
Osteomyelitis, retained tooth root.

Code
031.X1

Gingival Disease, Inflammatory (IV-9)

Code
034.X2

Toothache, Cause Unknown (IV-10)

Code
034.X8f

Diseases of the Jaw, Inflammatory Conditions (IV-11)

Code
033.X2

Other and Unspecified Pain in Jaws (IV-12)

Code
03X.X8d

Frostbite of Face (IV-13)

Code
022.X1

GROUP V: PRIMARY HEADACHE SYNDROMES, VASCULAR DISORDERS, AND CEREBROSPINAL FLUID SYNDROMES

Classic Migraine (Migraine with Aura) (V-1)

Definition
Throbbing head pain in attacks, often with a prodromal state and usually preceded by an aura which frequently contains visual phenomena. The pain is typically unilateral but may be bilateral. Nausea, vomiting, photophobia, and phonophobia often accompany the pain. Clear female predominance.

Site
Typically unilateral, but may be bilateral. Pain mostly begins in the fronto-temporal area and is most marked in this area, even at maximum, when it may involve the whole hemicranium. The side typically changes in different attacks or even during single attacks.

System
Unknown: vascular disturbances have been emphasized; central nervous system changes may be fundamental. The coding below accepts the latter.

Main Features
Frequent positive family history of migraine-like type of headache. *Prevalence:* high, but less frequent than common migraine. *Sex Ratio:* females more than males. *Onset:* from childhood to about 35. In most cases, attacks have started by late puberty. Onset of solitary attacks may be associated with emotional stress, relaxation, "anxiety," dietary causes (chocolate, cheese, citrus fruits, etc.), flashing lights, atmospheric changes, etc. *"Premonitory" Phase:* may last for hours to one or two days and precedes the aura phase, often with mood changes, weight gain. *The Aura* usually precedes the pain phase but may also occur both prior to and during it, and occasionally only during it. An aura may occur without subsequent pain, probably most frequently in male patients. In approximate order of frequency, the following phenomena occur during the aura phase: blurring of vision, flickering changes in the visual field, phenomena like a curtain or mist in parts of the field, fortification figures, scotomata and a variety of other visual changes (the visual changes usually have a homonymous distribution), paresthesias, mostly in the regions of the hand and mouth, mild paresis (the two last phenomena usually with a unilateral distribution), dysarthria, and aphasic disturbances. In extremely rare cases, there may be alloesthesia, micropsia, and macropsia, or distortions of perspective. If paresis, hemianopias, and sensory loss are prominent and longlasting,

they may be part of other migraine variants (V-3). *Duration of Aura Phase:* usually 20–25 minutes. *Pain:* the aura may overlap with the pain phase. Usually the pain succeeds the aura with or without a symptom-free interval. In occasional attacks in the classic migraineur, the pain starts without a preceding aura. The pain is throbbing, ranges from mild to severe in intensity, reaches a plateau, and usually lasts from 4 to 72 hours if unmodified by drugs. The pain may be global, but typically it is unilateral and alternates sides during an attack or between attacks. The pain typically starts in the frontal-temporal area. It may continue in that area or involve the entire hemicranium at a later stage. The pain is generally moderate to severe. Characteristically, the pulsating quality increases with moderate physical activity or stooping. *Frequency:* varies from a couple of attacks in a lifetime to several every week. The most usual pattern in clinical practice is 1–4 per month. Exacerbations often occur during episodes of anxiety, depressive illness, or personal conflict. The tendency to attacks is frequently markedly reduced in pregnancy. *Other Characteristics:* anorexia, nausea and vomiting, photophobia, and phonophobia are characteristic features of the attack.

Precipitating Factors
Numerous, may include stress, mood changes, relaxation, dietary factors.

Associated Symptoms and Signs
Anorexia, nausea, vomiting, photophobia, and phonophobia. With "complicated migraine," various deficiency symptoms and signs (e.g., hemiplegic migraine; see V-3).

Laboratory Findings
Fall in platelet serotonin during attacks. Changes in cerebral blood flow.

Relief
From ergot preparations, beta-blocking agents, calcium blocking agents, NSAIDs, and substances interfering with serotonin activity, in particular serotonin 1D receptor agonists like sumatriptan.

Usual Course
In time, interparoxysmal psychological changes if the headache is severe. Ergotamine dependence or other dependence on medication, even analgesic medication. Detoxification may be required to end a vicious circle of withdrawal headaches and medications.

Complications
Depression and related psychological changes if severe. Dependence on ergotamine or other medication.

Social and Physical Disability
Interruption of work in severe cases. Reduced efficiency for many.

Pathology
No definite, confirmed findings.

Essential Features
Presence of an aura phase, at least during the occasional attack. Pulsating headache. Usually unilateral headache. Nausea, vomiting, photophobia, and phonophobia.

Differential Diagnosis
Common migraine, migraine variants, cerebral angioma.

Code
004.X7a

References
Bille, S., Migraine in children and its prognosis, Cephalalgia, 1 (1981) 71–75.

Blau, J.N. (Ed.), Migraine, Chapman & Hall, London, 1987.

Graham, J.R., Seven common headache profiles, Neurology, 13 (1963) 16–23.

Selby, G., Migraine and Its Variants, ADIS Health Science Press, Sydney, 1983.

Common Migraine (Migraine without Aura) (V-2)

Common migraine generally has the same characteristics as the classic variety with some exceptions, of which the important ones are given below.

Definition
Repetitive, unilateral, and occasionally bilateral throbbing headache attacks, moderate to severe in intensity, often with a premonitory stage but without a distinct, clinically discernible aura, usually accompanied by nausea, vomiting, photophobia, and phonophobia. The pain alternates sides between attacks or even during an attack. The pain usually starts in the frontal areas.

Main Features
Prevalence: the prevalence is probably high. Estimates range from 1% to 31% depending on the criteria for definition of headache. Common migraine occurs much more often than classic migraine (the ratio of common to classic migraine is 2:1 or 3:1, depending upon the strictness of adherence to "classic" and to "common" criteria). *Aura:* absent. If the patient has had several attacks with aura, the majority being without an aura, the patient should still be classified under classic migraine. The complaints are clearly accentuated by minimal physical activity.

Other Features
Common migraine attacks usually last 1–2 days but may last longer, and at times may last only a few hours (lower limit: perhaps around 4 hours).

Relief
See Classic Migraine (V-1).

Complications
Drug abuse of analgesics and/or ergotamine. This is a frequent phenomenon. An improvement of the situation cannot be obtained unless detoxification is carried through.

Essential Features
The aura phase is lacking. The attack may seem to last longer than the classic migraine attack. Otherwise, grossly similar to classic migraine.

Differential Diagnosis
Tension headache, cervicogenic headache. Common migraine in general seems to be characterized by the absence of features characteristic of cervicogenic headache, such as reduced range of motion in the neck; ipsilateral, vague, nonradicular shoulder-arm pain; mechanical precipitation of attacks (see V-7.1).

Code
004.X7b

References
Blau, J.N. (Ed.), Migraine, Chapman & Hall, London, 1987.

Graham, J.R., Migraine: clinical aspects. In: P.J. Vinken and G.W. Bruyn (Eds.), Handbook of Clinical Neurology, North-Holland Publishing Co., Amsterdam, 1968, 5:45–58.

Selby, G. and Lance, J.W., Observations on 500 cases of migraine and allied vascular headache, J. Neurol. Neurosurg. Psychiatry, 23 (1960) 23–32.

Migraine Variants (V-3)

Hemiplegic migraine, migraine accompagnée, basilar migraine, ophthalmoplegic migraine, retinal migraine.

These variants are not described in detail. The neurological symptoms and signs are more pronounced than in "ordinary" migraine. The question of the nature of the underlying neurological disturbance may be more important than that of the differential diagnosis from other headache syndromes. Some of these terms (e.g., basilar migraine and retinal migraine) may be wrongly chosen, and it is uncertain whether they reflect separate entities.

"Migraine cervicale" is not grouped as a migraine variant, since it probably is not "migrainous" in nature. It may rather be a headache associated with neck disorders (see Cervicogenic Headache [VII-2]).

Differential Diagnosis
Classic and common migraine, Chiari malformations, arteriovenous malformations and other structural abnormalities, pseudotumor cerebri, etc., Tolosa-Hunt syndrome (painful ophthalmoplegia), and Raeder's syndrome.

Code
004.X7c

Note: See note on Cluster Headache (V-6).

Carotidynia (V-4)

Definition
Continuous dull aching pain, sometimes throbbing, near the upper portion of the carotid arteries and adjoining cranial regions, with features of migrainous exacerbation. A partly different picture has also been described, Roseman's variant, with a self-limited, relatively shortlasting course.

Site
Pain in the neck, frequently radiating to the face and head (temporal/mastoid area), usually on one side.

System
Vascular system, probably common and internal carotid arteries.

Main Features
Prevalence: occurrence unknown, depends somewhat upon the criteria used, probably rather rare. *Sex Ratio:* more prevalent in the female than the male except for Roseman's variant, where there seems to be no sex preponderance. *Age of Onset:* usually between 20 and 60 years of age. *Pain Quality:* the pain is constant and dull, aching or throbbing. *Time Pattern:* protracted course; dull, continuous neck pain with superimposed separate attacks of hours duration. Roseman's variant: 7–10 days to several weeks. Some patients seem to experience only one episode. There is, however, a tendency for the pain episodes to recur after a symptom-free interval. *Intensity:* moderate, not very severe; apparently less severe than migraine headache.

Precipitating Factors
Moving the head, swallowing, coughing, etc., may precipitate or aggravate the pain.

Associated Symptoms and Signs
Incapacity, nausea, and photophobia. Rarely vomiting. In Roseman's variant, few features in addition to the moderate pain. The carotid artery may on palpation appear enlarged, pulsating, and tender, and externally applied pressure against the common carotid artery may reproduce the pain in the neck and face. Regional muscles may also be tender.

Relief
The treatment of carotidynia is the same as that for migraine; prophylactic drugs (propranolol, methysergide) and ergotamine may help. Symptomatic treatment may also be of some avail. For Roseman's variant, no drugs have been found to be of specific use. It should be emphasized that in this variant the pain episode is self-limited and rather shortlasting. Success in treatment may, therefore, be confounded with the natural course of the disease.

Pathology
Unknown. The nosologic status of these headaches remains obscure.

Code
004.X7d

References
Roseman, D.M., Carotidynia, Arch. Otolaryngol., 85 (1967) 81–84.

Lovshin, L.L., Carotidynia, Headache, 17 (1977) 192–195.

Raskin, N.H. and Prusiner, S., Carotidynia, Neurology (Minneap.), 27 (1977) 43–46.

Murray, T.J., Carotidynia: a cause of neck and face pain, Can. Med. Assoc. J., 120 (1979) 441–443.

Mixed Headache (V-5)

Mixed headache in most cases probably refers either to migraine with interparoxysmal headache or to chronic tension headache, as described above. The headache should accordingly be categorized, whenever possible, as either migraine or chronic tension headache.

Code
003.X7b

Cluster Headache (V-6)

Definition
Unilateral, excruciatingly severe attacks of pain, principally in the ocular, frontal, and temporal areas, recurring in separate bouts with daily, or almost daily, attacks for weeks to months, usually with ipsilateral lacrimation, conjunctival injection, photophobia, and nasal stuffiness and/or rhinorrhea.

Site
Ocular, frontal, temporal areas: considerably less frequent in infraorbital area, ipsilateral upper teeth, back of the head, entire hemicranium, neck, or shoulder. The

maximum pain is usually in ocular, retro-ocular, or peri-ocular areas. Unilateral pain without alternation of sides is characteristic. The side *may*, however, change (in approximately 15% of the patients), even within a given cluster period.

System
Uncertain. The autonomic nervous system is activated. The vascular system is also involved. The pain may be neurogenic. The central nervous system may play a role.

Main Features
Prevalence: approximately 7 per 10,000 population. *Sex Ratio:* 85–90% male. *Age of Onset:* most frequently, headaches start between the ages of 18 and 40. *Pain Quality:* the pain is constant, stabbing, burning, or even throbbing. Patients characteristically pace the floor, bang their heads against the walls, etc., during attacks because of the vehement pain and are usually unable to lie down. *Time Pattern:* attacks grouped in bouts ("cluster periods") of several weeks' to months' duration (most often: 4–12 weeks, with a range from less than 1 week to 12 months), with intervals of some months' duration more or less free from attacks. Usually one cluster period occurs per 6–18 months. Usually, 1–3 attacks, lasting from half an hour to 2 hours each, occur per 24 hours in the cluster period. The maximum number of attacks is ordinarily 6–8 per 24 hours. Attacks may skip a day or two or more during the cluster period. Nocturnal attacks are typical. The patients tend to smoke and drink rather heavily. Sensitivity to alcohol occurs during bouts. *Intensity:* at maximum, excruciatingly severe. Abortive or mild attacks may nevertheless occur.

Precipitating Factors
Alcohol, during the bout. Longlasting stress may possibly predispose to bouts.

Associated Symptoms and Signs
Usually there is no nausea, but some may occur, probably with the more severe attacks or at the peak of attacks. Vomiting is less frequent than nausea. Ipsilateral miosis or ptosis associated with some attacks; occasionally they persist after attacks and sometimes permanently. Ipsilateral conjunctival injection, lacrimation, stuffiness of the nose, and/or rhinorrhea occur in most patients. Dysesthesia upon touching scalp hairs in the area of the ophthalmic division of the Vth cranial nerve and photophobia occur in most patients. A reduction in heart rate and irregular heart activity are features in some patients, especially during severe attacks.

Relief
From ergot preparations, oxygen, corticosteroids, lithium, verapamil, methysergide, etc. Serotonin 1D receptor agonists, like sumatriptan, have a convincing, beneficial effect.

Usual Course
Attacks, less than 1 to 3 per day, appearing in bouts of 4–12 weeks duration. Remissions last one-half to one and one-half years. The episodic form may eventually develop into a chronic form. Possibly, less activity of the disease process with age.

Complications
Suicide risk; peptic ulcer.

Social and Physical Disability
Considerable during bout. Many patients, nevertheless, manage to do their work between attacks.

Pathology
Unknown. Perhaps cavernous sinus changes or "central" changes.

Essential Features
Excruciatingly severe attacks of unilateral headache, appearing in bouts, lasting less than 1 year. Autonomic symptoms and signs on the symptomatic side. Male preponderance.

Differential Diagnosis
Sinusitis, chronic paroxysmal hemicrania, chronic cluster headache, cluster-tic syndrome, and migraine. Cervicogenic headache and tic douloureux ought not to present differential diagnostic problems.

Code
004.X8a

Note: Although cluster headache is grouped with migraine and similar disturbances, it is doubtful if vascular disturbances are the primary source of these events, and the second code digit refers to alternative possibilities for the origin of the pain.

References
Kudrow, L., Cluster Headache: Mechanism and Management, Oxford University Press, London, 1980.

Manzoni, G.W.C., Terzano, M.G., Bono, G., Micieli, G., Martucci, N. and Nappi, G., Cluster headache: clinical findings in 180 patients, Cephalalgia, 3 (1983) 21–30.

Russell, D., Studies of Autonomic Functions in the Cluster Headache Syndrome. Thesis, Oslo University, 1985.

Sjaastad, O., Cluster Headache Syndrome, WB Saunders, Philadelphia, 1992.

Chronic Paroxysmal Hemicrania (CPH) (Unremitting Form or Variety) (V-7.1)

Definition
Multiple daily attacks of severe to excruciating unilateral head pain, more frequently occurring in females than in males, and principally in ocular, frontal, and temporal areas by day and night, usually accompanied by ipsilateral lacrimation, conjunctival injection, and nasal stuffiness and/or rhinorrhea, and with absolute relief from indomethacin. Chronicity denotes an unremitting stage that has lasted more than a year.

Site
Ocular, frontal, and temporal areas; occasionally the infraorbital, aural, mastoid, occipital, and nuchal areas. Pain may also be felt in the ipsilateral part of the neck, arm, and upper part of the chest. There are only rare exceptions to the rule of unchanging unilaterality.

System
Uncertain. The pain may be neurogenic. The vascular and autonomic nervous systems are implicated during attacks. Central nervous system changes may play a role.

Main Features
Prevalence: probably rare. *Sex Ratio:* around 70% females. *Age of Onset:* average around 35 (more than 90% are aged 11–60). *Time Pattern:* at the top of the curve, attacks appear at a rate of 9 or more per 24 hours in more than 80% of the cases (range 4–40 attacks per 24 hours). Patients have attacks every day. Attacks may occur at relatively regular intervals all through day and night. Characteristically, there is marked fluctuation in the severity of attacks and their frequency. A period of 1–2 moderate attacks per day (occasionally even barely noticeable) is followed by a period with frequent, severe attacks, thus providing a "modified cluster pattern." Attacks usually last between 10 and 30 minutes (80% are less than 30 minutes in duration). *Pain Quality:* the pain is clawlike, throbbing, and occasionally boring, pressing, or like "dental" pain. Not infrequently, the patients are awakened by the nocturnal attacks. Some patients walk around during attacks, others sit quietly, still others curl up in bed. *Intensity:* at maximum, the pain attacks are excruciatingly severe, but there is marked fluctuation in severity.

Precipitating Factors
Attacks may be precipitated in the occasional patient (around 10%) by bending or rotating the head, particularly when at the peak of the attack curve ("mechanical precipitation of attacks").

Associated Symptoms and Signs
Ipsilateral conjunctival injection and lacrimation occur frequently, as do ipsilateral nasal stuffiness and/or rhinorrhea. Nausea is rare and vomiting very rare. Slight ipsilateral ptosis or miosis may occur during attacks, and rarely also edema of the upper lid. Photophobia and more rarely phonophobia are occasionally present during attacks. Tinnitus, hypersensitivity in the area of the ophthalmic division of the Vth cranial nerve, bradycardia, and extrasystoles occur in some patients during severe attacks.

Laboratory Findings
Increased nasal secretion and lacrimation (and partly also forehead sweating); increased intraocular pressure and corneal indentation pulse (CIP) amplitudes on the symptomatic side during attack.

Relief
Immediate, absolute, and permanent from continuous indomethacin treatment.

Usual Course
The chronic course may be *primary* chronic or it may develop from a remitting stage. Once chronic, the headache usually *remains* chronic. One case has been observed to revert to a remitting stage after many years of indomethacin treatment, and in a few cases, headache has virtually disappeared after a short course of indomethacin. Attacks frequently disappear partly or even completely during the greater part of pregnancy, to reappear immediately postpartum.

Complications
Possibly CPH "status." Untoward effects of chronic indomethacin therapy—peptic ulcer.

Social and Physical Disability
Considerable during the nontreated stage, including suicidal thoughts. In the worst cases, the patient does not function properly socially.

Pathology
Not identified yet.

Essential Features
Unremitting presence for at least one year of relatively shortlasting repetitive unilateral attacks, associated with ipsilateral autonomic symptoms and signs. Absolute response to indomethacin.

Differential Diagnosis
CPH, remitting form. Sinusitis, chronic cluster headache, cluster headache, cluster-tic syndrome, hemicrania continua.

Code
006.X8k

Note: See note on Cluster Headache (V-6).

References
Antonaci, F. and Sjaastad, O., Chronic paroxysmal hemicrania (CPH): a review of the clinical manifestations, Headache, 29 (1989) 648–656.

Sjaastad, O. and Dale, I., A new (?) clinical headache entity: "chronic paroxysmal hemicrania," Acta Neurol. Scand., 54 (1976) 140–159.

Sjaastad, O., Chronic paroxysmal hemicrania (CPH). In: P.J. Vinken, G.W. Bruyn, H. Klawans and F.C. Rose (Eds.), Handbook of Clinical Neurology 48 (rev. ser. 4), Elsevier, Amsterdam, 1986, pp. 257–266.

Sjaastad, O., Chronic paroxysmal hemicrania (CPH): nomenclature as far as the various stages are concerned, Cephalalgia, 9 (1989) 1–2.

Chronic Paroxysmal Hemicrania (CPH) (Remitting Form or Variety) (V-7.2)

The features of the remitting form are the same as for the chronic ("unremitting") form of CPH. The differences mainly concern the temporal pattern. Accordingly, for other details, the section on the unremitting variety (V-7.1) should be consulted. Absolute relief from indomethacin.

Definition
Attacks of unilateral severe or excruciating headache, occurring more frequently in females than in males, in the ocular, fronto-temporal area, and with the same attack characteristics as in the unremitting form. The periods of attacks last from a few days to many months (if a period exceeds 12 months, the chronic, unremitting stage has been reached). The remitting stage may seemingly go on indefinitely.

Main Features
The remitting form seems to be more rare than the unremitting. This is partly due to the not infrequent conversion of the remitting form to the chronic one. The diagnosis of the remitting form requires a duration of less than 1 year of a period of attacks.

Relief
Immediate, absolute, and permanent effect of indomethacin.

Essential Features
Frequently occurring, relatively shortlasting attacks of unilateral headache, not present continuously for as much as one year. Female preponderance. Absolute response to indomethacin.

Differential Diagnosis
CPH, unremitting form; cluster headache; sinusitis; cluster-tic syndrome; hemicrania continua.

Code
006.X8g

References
Antonaci, F. and Sjaastad, O., Chronic paroxysmal hemicrania (CPH): a review of the clinical manifestations, Headache, 29 (1989) 648–656.

Sjaastad, O., Chronic paroxysmal hemicrania (CPH): nomenclature as far as the various stages are concerned, Cephalalgia, 9 (1989) 1–2.

Sjaastad, O., Cluster Headache Syndrome, WB Saunders, Philadelphia, 1992.

Chronic Cluster Headache (V-8)

The main features of chronic cluster headache are the same as those for the episodic form of cluster headache, to which the reader is referred for further details (V-6). The differences mainly concern the temporal pattern.

Definition
Bouts of excruciatingly severe unilateral pain, usually in males, principally in the ocular, frontal, and temporal areas, usually occurring more frequently than twice a week and *for more than one year*.

Main Features
The chronic form may be *primary* chronic (i.e., the ordinary, episodic form has never existed) or *secondary* chronic (i.e., a further development from the episodic form). The chronic form of cluster headache is more rare than the episodic form (approximately 1:8); the diagnosis requires at least two or more attacks per week over a period of more than one year. Occasionally, however, even longer attack-free intervals may occur.

Relief
The same measures are effective as for cluster headache, but generally the chronic form is more difficult to treat. Surgical procedures (e.g., radio-frequency treatment of the Gasserian ganglion) may be more justifiable in the chronic than in the episodic case.

Essential Features
The unremitting presence of unilateral, relatively shortlasting, and excruciatingly severe attacks for at least one year. Autonomic symptoms and signs on the symptomatic side.

Differential Diagnosis
Sinusitis, chronic paroxysmal hemicrania, cluster headache (episodic form), cluster-tic syndrome, migraine.

Code
004.X8b

Note: See note on Cluster Headache (V-6).

References

Mathew, N. and Hurt, W., Percutaneous radio-frequency trigeminal gangliorhizolysis in intractable cluster headache, Headache, 28 (1988) 328–331.

Onofrio, B.M. and Campbell, J.K., Surgical treatment of chronic cluster headache, Mayo Clin. Proc., 61 (1986) 537–544.

Sjaastad, O., Cluster Headache Syndrome, WB Saunders, Philadelphia, 1992.

Cluster-Tic Syndrome (V-9)

Definition
The coexistence of the features of cluster headache and tic douloureux (trigeminal neuralgia), whether the two entities occur concurrently or separated in time.

Site
Pain limited to the head and face; the two parts of the syndrome generally appear on the same side. The cluster headache element is located in the ocular area as is usual in cluster headache. The most common site of the tic pain is the second or third divisions of the trigeminal nerve.

System
Nervous system.

Main Features
Prevalence: rare. *Sex Ratio:* approximately equal. *Age of Onset:* usually middle age; more rarely in the elderly. *Quality:* a combination of the following: cluster headache pain which includes agonizingly severe, longlasting, burning or throbbing pain, and, concurrently or separated in time, sharp, agonizing, electric shock–like stabs of pain felt superficially in the skin or buccal mucosa, triggered by light tactile stimuli from a restricted trigger point (the features of trigeminal neuralgia). *Time Pattern:* Paroxysms of brief pains occur many times a day with periods of freedom from pain. The attack is often precipitated by speaking, swallowing, washing the face, or shaving. This happens concurrently with, or temporally separated from, the features of cluster headache. The latter comprises severe episodes of steady pain lasting 10–120 minutes, frequently occurring at night, and characteristically occurring in cluster periods lasting 4–8 weeks, once or twice a year, but at times entering a more chronic phase and occurring daily for months. *Intensity:* Extremely severe; both elements of the combined syndrome are among the most severe pains.

Precipitating Factors
For the "tic component," a "trigger phenomenon," as with tic douloureux (see II-1). For the "cluster component," alcohol.

Associated Symptoms
Prominent autonomic features with the cluster-type pain, i.e., ipsilateral nasal obstruction or discharge, or both, ipsilateral lacrimation and conjunctival injection, facial flushing, facial diaphoresis, and agitation.

Signs and Laboratory Findings
Occasionally the presence of a Horner's syndrome is noted, presumably as a residuum from the attacks of cluster headache. No sensory deficit is present over the face.

Relief
The most successful treatment appears to be the use of carbamazepine or baclofen, or both, rather than the conventional drugs used for cluster headache.

Usual Course
The attacks of cluster headache and tic douloureux may start concurrently, or the attacks of tic douloureux may precede those of cluster headache. Cluster headache seems to precede tic douloureux only rarely.

Complications
Depression.

Social and Physical Disabilities
Usually profound during the attacks.

Pathology
Unknown.

Essential Features
Coexistence of features of cluster headache and tic douloureux. These two components of the syndrome may appear simultaneously or separated in time.

Differential Diagnosis
Sinusitis, chronic paroxysmal hemicrania. A careful neurological examination and appropriate tests such as CT scans may be necessary to rule out tumors in the cerebello-pontine region.

Code
006.X8h

References

Green, M. and Apfelbaum, R.J., Cluster-tic syndrome, Headache, 18 (1978) 112.

Solomon, S., Apfelbaum, R.I. and Guglielmo, K., The cluster-tic syndrome and its surgical therapy, Cephalalgia, 25 (1985) 123–126.

Post-traumatic Headache (V-10)

Definition
Continuous or nearly continuous diffusely distributed head pain associated with personality changes involving irritability, loss of concentration ability, dizziness, visual accommodation problems, change in tolerance to ethyl alcohol, loss of libido, and depression, and with or without post-traumatic stress disorder, following head injury.

Site
Head.

System
Nervous system.

Main Features
Prevalence: unknown. *Sex Ratio:* males more than females. *Onset:* difficult to recognize in children, particularly during rebellious age. *Pain Quality:* nonspecific, generalized, nonthrobbing, without aura, and without autonomic dysfunction such as nausea, vomiting, or diarrhea. *Time Pattern:* nearly constant. *Intensity:* mild (relative to migraine), but can be severe.

Associated Symptoms
Personality change involving irritability, inability to concentrate on relatively trivial matters such as balancing a checkbook, lightheadedness or vertigo, intermittent visual accommodation error, change in tolerance, usually intolerance of ethyl alcohol, and loss of libido with or without depression and with or without post-traumatic stress disorder.

Signs and Laboratory Findings
Any objective abnormality including MMPI changes, EEG abnormalities, clinical convulsions, focal neurologic findings, and organic brain syndrome usually absent and if present markedly limits the prognosis.

Usual Course
Without treatment, weeks to months, and in the presence of focal neurologic abnormalities, convulsions, or organic brain syndrome, indefinite.

Complications
Loss of victim's will to combat the illness.

Social and Physical Disabilities
At worst, left untreated, loss of gainful employment and family and social status to the point of complete destitution.

Pathology
Disruption of central axons and boutons due to angular positive or negative acceleration of the brain (unproven hypothesis). Damage to labyrinth is often postulated as well, and soft-tissue lesions from cervical sprain syndrome.

Differential Diagnosis
The word concussion is to be avoided because of lack of agreement in definition of term. Confusion with possible accompanying depression, post-traumatic stress disorder, and other accompanying or complicating psychiatric organic brain dysfunction disorders is to be avoided. In the presence of focal neurologic findings, convulsions, or organic brain syndrome, it is necessary to rule out subdural hematoma and other space-occupying lesions. It is difficult or impossible to distinguish from tension headache. The spouse or family is much more likely to be aware of the irritability of the victim.

Code
002.X1b

References
Brenner, C., Friedman, A.P., Merritt, H.H. and Denny-Brown, D.E., Post-traumatic headache, J. Neurol., 1 (1944) 379.

Merskey, H., Psychiatry and the cervical sprain syndrome (editorial), Can. Med. Assoc. J., 130 (1984) 1119–1121.

Tyler, G.S., NcNeely, H.E. and Dick, M.L., Treatment of post-traumatic headache with amitriptyline, Headache, 20, 4 (1980) 213.

Trimble, M.R., Post-traumatic Neurosis, John Wiley & Sons, Chichester, 1981.

The Syndrome of "Jabs and Jolts" (V-11)

("Ice-Pick Pain" [Raskin]; "Multiple Jabs" [Mathew]; "Idiopathic Stabbing Headache" [nomenclature of the International Headache Society])

Definition
Shortlasting (mostly "ultra-short") paroxysms of head pain, with varying localization, even in the same patient; most often unilateral; in one or more locations. Highly varying frequency even in the same person, usually of moderate severity.

Site
In any region of the head. During one period, the pain may be situated in one area, only to move to another one during another period. Usually unilateral at a given time; in the rare case, bilateral. When associated with hemicrania continua, etc., it frequently occurs in the painful area. In the preheadache phase of chronic paroxysmal hemicrania, it may appear on the side opposite that of the pain.

System
Nervous system.

Main Features

Prevalence: probably common, since it appears both on its own and in many combinations. Frequently associated with various types of unilateral headache, such as chronic paroxysmal hemicrania, cluster headache, migraine, temporal arteritis (giant cell arteritis), hemicrania continua, and probably also tension headache. *Sex Ratio:* both sexes. *Age of Onset:* any age (except perhaps childhood). Since several of the headache forms with which it is combined have a clear female preponderance (see above), it is likely that within some of them there is a female preponderance also of Jabs and Jolts. *Pain Quality:* Sharp, shortlasting, superficial, neuralgiform ("knife-like") pain, superimposed upon the preexisting pain if it occurs in conjunction with another specific headache. Under such circumstances jabs and jolts seem to increase at the time of the symptomatic episodes and in the related areas. The Syndrome of Jabs and Jolts also seems to be a headache per se, unassociated with any of the above-mentioned headaches. Can usually not be triggered from any palpable trigger point. May occasionally be triggered by neck movements, change of position, etc. Most paroxysms occur unprovoked. *Time Pattern:* Extremely unpredictable paroxysms from a temporal point of view, but may appear in bouts (cycles); even within such periods, irregular appearance, from less than once per day to multiple times per hour; the jabs usually appear together with the associated headache. May appear as solitary paroxysms or in volleys. Each paroxysm may last 1–2 seconds, but may occasionally last up to 1 minute (partly as lingering pain after the severe pain). A bout may last a day or two or months. Usually no nocturnal appearance. *Intensity:* Usually moderate, but can in periods be more severe. It may be so severe as to cause a jolt.

Precipitating Factors

Neck movements, change of body position, etc. Underlying mechanism: occasionally perhaps, mechanical irritation from enlarged lymph nodes.

Associated Symptoms and Signs

Few, if any, except for those of accompanying conditions.

Relief

Usually self-limiting. In some patients there is a good, incomplete effect from indomethacin (150 mg a day). The erratic spontaneous course of this headache makes the assessment of drug therapy a most difficult task.

Usual Course

Sporadic paroxysms, or bouts with accumulation of paroxysms, the bouts being of extremely varying duration, from less than one per day to many daily for months. Most frequently bouts recur.

Complications

Probably none.

Social and Physical Disability

In periods with accumulated jabs, the patient may be transitorily handicapped.

Pathology

Unknown, but nerve fibers are the likely source.

Essential Features

Ultrashort paroxysms in the cephalic area, in multiple sites, with no *fixed* location, and with very varying frequency, often occurring in bouts. Occurs sporadically or in conjunction with other headaches, such as chronic paroxysmal hemicrania, migraine, etc.

Differential Diagnosis

Trigeminal neuralgia, SUNCT syndrome.

Code

006.X8i

References

Lance, J.W. and Anthony, M., Migrainous neuralgia or cluster headache? J. Neurol. Sci., 13 (1971) 401–404.

Mathew, N., Indomethacin responsive headache syndromes, Headache, 21 (1981) 147–150.

Raskin, N.H. and Schartz, R.K., Icepick-like pain, Neurology (Minneap.), 30 (1980) 203–205.

Sjaastad, O., Chronic paroxysmal hemicrania (CPH): the clinical picture, Proc. Scand. Migraine Soc., 10 (1979).

Temporal Arteritis (Giant Cell Arteritis) (V-12)

Definition

Unilateral or bilateral headache, mainly continuous with aching or throbbing pain, sometimes very intense, usually in the elderly, with signs of temporal artery involvement—and occasionally more extensive cranial arterial involvement. Commonly associated with muscular aching ("polymyalgia rheumatica") and systemic disturbances like malaise, low-grade fever, and weight loss.

Site

The pain is maximal in the temporal area on one or both sides, from which it may spread to neighboring areas.

System

Vascular system.

Main Features

Prevalence: relatively rare; annual incidence 3–9 per 100,000. *Sex Ratio:* more common in the female. *Age of*

Onset: mostly after fifth decade. *Pain Quality:* varying severity from dull aching to intense pain, more or less continuous, at times pulsating headache. *Time Pattern:* usually a rather protracted course if untreated. The disorder may manifest itself with a repetitive pattern. May be particularly severe at night. *Intensity:* Moderate to severe, probably never excruciatingly severe.

Precipitating Factors
Mastication may produce an effect of intermittent claudication.

Associated Symptoms and Signs
The temporal artery on the symptomatic side may be bulging and irregular in its appearance. The eyesight may fail on the symptomatic side or both sides, and chewing may become deficient during the later part of meals. No deficiency signs from the Vth cranial nerve at rest.

Laboratory Findings
The temporal artery may be pulseless, tender to palpation, and clearly irregular in its shape. A temporal artery biopsy may reveal giant cell arteritis; to some extent this depends upon the stage of disease and whether or not the biopsy is representative.

Visual acuity may fade as a consequence of the disease process. This usually occurs in the early stage of disease; it is an "alarm" situation and necessitates immediate therapeutic action (corticosteroid therapy). Involvement of the other eye may occur after a short time. Arterial involvement is demonstrable with, for example, angiography and ocular dynamic tonometry (reduced corneal indentation pulse [CIP] amplitudes). The erythrocyte sedimentation rate is frequently clearly raised.

Relief
From corticosteroid and immunosuppressive therapy, e.g., azathioprine therapy.

Usual Course
The prognosis has changed drastically with the advent of corticosteroids. The early start of steroid therapy is essential. Once blindness has appeared, the prognosis for this phenomenon is poor. Relapse may occur in the early stage. Late deaths are more likely to be due to complications of steroid therapy than to the arteritis.

Complications
Fading vision or blindness (see Laboratory Findings). Impaired chewing in late phase of meals—probably due to masticatory muscle ischemia, caused by the same disease process in the appropriate arteries. Ocular palsy; arteritis in other vessels, e.g., coronary arteries and aorta; cerebral infarction. Complications may also arise as a consequence of steroid therapy.

Social and Physical Disability
Considerable during the acute stage, and in the case of complications like blindness.

Pathology
Fibrous tissue formation (giant cell arteritis) in the arterial wall. Relationship to polymyalgia rheumatica.

Essential Features
Acute pain, not infrequently unilateral, in the temporal area in an elderly person, with tenderness and irregular shape of the ipsilateral temporal artery and, usually, raised erythrocyte sedimentation rate. Various complications may arise, such as blindness.

Differential Diagnosis
Other acute unilateral headaches, such as the Tolosa-Hunt syndrome and Raeder's paratrigeminal neuralgia *in the early stages*; carotidynia; hemicrania continua; temporomandibular joint dysfunction (Costen's syndrome); auriculotemporal nerve neuralgia; polymyalgia rheumatica.

Code
023.X3

References
Horton, B.T. and Magath, T.B., An undescribed form of arteritis of the temporal vessels, Mayo Clin. Proc., 7 (1923) 700–701.

Ross Russell, R.W., Giant cell (cranial) arteritis. In: P.J. Vinken, G.W. Bruyn, H.L. Klawans and F.C. Rose (Eds.), Handbook of Clinical Neurology 48 (rev. ser. 4), Elsevier, Amsterdam, 1986, pp. 309–328.

Headache Associated with Low CSF Pressure (V-13)
(Spontaneous Low CSF Pressure Headache)

Definition
Dull aching or throbbing headache associated with low CSF pressure occurring spontaneously or after a minor incident.

Site
May be frontal, occipital, or global, and not infrequently unilateral.

System
Probably vascular or meningeal, or both.

Main Features
Prevalence: probably rare. *Sex Ratio:* probably a female preponderance. *Age of Onset:* most cases described have been more than 30 years old. *Pain Quality:* usually dull or aching, but may be throbbing. *Intensity:* from mild to rather severe, probably never excruciating. *Precipitating*

Factors: the pain is positional, markedly exacerbated or only present when the patient is sitting or standing, and usually relieved by lying down. *Time Pattern:* onset is usually insidious, but may occur after a mild trauma, sneezing, sudden strain, or orgasm. Individual headache episodes usually last as long as the patient remains in the upright position.

Associated Symptoms and Signs
Pain and stiffness in the neck, nausea, vomiting, tinnitus, dizziness, blurred vision, and VIth cranial nerve palsy have all been reported.

Laboratory Findings
A low CSF pressure, usually ≤ 60 mm H_2O, is found on lumbar puncture with the patient lying horizontally.

Usual Course
Most cases improve spontaneously after a few weeks and within three months. Recurrences seem to be rare. In some cases, the headache may last for years.

Relief
Lying down. *Treatment:* Epidural blood patch, epidural saline infusion, high dose corticosteroids have been used with success in a few patients.

Complications
Usually none.

Social and Physical Disability
Inability to sit or stay in the upright position because of the pain.

Pathology
Low CSF pressure demonstrated during spinal tap is essential for diagnosis. Lumbar isotope cisternography has given indications of a leakage through a nerve root sheath tear or hyperabsorption of CSF as possible causes of the low CSF pressure in a few patients. However, this can not be used as a diagnostic test.

Essential Features
Positional headache due to low CSF pressure occurring spontaneously or after mild incidents.

Differential Diagnosis
Low CSF pressure due to CSF leaks after major head trauma.

Code
023.X1a

References
Fernandez, E., Headaches associated with low spinal fluid pressure, Headache, 30 (1990) 122–138.

Molins, A., Alvarez, J., Titus, F. and Codina, A., Cisternographic pattern of spontaneous liquoral hypotension, Cephalalgia, 10 (1990) 59–65.

Gaukroger, P.B. and Brownridge, P., Epidural blood patch in the treatment of low CSF pressure headache, Pain, 29 (1987) 119–122.

Post–Dural Puncture Headache (V-14)

Definition
Dull, aching, or throbbing positional pain in the head occurring after dural puncture, most often in the lumbar region

Site
Frontal, occipital, or global. May be unilateral.

System
Probably vascular and/or meningeal.

Main Features
Prevalence: occurs in 15–30% of patients who have been subject to lumbar puncture. *Sex Ratio:* women are affected twice as often as men. *Age of Onset:* relatively reduced frequency under 13 years and over 60 years. *Pain Quality:* usually dull or aching, but may be throbbing. *Precipitating Factors:* the pain is positional, markedly exacerbated or only present when the patient is sitting or standing, usually relieved by lying down. *Intensity:* from mild to rather severe, probably never excruciating. *Time Pattern:* headache usually starts within 48 hours after lumbar puncture, but it may be delayed up to 12 days.

Associated Symptoms and Signs
Frequently, the patient will have pain and stiffness in the neck and the low back. Nausea is also fairly common, whereas blurred vision, tinnitus, and vomiting occur more rarely.

Laboratory Findings
Often, but not invariably, a low CSF pressure (≤ 60 mm H_2O) is found, provided a second lumbar puncture with the patient lying horizontally is carried out during a symptomatic period.

Usual Course
On average, symptoms persist for four days, but in some cases, the headache may be protracted (lasting even up to years).

Relief
Lying down. *Treatment:* Intravenous caffeine sodium benzoate, epidural blood patch, epidural saline infusion, surgical closure of dural leak.

Complications
Subdural hematoma or hygroma may rarely occur.

Social and Physical Disability

The patient may be unable to sit or stay in the upright position because of the pain.

Pathology

Sudden drop in CSF volume, usually, but not always, resulting in a low CSF pressure.

Continuous leakage of CSF probably also plays a role.

Essential Features

Positional headache occurring after lumbar puncture.

Differential Diagnosis

Meningitis (bacterial or aseptic) occurring after lumbar puncture.

Code

023.X1b

References

Tourtellotte, W.W., Haerer, A.F., Heller, G.L. and Somers, J.E., Post-Lumbar Puncture Headaches, CC Thomas Publisher, Springfield, 1964.

Vilming, S.T., Schrader, H. and Monstad, I., The significance of age, sex and cerebrospinal fluid pressure in post-lumbar-puncture headache, Cephalalgia, 9 (1989) 99–106.

Hemicrania Continua (V-15)

Definition

Unilateral dull pain, occasionally throbbing, initially intermittent but later frequently a continuous headache of moderate to severe degree, sometimes with superimposed stabbing pains. Usually, there are some autonomic symptoms and signs. There is a clear female preponderance, and the headache responds completely to indomethacin.

Site

The headache is strictly unilateral, and in general without change of side. The maximum pain is usually in the ocular and fronto-temporal areas.

System

Unknown.

Main Features

Prevalence: not known, probably not frequent but may be more frequent than the other headache, completely responsive to indomethacin, i.e., chronic paroxysmal hemicrania (CPH). *Sex Ratio:* female to male about 5:1. *Age of Onset:* mean about 35, range 11–57 years of age. *Pain Quality:* dull, during exacerbations, occasionally throbbing. Considerable fluctuations in pain, even during the late, nonremitting stage. Most patients experience occasional or more frequent "jabs and jolts." *Time Pat-*

tern: the chronic, nonremitting stage so typical of this headache is frequently preceded by a remitting stage (in approximately half the cases) of varying duration. During the remitting stage, there may be repetitive, separate attacks lasting hours or days. During the nonremitting stage, when the pain is more or less continuous, exacerbations occur, lasting a few hours to 4–5 days. *Intensity:* usually moderate to severe, with rather marked fluctuations; patients are usually able to cope with daily chores. Occasional nighttime awakening due to pain.

Precipitating Factors

Attacks or exacerbations are not known to be precipitated mechanically.

Associated Symptoms and Signs

Photophobia, phonophobia, nausea, conjunctival injection, and lacrimation (the last two on the symptomatic side) occur in up to half the cases, but these symptoms and signs generally are mild and usually only become clinically apparent during exacerbations.

Relief

Immediate, absolute, and permanent relief from continued indomethacin administration in adequate dosages.

Usual Course

The unremitting course may apparently continue for a long time, perhaps indefinitely. Once the chronic stage has been reached, no exceptions to this rule have been observed so far.

Complications

In a few instances, suicide attempts due to headache.

Social and Physical Disability

Considerable during exacerbations.

Pathology

Not known. "Symptomatic" cases have been observed, e.g., with tumor of osseous structures. When atypical features occur or when the indomethacin effect is incomplete or fading, such a possibility should be suspected.

Essential Features

Remitting or nonremitting unilateral headache, occurring mostly in the female, with the pain maximum in the oculo-fronto-temporal area, the pain being of moderate to severe degree. There may be moderate autonomic signs. Absolute and permanent indomethacin effect.

Differential Diagnosis

The other unilateral headache with absolute indomethacin response, CPH; other unilateral headaches such as Costen's syndrome, sinusitis, dental pain, and earache (in the remitting stage of hemicrania continua); cervicogenic headache. (Note the following points of differential diagnostic importance. HC: *complete* indomethacin response. Cervicogenic headache: reduced range of motion in the neck; ipsilateral, diffuse, nonradicular shoulder/arm symptoms; mechanical precipitation of attacks; absolute effect of major occipital nerve blockade.)

Code
093.X8

References
Bordini, C., Antonaci, F., Stovner, L.J., Schrader, H. and Sjaastad, O., Hemicrania continua: a clinical review, Headache, 31 (1991) 20–26.

Sjaastad, O. and Spierings, E.L.H., "Hemicrania continua": another headache absolutely responsive to indomethacin, Cephalalgia, 4 (1984) 65–70.

Headache Not Otherwise Specified (V-16)

Code
00X.X8f

HEADACHE CROSSWALK

The classification of headache of the International Headache Society appeared in 1988 (International Headache Society, Classification and diagnostic criteria for headache disorders, cranial neuralgias and facial pain, Cephalalgia, 8, Suppl. 7 [1988]). That system differs from the IASP classification in several respects. This list, which follows the first six sections (Groups II through VII) in which headache specifically appears in this volume, refers also to Groups IX-1 (IX-1.7 to IX-1.11) and IX-8. It is intended to provide a statement, where possible, of the correspondence between the categories of the IHS system and the IASP system. Because the structures of the two systems differ significantly, correspondence is often not easy to determine or is definitely not available. The principal feature of the structures which provides this problem is that the IASP system for head, face, and neck, follows the same pattern as that used in other parts of the body, i.e., proceeding through neurological, musculoskeletal, and visceral disorders as well as miscellaneous conditions. Some phenomena are also described in relation to the cervical spine. The IHS system also includes a number of acute categories that are lacking by design in the IASP system, and the IASP system contains categories that were not adopted by the IHS in 1988, but which should be adopted at this point and have no exact IHS equivalent.

All the IASP categories are printed in bold, as are those IHS syndromes for which the correspondence appears to be fairly good. The crosswalk is from the IASP system to the IHS system and not in reverse. Where the only corresponding item is a "catch-all" or residual category, an entry is not necessarily made.

IASP		IHS	
I-6	**Central Pain (if confined to head and face)**	12.7.2	**Thalamic pain**

IASP		IHS	
II-1	**Trigeminal neuralgia (tic douloureux)**	12.2.1	
II-2	**Secondary neuralgia (trigeminal) from central nervous system lesions (tumor or aneurysm)**	12.2.2.2	**Symptomatic trigeminal neuralgia: central lesions**
II-3	**Secondary trigeminal neuralgia from facial trauma**	12.2.2	**Symptomatic trigeminal neuralgia**
II-4	**Acute herpes zoster (trigeminal)**	12.1.4.1	**Herpes zoster**
II-5	**Postherpetic neuralgia (trigeminal)**	12.1.4.2	**Chronic postherpetic neuralgia**
II-6	**Geniculate neuralgia (VIth cranial nerve): Ramsay Hunt syndrome**	12.1.4.1	**Herpes zoster**
II-8	**Glossopharyngeal neuralgia (IXth cranial nerve)**	12.3.1 / 12.3.2	**Idiopathic glossopharyngeal neuralgia** / *Symptomatic glossopharyngeal neuralgia*
II-9	**Neuralgia of the superior laryngeal nerve (vagus nerve neuralgia)**	12.5	**Superior laryngeal neuralgia**
II-10	**Occipital neuralgia**	12.6	**Occipital neuralgia**
II-11	**Hypoglossal neuralgia**	12.1.7	*Other causes of persistent pain of cranial nerve origin*
II-12	**Glossopharyngeal pain from trauma**	12.3.2	**Symptomatic glossopharyngeal neuralgia**
II-12	**Hypoglossal pain from trauma**	12.1.7	*Other causes of persistent pain of cranial nerve origin*
II-14	**Tolosa-Hunt syndrome (painful ophthalmoplegia)**	12.1.5	**Tolosa-Hunt syndrome**

IASP		IHS	
III-2	Tension headache: chronic form (scalp muscle contraction headache	2.2	Chronic tension-type headache
		2.3	Headache of the tension type
III-3	Temporomandibular pain and dysfunction syndrome	2.3.2	*Headache of the tension type with oromandibular dysfunction*
III-5	Rheumatoid arthritis of the temporomandibular joint	11.7	*Temporomandibular joint disease*

IASP		IHS	
IV-1	Maxillary sinusitis	11.5.1	Acute sinus headache
IV-2 through IV-5	Types of odontalgia	11.6	*Headache or facial pain associated with disorder of teeth, mouth, or other facial or cranial structures*
IV-6	Glossodynia and sore mouth	11.6	*Headache or facial pain associated with disorder of teeth, mouth, or other facial or cranial structures*
IV-7	Cracked tooth syndrome	11.6	*Headache or facial pain associated with disorder of teeth, mouth, or other facial or cranial structures*
IV-8	Dry socket	11.6	*Headache or facial pain associated with disorder of teeth, mouth, or other facial or cranial structures*
IV-9	Gingival disease, inflammatory	11.6	*Headache or facial pain associated with disorder of teeth, mouth, or other facial or cranial structures*
IV-10	Toothache, cause unknown	11.6	*Headache or facial pain associated with disorder of teeth, mouth, or other facial or cranial structures*
IV-11	Diseases of the jaw, inflammatory conditions	11.6	*Headache or facial pain associated with disorder of teeth, mouth, or other facial or cranial structures*
IV-12	Other and unspecified pain in jaws	11.6	*Headache or facial pain associated with disorder of teeth, mouth, or other facial or cranial structures*

IASP		IHS	
V-1	Classic migraine (migraine with aura)	1.2.1	Migraine with aura
		1.2.2	
		1.2.6	
		1.6.1	
V-2	Common migraine (migraine without aura)	1.1	Migraine without aura
V-3	Migraine variants	1.2.3	Familial hemiplegic migraine
		1.2.4	Basilar migraine
		1.3	Ophthalmoplegic migraine
		1.4	Retinal migraine
V-5	Mixed headache	1.1	Migraine without aura
		2.2	Chronic tension type headache
V-6	Cluster headache	3.1.1	Cluster headache, periodicity undetermined
		3.1.2	Episodic cluster headache

IASP		IHS	
V-7.1	Chronic paroxysmal hemicrania: unremitting form or variety	3.2	Chronic paroxysmal hemicrania
V-7.2	Chronic paroxysmal hemicrania: remitting form or variety	3.2	*Chronic paroxysmal hemicrania*
V-8	Chronic cluster headache	3.1.3	Chronic cluster headache
V-10	Post-traumatic headache	5.2.1	Chronic post-traumatic headache with significant head trauma or confirmatory signs
		5.2.2	Minor head trauma with no confirmatory signs
V-11	Syndrome of "jabs and jolts"	4.1	*Idiopathic stabbing headaches*
V-12	Temporal arteritis (giant cell arteritis)	6.5.1	Giant cell arteritis
V-13	Headache associated with low cerebrospinal fluid pressure	7.2.2	*Cerebrospinal fluid fistula headache*
V-14	Post–dural puncture headache	7.2.1	Post lumbar puncture headache
V-16	Headache not otherwise specified	13.0	Headache, not classifiable

IASP		IHS	
VI-2	Hysterical or hypochondriacal pain in the head, face, and neck	2.3.3	*Headache of the tension type, not fulfilling above criteria*
VI-3	Headache of psychological origin in the head, face, and neck associated with depression	2.3.3	*Headache of the tension type, not fulfilling above criteria*

IASP		IHS	
VII-2	Cervicogenic headache	11.2.1	*Headache or facial pain associated with disorder of cranium, neck, etc.*

IASP		IHS	
IX-1	Cervical spinal or radicular pain attributable to a fracture	11.2.1	*Headache or facial pain associated with disorder of cranium, neck, etc.*
IX-1.7	Fracture of lamina	11.2.1	*Headache or facial pain associated with disorder of cranium, neck, etc.*
IX-1.9	Fracture of the anterior arch of the atlas	11.2.1	*Headache or facial pain associated with disorder of cranium, neck, etc.*
IX-1.10	Fracture of the posterior arch of the atlas	11.2.1	*Headache or facial pain associated with disorder of cranium, neck, etc.*
IX-1.11	Burst fracture of the atlas	11.2.1	*Headache or facial pain associated with disorder of cranium, neck, etc.*
NOTE:	Other items in the neck are not included, although they may potentially cause headache; if they do, they can be entered in the relevant section of the cervical spinal items		
IX-8	Acceleration-deceleration injury of the neck (cervical sprain)	5.2.2	*Minor head trauma with no confirmatory signs*

GROUP VI: PAIN OF PSYCHOLOGICAL ORIGIN IN THE HEAD, FACE, AND NECK

As for I-16 with local distribution.

Delusional or Hallucinatory Pain (VI-1)

Differential diagnosis from local and general conditions.

Code
01X.X9e   Head or face
11X.X9e   Neck

Hysterical, Conversion, or Hypochondriacal Pain (VI-2)

Distribution possibly more often on the left, except in cases with lesions or compensation claims. Differential diagnosis from local conditions (see above) and general conditions, e.g., hypothyroidism, polyarthralgia, etc., which cause diffuse symptoms.

Code
01X.X9f   Head or face
11X.X9f   Neck

Associated with Depression (VI-3)

Code
01X.X9g   Head or face
11X.X9g   Neck

GROUP VII: SUBOCCIPITAL AND CERVICAL MUSCULOSKELETAL DISORDERS

(See also Group IX; for Cervical Sprain see IX-8, Acceleration-Deceleration Injury of the Neck.)

Stylohyoid Process Syndrome (Eagle's Syndrome) (VII-1)

Definition
Pain following trauma in the region of a calcified stylohyoid ligament.

Site
Mandible, floor of mouth, lateral pharynx.

System
Musculoskeletal system.

Main Features
Prevalence: among patients with calcified stylohyoid ligament and history of trauma to mandible and/or neck. *Sex Ratio:* no predilection. *Age of Onset:* 40–50 years. *Start:* evoked by swallowing, opening mandible, turning head toward pain and down, with palpation of stylohyoid ligament. *Pain Quality:* throbbing, deep. *Occurrence:* with function. *Intensity:* mild to moderate. *Duration:* seconds to minutes.

Associated Symptoms
Dizziness, tenderness on palpation of the carotid trunk and branches.

Signs
Carotid bruit, transient ischemic episodes.

Radiologic Findings
Calcified stylohyoid process.

Usual Course
Benign, intractable if styloid process not excised or fractured, partial relief from stellate ganglion local anesthetic infiltration, and acetylsalicylic acid.

Complication
Secondary carotid arteritis and cerebral ischemia.

Social and Physical Disability
Interference with speech and mastication.

Pathology

Calcified stylohyoid ligament, carotid—external carotid branch arteritis.

Summary of Essential Features and Diagnostic Criteria

Presence of calcified stylohyoid ligament, tenderness of superficial vessels, history of trauma.

Differential Diagnosis

Myofascial pain dysfunction, carotid arteritis, glossopharyngeal neuralgia, tonsillitis, parotitis, mandibular osteomyelitis.

Code

036.X6

Cervicogenic Headache (VII-2)

Definition

Attacks of moderate or moderately severe unilateral head pain without change of side, ordinarily involving the whole hemicranium, usually starting in the neck or occipital area, and eventually involving the forehead and temporal areas, where the maximal pain is frequently located. The headache usually appears in episodes of varying duration in the early phase, but with time the headache frequently becomes more continuous, with exacerbations and remissions. Symptoms and signs such as mechanical precipitation of attacks imply involvement of the neck.

Site

Whole hemicranium. The pain usually starts in the neck or back of the head but soon moves to the frontal and temporal areas. It occasionally extends into the infraorbital area. Unilaterality without alternation of sides is typical, but occasionally moderate involvement of the opposite side occurs during the most severe attacks. Bilateral cases certainly exist and may be quite frequent. At the present time, however, scientific studies should preferably include only unilateral cases. Frequently, diffuse ("nonradicular") pain or discomfort occurs in the ipsilateral shoulder and arm.

System

Probably the peripheral nervous system. Musculoskeletal system is probably also involved.

Main Features

Prevalence: probably rather frequent, but exact figures are lacking. *Sex Ratio:* probably less than 3/4 of the patients are female. *Age of Onset:* young adult or middle age. Many of the patients have sustained neck trauma a relatively short time prior to the onset. *Pain Quality:* constant, deep, dull, steady, not excruciating pain. Pain seemingly identical, may be triggered by neck movements or by external pressure over the greater occipital nerve (GON). *Time Pattern:* pain episodes are of greatly varying duration, from hours to weeks, even intra-individually, the usual duration being one to a few days. The varying duration of attacks is a characteristic feature of this headache. Interval between pain episodes: days to weeks. In the later phase, there is characteristically a protracted or continuous, low-intensity pain, with superimposed exacerbations. *Intensity:* moderate to severe pain.

Precipitating Factors

Pain similar to that of the "spontaneous" pain episodes or even attacks may be precipitated by awkward neck movements or awkward positioning of the head during sleep. Also by external pressure over the GON on the symptomatic side.

Associated Symptoms

More rarely the symptoms include: nausea, vomiting, phonophobia and photophobia (usually of a low degree), dizziness, "blurred vision" (longlasting) on the symptomatic side, and difficulties in swallowing.

Signs

Reduced range of motion in the neck, in one or more directions. Occasionally, edema and redness of the skin below the eye on the symptomatic side.

Tests and Laboratory Findings

A blockade of the greater occipital nerve (GON), the minor occipital nerve, the so-called IIIrd occipital nerve, or the cervical nerve roots should be carried out on the symptomatic side. Such blockades reduce or take away the pain transitorily, not only in the anesthetized area (the innervation area of the respective nerve) but also in the nonanesthetized, painful Vth nerve area. This represents a diagnostic test.

Relief

Repeated corticosteroid injections along the GON may provide relief of some duration. Neurolysis ("liberation operation") of GON may provide longlasting relief (1/3 to more than 2 years), but it rarely, if ever, provides *permanent* relief. There are reasons to believe that denervation of the periosteum of the occipital area on the symptomatic side may provide permanent relief in a high percentage of the cases.

Usual Course

Persistence and intensification of the pain syndrome over time.

Complications

Combination with root pain into shoulder/arm.

Social and Physical Disability
Patients can frequently do some routine work during symptomatic periods. In the worst periods, total disability.

Pathology
Probably related to various structures in the neck or posterior part of the scalp on the symptomatic side (C2/C3 innervation area), but cannot at present be precisely identified. Although the clinical picture is identifiable and rather stereotyped, the pathology varies in that pathology in the lower part of the neck may also be the underlying cause.

Essential Features
Combination of unilateral headache, ipsilateral diffuse shoulder or arm pain, reduced range of motion in the neck, presence of mechanical precipitation mechanisms, and discontinuation of the pain upon anesthetic blockades (GON, C2, etc.) in the typical case. Frequently there is a history of neck injury.

Differential Diagnosis
Common migraine, hemicrania continua, spondylosis of the cervical spine. Other unilateral headaches, such as cluster headache, are less important in this respect. Tension headache (as regards the bilateral variant of cervicogenic headache).

Code
033.X6b

References
Bogduk, N. and Marsland, H., On the concept of third occipital headache, J. Neurol. Nurosurg. Psychiatry, 49 (1986) 775–780.

Fredriksen, T.A., Studies on Cervicogenic Headache: Clinical Manifestation and Differentiation from Other Unilateral Headache Forms (thesis), Tapir, Trondheim, 1989.

Sjaastad, O., Sante, C., Hovdal, H., Breivik, H. and Gronbaek, E., "Cervicogenic" headache: an hypothesis, Cephalalgia, 3 (1983) 249–256.

Sjaastad, O., Fredriksen, T.A. and Pfaffenrath, V., Cervicogenic headache: diagnostic criteria, Headache, 30 (1990) 725–726.

Superior Pulmonary Sulcus Syndrome (Pancoast Tumor) (VII-3)

Definition
Progressively intense pain in the shoulder and ulnar side of the arm, associated with sensory and motor deficits and Horner's syndrome due to neoplasm.

Continuous aching pain in the paraspinal region, shoulder, or elbow, in time expanding to the whole ulnar side of the arm. Exacerbations of sharp lancinating pain in the region of the lower brachial plexus. Often radiological evidence of a tumor in the apex of the lung.

Site
Shoulder and upper limb.

System
Nervous system.

Main Features
Sex Ratio: males more than females. *Age of Onset:* usually in the decades corresponding with the occurrence of carcinoma of the lung. *Pain Quality:* the pain is continuous, involving the root of the neck and ulnar side of the upper limb. It is usually progressive, requiring narcotics for relief, and becomes excruciating unless properly managed. The lesion is involvement of the VIIIth cervical and Ist thoracic roots. The pain is a severe aching and burning associated with sharp lancinating exacerbations. There is paralysis and atrophy of the small muscles of the hand and a sensory loss corresponding to the pain distribution.

Associated Symptoms
The cervical sympathetic is involved with a Horner's syndrome.

Signs and Laboratory Findings
Atrophy of the small muscles of the hand, ulnar sensory loss, ulnar paresthesias and pain, and Horner's syndrome. The diagnosis is made on chest X-ray by the appearance of a tumor in the superior sulcus. Electromyography will demonstrate denervation in the appropriate distribution.

Usual Course
The course is generally relentless and the prognosis poor.

Complications
Occasional infiltration of spinal cord with compression. Occasional hoarseness from infiltration of the laryngeal nerves.

Social and Physical Disability
Those related to the neurological loss, unemployment, and family stress.

Pathology or Other Contributory Factors
Virtually always carcinoma of the lung, though any tumor metastatic to the area may give identical findings.

Summary of Essential Features and Diagnostic Criteria
The essential features are unremitting, aching pain of increasing severity, in time expanding to the ulnar side of the arm with exacerbations of sharp lancinating pain in the distribution of the lower brachial plexus. Horner's syndrome occurs associated with damage to T1 and C8

and occasional neurological loss; the diagnosis is made by chest X-ray demonstrating tumor at the apex of the lung, and the biopsy is made by tumor.

Code
102.X4a

Reference
Bonica, J.J., Ventafridda, V. and Pagni, C.A., Management of superior pulmonary sulcus syndrome (Pancoast syndrome). In: J.J. Bonica, V. Ventafridda and C.A. Pagni, (Eds.), Advances in Pain Research and Therapy, Vol. 4, Raven Press, New York, 1982.

Thoracic Outlet Syndrome (VII-4)
(includes Scalenus Anticus Syndrome, Cervical Rib Syndrome)

Definition
Pain in the root of the neck, head, shoulder, radiating down the arm into the hand. Due to compression of the brachial plexus by hypertrophied muscle, congenital bands, post-traumatic fibrosis, cervical rib or band, or malformed first thoracic rib.

Site
Ipsilateral side of head, neck, arm, and hand.

System Involved
Musculoskeletal system.

Main Features
Sex Ratio: there is no sexual predilection. *Age of Onset:* the thoracic outlet syndrome is characteristically found in young to middle-aged adults but may affect older adults also. *Pain Quality:* typically, pain begins in the root of the neck, or shoulder, and radiates down the arm, but it may also affect the head. The ulnar aspect of the arm is the most commonly involved, but the pain may affect the entire arm. Paresthesias are common in the same distribution. The pain occurs irregularly, usually with activity. The pain in the hand or the arm is not usually intense, but the associated headache may be severe. When the pain occurs, it usually diminishes with rest.

The distribution of the paresthesias or pain in the shoulder or arm is varied and can be associated with a particular nerve root, or with many nerve roots. Often it is rather baffling in that it cannot readily be related to specific nerves or nerve roots.

Associated Symptoms
Raynaud's phenomenon involving the same extremity is common. Hemiplegia from stroke secondary to vascular thrombosis and propagation of the clot may occur. The pain is generally aggravated by exercise and relieved by rest. A dystrophic sympathetic change may also occur.

Rarely, peripheral vascular insufficiency syndromes are found, and occasionally, the subclavian axillary vein complex can be compressed, and the patient presents with swelling and blueness consistent with symptoms of venous obstruction.

Signs and Laboratory Findings
Postural abnormalities are common. Three physical findings are frequent: pain on pressure over the brachial plexus, just lateral to the scalenus anticus muscle; pain mimicked by abduction and external rotation of the arm; and pain when the brachial plexus is stretched by tipping the head to the opposite side. Color change may also appear with other maneuvers, e.g., bracing back the shoulders. The classic sign is Adson's maneuver. This is performed by maximal extension of the chin and deep inspiration with the shoulders relaxed forward and the head turned towards the suspected side of abnormality. Obliteration of the pulse, or at least diminution, should occur. This sign is not always found and may occur in normal individuals also.

Laboratory findings are often not helpful. Angiograms are indicated when there is an arterial or venous obstruction but are very poor diagnostic maneuvers, the milder forms of the thoracic outlet syndrome only affecting neurological symptoms. Electromyography may demonstrate evidence of nerve root compression across the thoracic outlet and denervation distally in the arm, but often fails to do so.

Usual Course
The usual course is one of continued persistent discomfort. Physiotherapy may strengthen the shoulder girdle and relieve symptoms, and this should be tried at first, but ordinarily symptoms will persist until the entrapment of the plexus is relieved.

Complications
Complications include arterial compression with thrombosis and an ischemic arm. Axillary subclavian vein thrombosis may also occur separately, or in addition.

Pathology
A variety of anatomical abnormalities will compress the neurovascular bundle at the thoracic outlet and may cause this syndrome. It may be precipitated in predisposed individuals by flexion-extension injuries of the cervical spine with consequent postural or other change. This is a late sequel of such injuries.

Social and Physical Disabilities
The patients are often unable to work because of dysfunction of the extremity involved.

Summary of Essential Features and Diagnostic Criteria

Patients with this syndrome suffer from compression of the brachial plexus for which many causes exist. Characteristically, they develop pain and paresthesias in the upper extremity, sometimes associated with headache. The most common diagnostic criteria are tenderness over the brachial plexus in the neck, reproduction of the pain by the maneuver of abduction and external rotation of the arm, and pain on stretching the brachial plexus.

Differential Diagnosis

Differential diagnosis includes cervical rib, cervical osteoarthritis, Pancoast's tumor, aneurysm of the subclavian artery, tumors of the brachial plexus, cervical disk, adenopathy or tumor of other supraclavicular structures, metastatic cancer to the cervical spine.

Code

133.X6d
233.X6a

Cervical Rib or Malformed First Thoracic Rib (VII-5)

It is impossible to differentiate the scalenus anticus syndrome (VII-4) from cervical or malformed first thoracic rib, except by X-ray. The presentations are identical. The diagnosis and differential diagnoses are the same. The only variation from the scalenus anticus syndrome is the finding of the abnormal or deformed rib on X-ray. The code is the same and the reference for this syndrome is the same.

Pain of Skeletal Metastatic Disease of the Neck, Arm, or Shoulder Girdle (VII-6)

Definition

Dull aching pain in the shoulder girdle or upper extremity due to tumor infiltration of bone.

Site

Clavicle, scapula, humerus.

System

Skeletal system.

Main Feature

Age of Onset: usually in the fifth, sixth, and seventh decades—corresponding to the occurrence of carcinoma of the lung, breast, and prostate. *Pain Quality:* The pain is usually described as a continuous dull ache or a constant throb. It may radiate up into the neck or down into the anterior chest wall. An expanding lesion in the humerus may radiate into the forearm. The cardinal feature is acute exacerbation of the pain by any movement of the shoulder girdle.

Associated Symptoms

Pain at rest usually responds to nonsteroidal anti-inflammatory drugs and narcotic analgesics. Pain secondary to movement is sometimes relieved by internal fixation. Both types of pain may respond to radiation therapy.

Signs and Laboratory Findings

The active range of movement of the shoulder girdle is usually much more limited than the passive range of movement. Well-localized bony tenderness is common. Neurological signs are unusual. A radioisotope bone scan is usually positive before a plain X-ray. However, both of these tests may be normal in the setting of severe pain.

Complications

The tendency to keep the upper extremity immobilized may result in a "frozen shoulder," with secondary pain on that basis. A pathological fracture in the shaft of the humerus severely exacerbates pain on movement, and this usually requires treatment with internal fixation.

Social and Physical Disability

There may be loss of use of the involved upper extremity.

Summary of Essential Features and Diagnostic Criteria

Continuous aching pain, exacerbation of the pain by movement, localized bony tenderness at the site of metastatic deposit.

Differential Diagnosis

It is important to rule out referred pain to the shoulder girdle and upper extremity due to tumor infiltration of the cervical roots and brachial plexus.

Code

133.X4j
233.X4

GROUP VIII: VISCERAL PAIN IN THE NECK

Carcinoma of Thyroid (VIII-1)

Definition
Pain in the thyroid gland, aggravated by palpation and associated with an adherent neoplastic mass.

Site
Throat and anterior neck area, spreading to the ear.

System
Endocrine system.

Main Features
Localized sharp or dull, aching or burning, occasionally stabbing if superior laryngeal nerve involved.

Associated Symptoms
Mass in neck, dysphagia, dyspnea or stridor, symptoms from secondary deposits.

Signs
Neck swelling, fixation of thyroid, stridor.

Laboratory Findings
Cold nodule on scan.

Complications
Local—dysphagia; stridor.

Code
172.X4

Carcinoma of Larynx (VIII-2)

Definition
An aching soreness in the throat, aggravated by swallowing, with hoarseness and dysphagia.

Site
Larynx and adjoining portions of neck.

System
Respiratory system.

Main Features
Initially, there is a complaint of sore throat, with irritation, which becomes a severe soreness. Later, pain may develop on swallowing. The pain spreads to the ear (otalgia), possibly because of the involvement of the vagus nerve. The pain is usually moderately severe, dull, aching, burning in character, occasionally sharp, stabbing, or lancinating if the superior laryngeal nerve is involved.

Associated Symptoms
Hoarseness; dysphagia, when local spread has occurred.

Signs
Tumor on inspection of larynx.

Complications
Stridor progressing to respiratory obstruction; dysphagia, when local spread has occurred.

Social and Physical Disability
Loss of voice following surgical treatment.

Essential Features
Persistent hoarseness, with soreness or pain supervening.

Code
122.X4

Tuberculosis of Larynx (VIII-3)

Definition
A painful irritation in the throat on air flow during breathing, coughing, and swallowing due to tuberculous lesions.

Site
Larynx and adjoining regions of neck.

System
Respiratory system.

Main Features
Now rare. Local in larynx; spreads to ear (otalgia); continuous, dull, aching, burning, stabbing, or lancinating if superior laryngeal nerve involved. Worse on swallowing. N.B.: In early stage is pain free. In advanced cases there is severe pain in the laryngeal and pharyngeal area, which may radiate to the ear.

Associated Symptoms
Hoarseness; cough; purulent sputum; night sweats and fever; weight loss.

Signs
Inflammation of larynx; ulceration of larynx; chest signs.

Pathology
Infection with *Mycobacterium tuberculosis*.

Summary of Essential Features and Diagnostic Criteria

Hoarseness in someone with tuberculosis of chest, i.e., cough, sputum, night sweats, and weight loss, with pain supervening.

Differential Diagnosis

Cancer of larynx.

Code

123.X2

Chronic Pharyngitis (VIII-4)

Code

151.X5	If known
151.X8	Alternative

Carcinoma of Pharynx (VIII-5)

Code

153.X4

C. SPINAL PAIN, SECTION 1: SPINAL AND RADICULAR PAIN SYNDROMES

For a discussion of spinal and radicular pain syndromes, please see pages 11–16.

D. SPINAL PAIN, SECTION 2: SPINAL AND RADICULAR PAIN SYNDROMES OF THE CERVICAL AND THORACIC REGIONS

N.B. For explanatory material on this section and on section G, Spinal and Radicular Pain Syndromes of the Lumbar, Sacral, and Coccygeal Regions, see pp. 11–16 in the list of Topics and Codes. Please also note the comments on coding on p. 17.

GROUP IX: CERVICAL OR RADICULAR SPINAL PAIN SYNDROMES

Cervical Spinal or Radicular Pain Attributable to a Fracture (IX-1)

Definition
Cervical spinal pain occurring in a patient with a history of injury in whom radiography or other imaging studies demonstrate the presence of a fracture that can reasonably be interpreted as the cause of the pain.

Clinical Features
Cervical spinal pain with or without referred pain.

Diagnostic Features
Radiographic or other imaging evidence of a fracture of one of the osseous elements of the cervical vertebral column.

Schedule of Fractures
IX-1.1(S)(R)
> Fracture of a Vertebral Body
> Code 133.X1eS/C 233.X1eR

IX-1.2(S)
> Fracture of a Spinous Process (Synonym: "clay-shovelers fracture")
> Code 133.X1fS

IX-1.3(S)(R)
> Fracture of a Transverse Process
> Code 133.X1gS/C 233.X1fR

IX-1.4(S)(R)
> Fracture of an Articular Pillar
> Code 133.X1hS/C 233.X1gR

IX-1.5(S)(R)
> Fracture of a Superior Articular Process
> Code 133.X1iS/C 233.X1hR

IX-1.6(S)(R)
> Fracture of an Inferior Articular Process
> Code 133.X1jS/C 233.X1iR

IX-1.7(S)(R)
> Fracture of Lamina
> Code 133.X1kS/C 233.X1uR

IX-1.8(S)(R)
> Fracture of the Odontoid Process
> Code 133.X1lS/C 233.X1vR

IX-1.9(S)(R)
> Fracture of the Anterior Arch of the Atlas
> Code 133.X1mS/C 233.X1pR

IX-1.10(S)(R)
> Fracture of the Posterior Arch of the Atlas
> Code 133.X1nS/C 233.X1qR

IX-1.11(S)(R)
> Burst Fracture of the Atlas
> Code 133.X1oS/C 233.X1wR

Cervical Spinal or Radicular Pain Attributable to an Infection (IX-2)

Definition
Cervical spinal pain occurring in a patient with clinical or other features of an infection, in whom the site of infection can be specified and which can reasonably be interpreted as the source of the pain.

Clinical Features
Cervical spinal pain with or without referred pain, associated with pyrexia or other clinical features of infection.

Diagnostic Features
A presumptive diagnosis can be made on the basis of an elevated white cell count or other serological features of infection, together with imaging evidence of the presence of a site of infection in the cervical vertebral column or its adnexa. Absolute confirmation relies on histological and/or bacteriological confirmation using material obtained by direct or needle biopsy.

Schedule of Sites of Infection
IX-2.1(S)(R)
> Infection of a Vertebral Body (Osteomyelitis)
> Code 132.X2aS/C 232.X2iR

IX-2.2(S)(R)
> Septic Arthritis of a Zygapophysial Joint
> Code 132.X2bS/C 232.X2jR

IX-2.3(S)(R)
> Septic Arthritis of an Atlanto-Axial Joint
> Code 132.X2cS/C 232.X2cR

IX-2.4(S)(R)
> Infection of the Prevertebral Muscles or Space
> Code 132.X2dS/C 232.X2kR

IX-2.5(S)(R)
> Infection of an Intervertebral Disk (Diskitis)
> Code 132.X2eS/C 232.X2lR

IX-2.6(S)(R)
> Infection of an Interbody Graft
> Code 132.XtS/C 232.X2mR

IX-2.7(S)(R)
> Infection of a Posterior Fusion
> Code 132.X2gS/C 232.X2nR

IX-2.8(S)(R)
> Infection of the Epidural Space
> (Epidural Abscess)
> Code 132.X2hS/C 232.X2oR

IX-2.9(S)(R)
> Infection of the Spinal Meninges (Meningitis)
> Code 103.X2cS/C 203.X2cR

IX-2.10(S)(R)
> Herpes Zoster Acute
> Code 103.X2dS/C 203.X2dR

IX-2.11(S)(R)
> Postherpetic Neuralgia
> Code 103.X2eS/C 203.X2eR

IX-2.12(S)(R)
> Syphilis: Tabes Dorsalis and Hypertrophic
> Pachymeningitis
> Code 107.X2*S/C 207.X2*R

IX-2.13(S)(R)
> Other Syphilitic Changes, Including Gumma
> (No Code)

Cervical Spinal or Radicular Pain Attributable to a Neoplasm (IX-3)

Definition
Cervical spinal pain associated with a neoplasm that can reasonably be interpreted as the source of the pain.

Clinical Features
Cervical spinal pain with or without referred pain.

Diagnostic Features
A presumptive diagnosis may be made on the basis of imaging evidence of a neoplasm that directly or indirectly affects one or other of the tissues innervated by cervical spinal nerves. Absolute confirmation relies on obtaining histological evidence by direct or needle biopsy.

Schedule of Neoplastic Diseases
IX-3.1(S)(R)
> Primary Tumor of a Vertebral Body
> Code 133.X4aS/C 233.X4aR

IX-3.2(S)(R)
> Primary Tumor of Any Part of a Vertebra Other than Its Body
> Code 133.X4bS/C 233.X4bR

IX-3.3(S)(R)
> Primary Tumor of a Zygapophysial Joint
> Code 133.X4cS/C 233.X4cR

IX-3.4(S)(R)
> Primary Tumor of an Atlanto-Axial Joint
> Code 133.X4dS/C 233.X4dR

IX-3.5(S)(R)
> Primary Tumor of a Paravertebral Muscle
> Code 133.X4eS/C 233.X4eR

IX-3.6(S)(R)
> Primary Tumor of Epidural Fat (e.g., lipoma)
> Code 133.X4fS/C 233.X4yR

IX-3.7(S)(R)
> Primary Tumor of Epidural Vessels
> (e.g., angioma)
> Code 133.X4gS/C 233.X4gR

IX-3.8(S)(R)
> Primary Tumor of Meninges (e.g., meningioma)
> Code 103.X4aS/C 203.X4aR

IX-3.9(R)
> Primary Tumor of Spinal Nerves
> (e.g., neurofibroma, schwannoma, neuro-
> blastoma)
> Code 203.X4bR

IX-3.10(S)(R)
> Primary Tumor of Spinal Cord (e.g., glioma)
> Code 103.X4cS/C 203.X4cR

IX-3.11(S)(R)
> Metastatic Tumor Affecting a Vertebra
> Code 133.X4hS/C 233.X4gR

IX-3.12(S)(R)
> Metastatic Tumor Affecting the Vertebral Canal
> Code 133.X4iS/C 233.X4uR

IX-3.13(S)(R)
> Other Infiltrating Neoplastic Disease of a
> Vertebra (e.g., lymphoma)
> Code 133.X4jS/C 233.X4qR

Cervical Spinal or Radicular Pain Attributable to Metabolic Bone Disease (IX-4)

Definition
Cervical spinal pain associated with a metabolic bone disease that can reasonably be interpreted as the source of the pain.

Clinical Features
Cervical spinal pain with or without referred pain.

Diagnostic Features

Imaging or other evidence of metabolic bone disease affecting the cervical vertebral column, confirmed by appropriate serological or biochemical investigations and/or histological evidence obtained by needle or other biopsy.

Schedule of Metabolic Bone Diseases

IX-4.1(S)(R)
>Osteoporosis of Age
>Code 132.X5aS/C 232.X5gR

IX-4.2(S)(R)
>Osteoporosis of Unknown Cause
>Code 132.X5bS/C 232.X5hR

IX-4.3(S)(R)
>Osteoporosis of Some Known Cause
>Other than Age
>Code 132.X5cS/C 232.X5iR

IX-4.4(S)(R)
>Hyperparathyroidism
>Code 132.X5dS/C 232.X5jR

IX-4.5(S)(R)
>Paget's Disease of Bone
>Code 132.X5eS/C 232.X5kR

IX-4.6(S)(R)
>Metabolic Disease of Bone Not
>Otherwise Classified
>Code 132.X5fS/C 232.X5lR

Cervical Spinal or Radicular Pain Attributable to Arthritis (IX-5)

Definition

Cervical spinal pain associated with arthritis that can reasonably be interpreted as the source of the pain.

Clinical Features

Cervical spinal pain with or without referred pain.

Diagnostic Features

Imaging or other evidence of arthritis affecting the joints of the cervical vertebral column.

Schedule of Arthritides

IX-5.1(S)(R)
>Rheumatoid Arthritis
>Code 132.X3aS/C 232.X3aR

IX-5.2(S)(R)
>Ankylosing Spondylitis
>Code 132.X8aS/C 232.X8aR

IX-5.3(S)(R)
>Osteoarthritis
>Code 138.X6aS/C 238.X6aR

IX-5.4(S)(R)
>Seronegative Spondylarthropathy Not
>Otherwise Classified
>Code 123.X8aS/C 232.X8aR

Remarks

Osteoarthritis is included in this schedule with some hesitation because there is only weak evidence that indicates that this condition as diagnosed radiologically is causally associated with spinal pain.

The alternative classification to "cervical pain due to osteoarthrosis" should be "cervical zygapophysial joint pain" if the criteria for this diagnosis are satisfied (see IX-11) or "cervical spinal pain of unknown or uncertain origin" (see IX-7).

The condition of "spondylosis" is omitted from this schedule because there is no significant positive correlation between the radiographic presence of this condition and the presence of spinal pain (Friedenberg and Miller 1963; Heller et al. 1983). There is no evidence that this condition represents anything more than age-changes in the vertebral column.

References

Friedenberg, Z.B. and Miller, W.T., Degenerative disk disease of the cervical spine, J. Bone Joint Surg., 45A (1963) 1171-1178.

Heller, C.A., Stanley, P., Lewis-Jones, B. and Heller, R.F., Value of X-ray examinations of the cervical spine, Br. Med. J., 287 (1983) 1276-1279.

Cervical Spinal or Radicular Pain Associated with a Congenital Vertebral Anomaly (IX-6)

Definition

Cervical spinal or radicular pain associated with a congenital vertebral anomaly.

Clinical Features

Cervical spinal pain with or without referred pain.

Diagnostic Features

Imaging evidence of a congenital vertebral anomaly affecting the cervical vertebral column.

Remarks

There is no evidence that congenital anomalies per se cause pain. Although they may be associated with pain, the specificity of this association is unknown. This classification should be used only when the cause of pain cannot be otherwise specified and there is a perceived need to highlight the presence of the congenital anomaly, but should not be used to imply that the congenital anomaly is the actual source of pain.

Code
123.X0*S/C
223.X0R

Cervical Spinal Pain of Unknown or Uncertain Origin (IX-7)

Definition
Cervical spinal pain occurring in a patient whose clinical features and associated features do not enable the cause and source of the pain to be determined, and whose cause or source cannot be or has not been determined by special investigations.

Clinical Features
Cervical spinal pain with or without referred pain.

Diagnostic Features
Cervical spinal pain for which no other cause has been found or can be attributed.

Pathology
Unspecified.

Remarks
This definition is intended to cover those complaints that for whatever reason currently defy conventional diagnosis. It does not encompass pain of psychological origin. It presupposes an organic basis for the pain, but one that cannot be or has not been established reliably by clinical examination or special investigations such as imaging techniques or diagnostic blocks.

This diagnosis may be used as a temporary diagnosis. Patients given this diagnosis could in due course be accorded a more definitive diagnosis once appropriate diagnostic techniques are devised or applied. In some instances, a more definitive diagnosis might be attainable using currently available techniques, but for logistic or ethical reasons these may not have been applied.

Upper Cervical Spinal Pain of Unknown or Uncertain Origin (IX-7.1)

Definition
As for IX-7, but the pain is located in the upper cervical region.

Clinical Features
Spinal pain located in the upper cervical region.

Diagnostic Criteria
As for IX-7, save that the pain is located in the upper cervical region.

Pathology
Unspecified.

Remarks
As for IX-7.

Code
13X.X8cS/C
23X.X8cR

Lower Cervical Spinal Pain of Unknown or Uncertain Origin (IX-7.2)

Definition
As for IX-7, but the pain is located in the lower cervical region.

Clinical Features
Spinal pain located on the lower cervical region.

Diagnostic Criteria
As for IX-7, save that the pain is located in the lower cervical region.

Pathology
Unspecified.

Remarks
As for IX-7.

Code
13X.X8dS/C
23X.X8dR

Cervico-Thoracic Spinal Pain of Unknown or Uncertain Origin (IX-7.3)

Definition
As for IX-7, but the pain is located in the cervico-thoracic region.

Clinical Features
Spinal pain located in the cervico-thoracic region.

Diagnostic Criteria
As for IX-7, save that the pain is located in the cervico-thoracic region.

Pathology
Unspecified.

Remarks
As for IX-7.

Code
13X.X8eS/C
23X.X8eR

Acceleration-Deceleration Injury of the Neck (Cervical Sprain) (IX-8)

Definition
Cervical spinal pain precipitated by an event involving sudden acceleration or deceleration of the head and neck with respect to the trunk.

Clinical Features
The pain is aggravated by motion of the cervical spine, tension, sitting, or reading and is often accompanied by muscle spasm and trigger points in one or more muscles of the occiput or neck. Prolonged or repetitive use of the shoulder girdle muscles, e.g., carrying dishes or washing them, may induce radiation of pain in the upper extremity. Push/pull activities, e.g., vacuum cleaning, may aggravate pain also. Cervical spinal pain with or without referred pain in a patient describing a history of sudden acceleration or deceleration of the head and neck of a magnitude sufficient to be presumed to have injured one or more of the components of the cervical spine.

Diagnostic Criteria
The presence of clinical features described above.

Pathology
No single pathologic entity can be ascribed to this condition. The spinal pain can be caused by any of a variety of injuries that may befall the cervical spine.

Remarks
The use of the term "whiplash" is not recommended.

This classification is essentially a clinical diagnosis. A more specific diagnosis could be entertained if the appropriate diagnostic criteria could be satisfied, for example sprain of an anulus fibrosus, zygapophysial joint pain, muscle sprain, muscle spasm. Certain associated features such as dizziness, tinnitus, and blurred vision occur in some cases, often those which are relatively severe. Sleep disturbance and mood disturbance often appear for months or longer in the more severe cases, but these are a minority of all cases. These associated features may be coincidental or expressions of an anxiety state or a secondary response to chronic pain. Their

presence or absence is immaterial to the formulation of the diagnosis.

Code
133.X1aS/C
233.X1aS/C
233.X1aR

References
Bogduk, N., The anatomy and pathophysiology of whiplash, Clin. Biomech., 1 (1986) 92–101.

Macnab, I., The whiplash syndrome, Clin. Neurosurg., 20 (1973) 232–241.

Mendelson, G., Not "cured by a verdict": effect of legal settlement on compensation claimants, Med. J. Aust., 2 (1982) 132–134.

Merskey, H., Psychiatry and the cervical sprain syndrome, Can. Med. Assoc. J., 130 (1984) 1119–1121.

Torticollis (Spasmodic Torticollis) (IX-9)

Definition
Cervical spinal pain associated with sustained rotatory deformity of the neck.

Clinical Features
Cervical spinal pain, with or without referred pain, occurring in a patient who maintains a rotated posture of the head and neck.

Diagnostic Criteria
Obvious rotated posture of the neck with or without compensatory rotation of the head.

As far as possible, the cause should be specified, but the clinical features of this condition are so distinctive that it can remain a clinical diagnosis.

Neurological causes induce spasmodic torticollis and should be distinguished from muscular or articular causes.

Pathology
1. Neurological: Torticollis may be a feature of a basal ganglia disorder, either primary or drug-induced. Pain may only be a result of secondary degenerative musculoskeletal effects.
2. Muscular: Sprain of a muscle may result in the patient assuming an antalgic, rotated posture that minimizes the strain on the affected muscle. Contracture can develop not susceptible to manipulation under anesthesia.
3. Articular: One of the synovial joints of the neck may be dislocated or subluxated so as to cause the rotatory deformity, and voluntary reduction is not possible

because of structural changes in the joint or because attempted reduction stresses periarticular or intraarticular structures and aggravates the patient's pain. This includes fixed atlanto-axial rotatory deformity and meniscus extrapment of a cervical zygapophysial joint.

4. Herniated nucleus pulposus: In the presence of a herniated nucleus pulposus, a patient may adopt a reflex or voluntary antalgic rotated posture of the neck to avoid the pain produced by the herniated nuclear material compromising a spinal nerve.

Relief
Torticollis due to neurologic disorder or muscle spasm may sometimes be relieved by repeated injections of the motor nerve supply with botulinum toxin.

Code
133.X0jS	Congenital
133.X1*S	Trauma
133.X2*S	Infection
133.X8fS	Unknown or other

Cervical Discogenic Pain (IX-10)

Definition
Cervical spinal pain, with or without referred pain, stemming from a cervical intervertebral disk.

Clinical Features
Spinal pain perceived in the cervical region, with or without referred pain to the head, anterior or posterior chest wall, upper limb girdle, or upper limb.

Diagnostic Criteria
The patient's pain may be shown conclusively to stem from an intervertebral disk by demonstrating

either   (1) that selective anesthetization of the putatively symptomatic intervertebral disk completely relieves the patient of the accustomed pain for a period consonant with the expected duration of action of the local anesthetic used;

or   (2) that selective anesthetization of the putatively symptomatic intervertebral disk substantially relieves the patient of the accustomed pain for a period consonant with the expected duration of action of the local anesthetic used, save that whatever pain persists can be ascribed to some other coexisting source or cause;

or   (3) provocation diskography of the putatively symptomatic disk reproduces the patient's accustomed pain, provided that provocation of at least two adjacent intervertebral disks clearly does not reproduce the patient's pain, and provided that

the pain cannot be ascribed to some other source innervated by the same segments that innervate the putatively symptomatic disk.

Pathology
Unknown, but presumably the pain arises as a result of chemical or mechanical irritation of the nerve endings in the outer anulus fibrosus, initiated by injury to the anulus, or as a result of excessive stresses imposed on the anulus by injury, deformity or other disease within the affected segment or adjacent segments.

Remarks
Provocation diskography alone is insufficient to establish conclusively a diagnosis of discogenic pain because of the propensity for false-positive responses either because of apprehension on the part of the patient or because of the coexistence of a separate source of pain within the segment under investigation. If analgesic diskography is not performed or is possibly false-negative, criterion 3 must be explicitly satisfied. Otherwise, the diagnosis of "discogenic pain" cannot be sustained, whereupon an alternative classification must be used.

Code
133.X1vS	Trauma
133.X6bS	Degeneration
133.X7*S	Dysfunction
233.X1bR	Trauma
233.X6*R	Degeneration
233.X7*R	Dysfunction

References
Cloward, R.B., Cervical diskography: a contribution to the aetiology and mechanism of neck, shoulder and arm pain, Ann. Surg., 130 (1959) 1052–1064.

Collins, H.R., An evaluation of cervical and lumbar discography, Clin. Orthop., 107 (1975) 133–138.

Kikuchi, S., Macnab, I. and Moreau, P., Localisation of the level of symptomatic cervical disc degeneration, J. Bone Joint Surg., 63B (1981) 272–277.

Roth, D.A., Cervical analgesic discography: a new test for the definitive diagnosis of the painful-disk syndrome, JAMA, 235 (1976) 1713–1714.

Simmons, E.H. and Segil, C.M., An evaluation of discography in the localisation of symptomatic levels in discogenic disease of the spine, Clin. Orthop., 108 (1975) 57–69.

Cervical Zygapophysial Joint Pain (IX-11)

Definition
Cervical spinal pain with or without referred pain stemming from one or more of the cervical zygapophysial joints.

Clinical Features
Cervical spinal pain with or without referred pain.

Diagnostic Criteria
No criteria have been established whereby zygapophysial joint pain can be diagnosed on the basis of the patient's history or by conventional clinical examination.

The condition can be firmly diagnosed only by the use of diagnostic intraarticular zygapophysial joint blocks. For the diagnosis to be declared, all of the following criteria must be satisfied.
1. The blocks must be radiologically controlled.
2. Arthrography must demonstrate that any injection has been made selectively into the target joint, and any material that is injected into the joint must not spill over into adjacent structures that might otherwise be the actual source of the patient's pain.
3. The patient's pain must be totally relieved following the injection of local anesthetic into the target joint.
4. A single positive response to the intra-articular injection of local anesthetic is insufficient for the diagnosis to be declared. The response must be validated by an appropriate control test that excludes false-positive responses on the part of the patient, such as:
   - no relief of pain upon injection of a nonactive agent;
   - no relief of pain following the injection of an active local anesthetic into a site other than the target joint; or
   - a positive but differential response to local anesthetics of different durations of action injected into the target joint on separate occasions.

Local anesthetic blockade of the nerves supplying a target zygapophysial joint may be used as a screening procedure to determine in the first instance whether a particular joint might be the source of symptoms, but the definitive diagnosis may be made only upon selective intraarticular injection of the putatively symptomatic joint.

Pathology
Still unknown. May be due to small fractures not evident on plain radiography or conventional computerized tomography, but possibly demonstrated on high-resolution CT, conventional tomography, or stereoradiography. May be due to osteoarthrosis, but the radiographic presence of osteoarthritis is not a sufficient criterion for the diagnosis to be declared. Zygapophysial joint pain may be caused by rheumatoid arthritis, ankylosing spondylitis, septic arthritis, or villo-nodular synovitis.

Sprains and other injuries to the capsule of zygapophysial joints have been demonstrated at post mortem and may be the cause of pain in some patients, but these types of injuries cannot be demonstrated in vivo using currently available imaging techniques.

Remarks
See also Cervical Segmental Dysfunction (IX-15).

Codes
133.X1pS	Trauma
133.X6cS	Degeneration
133.X7aS	Dysfunction

References
Abel, M.S., Occult traumatic lesions of the cervical vertebrae, CRC Crit. Rev. Clin. Radiol. Nucl. Med., 6 (1975) 469-553.

Binet, E.F., Moro, J.J., Marangola, J.P. and Hodge, C.J., Cervical spine tomography in trauma, Spine. 2 (1977) 163-173.

Bogduk, N. and Marsland, A., The cervical zygapophyseal joints as a source of neck pain, Spine, 13 (1988) 610-617.

Dwyer, A., Aprill, C. and Bogduk, N., Cervical zygapophyseal joint pain patterns I: a study in normal volunteers, Spine, 15 (1990) 453-457.

Dory, M.A., Arthrography of the cervical facet joints, Radiology, 148 (1983) 379-382.

Dussault, R.G. and Nicolet, V.M., Cervical facet joint arthrography, J. Can. Assoc. Radiol., 36 (1985) 79–80.

Hove, B. and Gyldensted, C., Cervical analgesic facet joint arthrography, Neuroradiology, 32 (1990) 456–459.

McCormick, C.C., Arthrography of the atlanto-axial (C1–C2) joints: technique and results, J. Intervent. Radiol., 2 (1987) 9–13.

Smith, G.R., Beckly, D.E. and Abel, M.S., Articular mass fracture: a neglected cause of post traumatic neck pain? Clin. Radiol., 27 (1976) 335–340.

Wedel, D.J. and Wilson, P.R., Cervical facet arthrography, Reg. Anesth., 10 (1985) 7-11.

Woodring, J.H. and Goldstein, S.J., Fractures of the articular processes of the cervical spine, AJR, 139 (1982) 341-344.

Cervical Muscle Sprain (IX-12)

Definition
Cervical spinal pain stemming from a lesion in a specified muscle caused by strain of that muscle beyond its normal physiological limits.

Clinical Features
Cervical spinal pain, with or without referred pain, associated with tenderness in the affected muscle and aggravated by either passive stretching or resisted contraction of that muscle.

Diagnostic Criteria
The following criteria must all be satisfied.
1. The affected muscle is specified.
2. There is a history of activities consistent with the affected muscle having been strained.
3. The muscle is tender to palpation.

4. (a)   Aggravation of the pain by any clinical test that can be shown to stress selectively the affected muscle, or

(b)   Selective infiltration of the affected muscle with local anesthetic completely relieves the patient's pain.

Pathology
Rupture of muscle fibers, usually near their myotendinous junction, that elicits an inflammatory repair response.

Remarks
This category has been included in recognition of its frequent use in clinical practice, and because a pattern of "muscle sprain" is readily diagnosed in injuries of the limbs.

Code
133.X1mS
233.X1k

Cervical Trigger Point Syndrome (IX-13)

Definition
Cervical spinal pain stemming from a trigger point or trigger points in one or more of the muscles of the cervical spine.

Clinical Features
Cervical spinal pain, with or without referred pain, associated with a trigger point in one or more muscles of the cervical vertebral column.

Diagnostic Criteria
The following criteria must all be satisfied.
1. A trigger point must be present in a muscle, consisting of a palpable, tender, firm, fusiform nodule or band orientated in the direction of the affected muscle's fibers.
2. The muscle must be specified.
3. Palpation of the trigger point reproduces the patient's pain and/or referred pain.
4. Elimination of the trigger point relieves the patient's pain. Elimination may be achieved by stretching the affected muscle, dry needling the trigger point, or infiltrating it with local anesthetic.

Pathology
Unknown. Trigger points are believed to represent areas of contracted muscle that have failed to relax as a result of failure of calcium ions to sequestrate. Pain arises as a result of the accumulation of algogenic metabolites.

Remarks
For the diagnosis to be accorded, the diagnostic criteria for a trigger point must be fulfilled. Simple tenderness in a muscle without a palpable band does not satisfy the criteria, whereupon an alternative diagnosis should be accorded, such as muscle sprain, if the criteria for that condition are fulfilled, or spinal pain of unknown or uncertain origin.

Trigger points in different muscles of the cervical spine allegedly give rise to distinctive pain syndromes differing in the distribution of referred pain, and in some instances differing in the nature of associated features. The wisdom of enunciating each and every syndrome, muscle by muscle, is questionable; there is no point attempting to define each syndrome by its allegedly distinctive pain patterns and associated features when the critical diagnostic feature is the identification of a trigger point.

Schedule of Trigger Point Sites
IX-13.1(S)
   Upper Sternocleidomastoid
   Code 132.X1aS
IX-13.2(S)
   Lower Sternocleidomastoid
   Code 132.X1bS
IX-13.3(S)
   Upper Trapezius
   Code 132.X1cS
IX-13.4(S)
   Middle Trapezius
   Code 132.X1dS
IX-13.5(S)
   Lower Trapezius
   Code 132.X1eS
IX-13.6(S)
   Splenius Capitis
   Code 132.X1fS
IX-13.7(S)
   Upper Splenius Cervicis
   Code 132.X1gS
IX-13.8(S)
   Lower Splenius Cervicis
   Code 132.X1hS
IX-13.9(S)
   Semispinalis Capitis
   Code 132.X1iS
IX-13.10(S)
   Levator Scapulae
   Code 132.X1jS

References
Simons, D.G., Myofascial pain syndromes: Where are we? Where are we going? Arch. Phys. Med. Rehab., 69 (1988) 207–212.

Travell, J.G. and Simons, D.G., Myofascial Pain and Dysfunction. The Trigger Point Manual, Williams & Wilkins, Baltimore, 1983.

Alar Ligament Sprain (IX-14)

Definition
Cervical spinal pain or referred pain to the head arising from an alar ligament as a result of sprain of that ligament.

Clinical Features
Upper cervical spinal pain, suboccipital pain, and/or headache, aggravated by contralateral rotation of the atlas, associated with hypermobility of the atlas in contralateral rotation.

Diagnostic Criteria
The patient's pain must clearly be aggravated by rotation of the atlas to the side opposite that of the putatively affected ligament, and hypermobility of the atlas must be evident on functional CT scan of the joint, both features being in the context of an appropriate mechanism of injury or some other reason for the ligament to have been injured.

Pathology
Unproven. Presumably the same as for sprains in ligaments of the appendicular skeleton.

Code
132.X1*S

References
Dvorak, J., Hayek, J. and Zehnder, R., CT-functional diagnostics of the rotatory instability of the upper cervical spine, part 2: an evaluation of healthy adults and patients with suspected instability, Spine 12 (1987) 726–731.

Cervical Segmental Dysfunction (IX-15)

Definition
Cervical spinal pain ostensibly due to excessive strains sustained by the restraining elements of a single spinal motion segment.

Clinical Features
Cervical spinal pain, with or without referred pain, that can be aggravated by selectively stressing a particular spinal segment.

Diagnostic Criteria
All the following criteria should be satisfied.
1. The affected segment must be specified.
2. The patient's pain is aggravated by clinical tests that selectively stress the affected segment.
3. Stressing adjacent segments does not reproduce the patient's pain.

Pathology
Unknown. Presumably involves excessive strain incurred during activities of daily living by structures such as the ligaments, joints, or intervertebral disk of the affected segment.

Remarks
This diagnosis is offered as a partial distinction from spinal pain of unknown origin, insofar as the source of the patient's pain can at least be narrowed to a particular offending segment. Further investigation of a patient accorded this diagnosis might result in the patient's condition being ascribed a more definitive diagnosis such as diskogenic pain or zygapophysial joint pain, but the diagnosis of segmental dysfunction could be applied if facilities for undertaking the appropriate investigations are not available, if the physician or patient does not wish to pursue such investigations, or if the pain arises from multiple sites in the same segment.

For this diagnosis to be sustained, the clinical tests used should be able to stress selectively the segment in question and have acceptable interobserver reliability.

Code
133.X1tS
233.X1cR

Radicular Pain Attributable to a Prolapsed Cervical Disk (IX-16)

Code
203.X6aR   Arm

Traumatic Avulsion of Nerve Roots (IX-17)

Code
103.X1aS/C
203.X1cR

GROUP X: THORACIC SPINAL OR RADICULAR PAIN SYNDROMES

Thoracic Spinal or Radicular Pain Attributable to a Fracture (X-1)

Definition
Thoracic spinal pain occurring in a patient with a history of injury, in whom radiography or other imaging studies demonstrate the presence of a fracture that can reasonably be interpreted as the cause of the pain.

Clinical Features
Thoracic spinal pain with or without referred pain.

Diagnostic Features
Radiographic or other imaging evidence of a fracture of one of the osseous elements of the thoracic vertebral column.

Schedule of Fractures
X-1.1(S)(R)
> Fracture of a Vertebral Body
> Code 333.X1eS/C 233.X1jR

X-1.2(S)
> Fracture of a Spinous Process
> Code 333.X1fS

X-1.3(S)(R)
> Fracture of a Transverse Process
> Code 333.X1gS/C 233.X1kR

X-1.4(S)
> Fracture of a Rib
> Code 333.X1hS

X-1.5(S)(R)
> Fracture of a Superior Articular Process
> Code 333.X1tS/C 233.X1lR

X-1.6(S)(R)
> Fracture of an Inferior Articular Process
> Code 333.X1jS/C 233.X1mR

X-1.7(S)(R)
> Fracture of Lamina
> Code 333.X1kS/C 233.X1nR

Thoracic Spinal or Radicular Pain Attributable to an Infection (X-2)

Definition
Thoracic spinal pain occurring in a patient with clinical and/or other features of an infection, in whom the site of infection can be specified and which can reasonably be interpreted as the source of the pain.

Clinical Features
Thoracic spinal pain with or without referred pain, associated with pyrexia or other clinical features of infection.

Diagnostic Features
A presumptive diagnosis can be made on the basis of an elevated white cell count or other serological features of infection, together with imaging evidence of the presence of a site of infection in the thoracic vertebral column or its adnexa. Absolute confirmation relies on histological and/or bacteriological confirmation using material obtained by direct or needle biopsy.

Schedule of Sites of Infection
X-2.1(S)(R)
> Infection of a Vertebral Body (osteomyelitis)
> Code 332.X2aS/C 232.X2iR

X-2.2(S)(R)
> Septic Arthritis of a Zygapophysial Joint
> Code 332.X2bS/C 232.X2jR

X-2.3(S)(R)
> Septic Arthritis of a Costo-Vertebral Joint
> Code 332.X2cS/C 232.X2cR

X-2.4(S)(R)
> Septic Arthritis of a Costo-Transverse Joint
> Code 332.X2dS/C 232.X2kR

X-2.5(S)(R)
> Infection of a Paravertebral Muscle
> Code 332.X2eS/C 232.X2lR

X-2.6(S)(R)
> Infection of an Intervertebral Disk (diskitis)
> Code 332.X2fS/C 232.X2mR

X-2.7(S)(R)
> Infection of a Surgical Fusion-Site
> Code 332.X2gS/C 232.X2nR

X-2.8(S)(R)
> Infection of the Epidural Space (epidural abscess)
> Code 332.X2hS/C 232.X2oR

X-2.9(S)(R)
> Infection of the Meninges (meningitis)
> Code 303.X2cS/C 203.X2fR

X-2.10(S)(R)
> Acute Herpes Zoster (code only)
> Code 303.X2aS/C 203.X2aR

X-2.11(S)(R)
> Postherpetic Neuralgia
> Code 303.X2bS/C 203.X2bR

Thoracic Spinal or Radicular Pain Attributable to a Neoplasm (X-3)

Definition

Thoracic spinal pain associated with a neoplasm that can reasonably be interpreted as the source of the pain.

Clinical Features

Thoracic spinal pain with or without referred pain.

Diagnostic Features

A presumptive diagnosis may be made on the basis of imaging evidence of a neoplasm that directly or indirectly affects one or other of the tissues innervated by thoracic spinal nerves. Absolute confirmation relies on obtaining histological evidence by direct or needle biopsy.

Schedule of Neoplastic Diseases

X-3.1(S)(R)
> Primary Tumor of a Vertebral Body
> Code 333.X4aS/C 233.X4vR

X-3.2(S)(R)
> Primary Tumor of Any Part of a Vertebra Other than Its Body
> Code 333.X4bS/C 233.X4lR

X-3.3(S)(R)
> Primary Tumor of a Zygapophysial Joint
> Code 333.X4cS/C 233.X4mR

X-3.4(S)(R)
> Primary Tumor of the Proximal End of a Rib
> Code 333.X4dS/C 233.X4nR

X-3.5(S)(R)
> Primary Tumor of a Paravertebral Muscle
> Code 333.X4eS/C 233.X4oR

X-3.6(S)(R)
> Primary Tumor of Epidural Fat (e.g., lipoma)
> Code 333.X4fS/C 233.X4pR

X-3.7(S)(R)
> Primary Tumor of Epidural Vessels (e.g., angioma)
> Code 333.X4gS/C 233.X4qR

X-3.8(S)(R)
> Primary Tumor of Meninges (e.g., meningioma)
> Code 303.X4aS/C 203.X4dR

X-3.9(S)(R)
> Primary Tumor of Spinal Nerves (e.g., neurofibroma, schwannoma, neuroblastoma)
> Code 303.X4bS/C 203.X4eR

X-3.10(S)(R)
> Primary Tumor of Spinal Cord (e.g., glioma, etc.)
> Code 303.X4cS/C 203.X4fR

X-3.11(S)(R)
> Metastatic Tumor Affecting a Vertebra
> Code 333.X4hS/C 233.X4hR

X-3.12(S)(R)
> Metastatic Tumor Affecting the Vertebral Canal
> Code 333.X4iS/C 233.X4iR

X-3.13(S)(R)
> Other Infiltrating Neoplastic Disease of a Vertebra (e.g., lymphoma)
> Code 333.X4jS/C 233.X4jR

Thoracic Spinal or Radicular Pain Attributable to Metabolic Bone Disease (X-4)

Definition

Thoracic spinal pain associated with a metabolic bone disease that can reasonably be interpreted as the source of the pain.

Clinical Features

Thoracic spinal pain with or without referred pain.

Diagnostic Features

Imaging or other evidence of metabolic bone disease affecting the thoracic vertebral column, confirmed by appropriate serological or biochemical investigations and/or histological evidence obtained by needle or other biopsy.

Schedule of Metabolic Bone Diseases

X-4.1(S)(R)
> Osteoporosis of Age
> Code 332.X5aS/C 232.X5gR

X-4.2(S)(R)
> Osteoporosis of Unknown Cause
> Code 332.X5bS/C 232.X5hR

X-4.3(S)(R)
> Osteoporosis of Some Known Cause Other than Age
> Code 332.X5cS/C 232.X5iR

X-4.4(S)(R)
> Hyperparathyroidism
> Code 332.X5dS/C 232.X5jR

X-4.5(S)(R)
> Paget's Disease of Bone
> Code 332.X5eS/C 232.X5kR

X-4.6(S)(R)
> Metabolic Disease of Bone Not Otherwise Classified
> Code 332.X5fS/C 232.X5lR

Thoracic Spinal or Radicular Pain Attributable to Arthritis (X-5)

Definition
Thoracic spinal pain associated with arthritis that can reasonably be interpreted as the source of the pain.

Clinical Features
Thoracic spinal pain with or without referred pain.

Diagnostic Features
Imaging or other evidence of arthritis affecting the joints of the thoracic vertebral column.

Schedule of Arthritides
X-5.1	Rheumatoid Arthritis	
	Code 334.X3aS/C 234.X3aR	
X-5.2	Ankylosing Spondylitis	
	Code 332.X8aS/C	
X-5.3	Osteoarthritis	
	Code 338.X6*S/C 238.X6bR	
X-5.4	Seronegative Spondylarthropathy Not Otherwise Classified	
	Code 323.X8*S/C 223.X8*R	

Remarks
Osteoarthritis is included in this schedule with some hesitation because there is only a weak relation between pain and this condition as diagnosed radiologically.

The alternative classification to "thoracic pain due to osteoarthrosis" should be "thoracic zygapophysial joint pain" if the criteria for this diagnosis are satisfied (see X-10), or "thoracic spinal pain of unknown or uncertain origin" (see X-8).

Similarly, the condition of "spondylosis" is omitted from this schedule because there is no positive correlation between the radiographic presence of this condition and the presence of spinal pain.

Thoracic Spinal or Radicular Pain Associated with a Congenital Vertebral Anomaly (X-6)

Definition
Thoracic spinal pain associated with a congenital vertebral anomaly.

Clinical Features
Thoracic spinal pain with or without referred pain.

Diagnostic Features
Imaging evidence of a congenital vertebral anomaly affecting the thoracic vertebral column.

Remarks
There is no evidence that congenital anomalies per se cause pain. Although they may be associated with pain, the specificity of this association is unknown. This classification should be used only when the cause of pain cannot be otherwise specified and there is a perceived need to highlight the presence of the congenital anomaly, but should not be used to imply that the congenital anomaly is the actual source of pain.

Code
323.X0*S/C
223.X0aR

Pain Referred from Thoracic Viscera or Vessels and Perceived as Thoracic Spinal Pain (X-7)

Definition
Thoracic spinal pain associated with disease of a thoracic viscus or vessel that reasonably can be interpreted as the source of pain.

Clinical Features
Thoracic spinal pain with or without referred pain, together with features of the disease affecting the viscus or vessel concerned.

Diagnostic Features
Imaging or other evidence of the primary disease affecting a thoracic viscus or vessel.

Schedule of Diseases
X-7.1	Pericarditis	
	Code 323.X2 (known infection);	
	Code 323.X3 (unknown infective cause);	
	Code 323.X1 (trauma);	
	Code 323.X4 (neoplasm);	
	Code 323.X5 (toxic)	
X-7.2	Aneurysm of the Aorta	
	Code 322.X6	
X-7.3	Carcinoma of the Esophagus	
	Code 353.X4	

Thoracic Spinal Pain of Unknown or Uncertain Origin (X-8)

Definition
Thoracic spinal pain occurring in a patient whose clinical features and associated features do not enable the cause and source of the pain to be determined, and in

whom the cause or source of the pain cannot be or has not been determined by special investigations.

Clinical Features
Thoracic spinal pain with or without referred pain.

Diagnostic Features
Thoracic spinal pain for which no other cause has been found or can be attributed.

Pathology
Unspecified.

Remarks
This definition is intended to cover those complaints that for whatever reason currently defy conventional diagnosis. It does not encompass pain of psychological origin. It presupposes an organic basis for the pain, but one that cannot be or has not been established reliably by clinical examination or special investigations such as imaging techniques or diagnostic blocks.

This diagnosis may be used as a temporary diagnosis. Patients given this diagnosis could in due course be accorded a more definitive diagnosis once appropriate diagnostic techniques are devised or applied. In some instances, a more definitive diagnosis might be attainable using currently available techniques, but for logistic or ethical reasons these may not have been applied.

Upper Thoracic Spinal Pain of Unknown or Uncertain Origin (X-8.1)

Definition
As for X-8, but the pain is located in the upper thoracic region.

Clinical Features
Spinal pain located on the upper thoracic region.

Diagnostic Criteria
As for X-8, save that the pain is located in the upper thoracic region.

Pathology
As for X-8.

Remarks
As for X-8.

Code
3XX.X8bS/C
2XX.X8fR

Midthoracic Spinal Pain of Unknown or Uncertain Origin (X-8.2)

Definition
As for X-8, but the pain is located in the middle thoracic region.

Clinical Features
Spinal pain located on the midthoracic region.

Diagnostic Criteria
As for X-8, save that the pain is located in the midthoracic region.

Pathology
As for X-8.

Remarks
As for X-8.

Code
3XX.X8cS/C
2XX.X8gR

Lower Thoracic Spinal Pain of Unknown or Uncertain Origin (X-8.3)

Definition
As for X-8, but the pain is located in the lower thoracic region.

Clinical Features
Spinal pain located on the lower thoracic region.

Diagnostic Criteria
As for X-8, save that the pain is located in the lower thoracic region.

Pathology
As for X-8.

Remarks
As for X-8.

Code
3XX.X8dS/C
2XX.X8hR

Thoracolumbar Spinal Pain of Unknown or Uncertain Origin (X-8.4)

Definition
As for X-8, but the pain is located in the thoracolumbar region.

Clinical Features
Spinal pain located on the thoracolumbar region.

Diagnostic Criteria
As for X-8, save that the pain is located in the thoracolumbar region.

Pathology
As for X-8.

Remarks
As for X-8.

Code
3XX.X8eS/C
2XX.X8iR

Thoracic Discogenic Pain (X-9)

Definition
Thoracic spinal pain, with or without referred pain, stemming from a thoracic intervertebral disk.

Clinical Features
Spinal pain perceived in the thoracic region, with or without referred pain.

Diagnostic Criteria
The patient's pain must be shown conclusively to stem from an intervertebral disk by demonstrating

either (1) that selective anesthetization of the putatively symptomatic intervertebral disk completely relieves the patient of the accustomed pain for a period consonant with the expected duration of action of the local anesthetic used;

or   (2) that selective anesthetization of the putatively symptomatic intervertebral disk substantially relieves the patient of the accustomed pain for a period consonant with the expected duration of action of the local anesthetic used, save that whatever pain persists can be ascribed to some other coexisting source or cause;

or   (3) that provocation diskography of the putatively symptomatic disk reproduces the patient's accustomed pain, provided that provocation of at least two adjacent intervertebral disks clearly does not reproduce the patient's pain, and provided that the pain cannot be ascribed to some other source innervated by the same segments that innervate the putatively symptomatic disk.

Pathology
Unknown, but presumably the pain arises as a result of chemical or mechanical irritation of the nerve endings in the outer anulus fibrosus, initiated by injury to the anulus, or as a result of excessive stresses imposed on the anulus by injury, deformity, or other disease within the affected segment or adjacent segments.

Remarks
Provocation diskography alone is insufficient to establish conclusively a diagnosis of discogenic pain because of the propensity for false-positive responses, either because of apprehension on the part of the patient or because of the coexistence of a separate source of pain within the segment under investigation. If analgesic diskography is not performed or is possibly false-negative, criterion 3 must be explicitly satisfied. Otherwise, the diagnosis of "discogenic pain" cannot be sustained, whereupon an alternative classification must be used.

Thoracic diskography is particularly hazardous because of the risk of pneumothorax. No publications have formally described this procedure or experience with it. Until its safety and clinical utility have been established, thoracic diskography should be restricted to centers capable of dealing with potential complications and prepared to determine its utility by way of formal study.

Code
333.X1lS   Trauma
333.X6aS   Degeneration
333.X7cS   Dysfunctional

Thoracic Zygapophysial Joint Pain (X-10)

Definition
Thoracic spinal pain, with or without referred pain, stemming from one or more of the thoracic zygapophysial joints.

Clinical Features
Thoracic spinal pain with or without referred pain.

Diagnostic Criteria
No criteria have been established whereby zygapophysial joint pain can be diagnosed on the basis of the patient's history or by conventional clinical examination.

The condition can be diagnosed only by the use of diagnostic intraarticular zygapophysial joint blocks. For the diagnosis to be declared, all of the following criteria must be satisfied.

1. The blocks must be radiologically controlled.
2. Arthrography must demonstrate that any injection has been made selectively into the target joint, and any material that is injected into the joint must not spill over into adjacent structures that might otherwise be the actual source of the patient's pain.

3. The patient's pain must be totally relieved following the injection of local anesthetic into the target joint.
4. A single positive response to the intraarticular injection of local anesthetic is insufficient for the diagnosis to be declared. The response must be validated by an appropriate control test that excludes false-positive responses on the part of the patient, such as:
   - no relief of pain upon injection of a nonactive agent;
   - no relief of pain following the injection of an active local anesthetic into a site other than the target joint; or
   - a positive but differential response to local anesthetics of different durations of action injected into the target joint on separate occasions.

Local anesthetic blockade of the nerves supplying a target zygapophysial joint may be used as a screening procedure to determine in the first instance whether a particular joint might be the source of symptoms, but the definitive diagnosis may be made only upon selective intraarticular injection of the putatively symptomatic joint.

Pathology
Unknown and unstudied.

Remarks
See also Thoracic Segmental Dysfunction (X-15).

Code
333.X1mS/C Trauma
333.X6bS/C Degeneration
333.X7tS/C Dysfunctional

Reference
Wilson, P.R., Thoracic facet syndrome: a clinical entity? Pain, Suppl. 4 (1987) S87.

Costo-Transverse Joint Pain (X-11)

Definition
Thoracic spinal pain, with or without referred pain, stemming from one or more of the costo-transverse joints.

Clinical Features
Thoracic spinal pain, with or without referred pain, aggravated by selectively stressing a costo-transverse joint.

Diagnostic Criteria
No criteria have been established whereby costo-transverse joint pain can be diagnosed on the basis of the patient's history or by conventional clinical examination. Stressing the putatively symptomatic joint by selectively gliding the related rib ventrad, cephalad, or caudad constitutes presumptive evidence that the joint may be symptomatic.

The condition can be firmly diagnosed only by the use of diagnostic local anesthetic blocks of the putatively symptomatic joint. For the diagnosis to be firmly sustained, all of the following criteria must be satisfied.

If intraarticular blocks are used,
1. The blocks must be radiologically controlled.
2. Arthrography must demonstrate that any injection has been made selectively into the target joint, and any material that is injected into the joint must not spill over into adjacent structures that might otherwise be the actual source of the patient's pain.
3. The patient's pain must be totally relieved following the injection of local anesthetic into the target joint.
4. A single positive response to the intraarticular injection of local anesthetic is insufficient for the diagnosis to be declared. The response must be validated by an appropriate control test that excludes false-positive responses on the part of the patient, such as:
   - no relief of pain upon injection of a nonactive agent;
   - no relief of pain following the injection of an active local anesthetic into a site other than the target joint; or
   - a positive but differential response to local anesthetics of different durations of action injected into the target joint on separate occasions.

If periarticular blocks are used, an injection of contrast medium of a volume identical to that of the volume of local anesthetic used must show that the dispersal of injectate does not embrace structures that might constitute alternative sources of the patient's pain. Otherwise criteria 3 and 4 for intraarticular blocks must apply.

Pathology
Unknown and unstudied.

Code
333.X1nS Trauma
333.X6cS Degeneration
333.X7eS Dysfunctional

Thoracic Muscle Sprain (X-12)

Definition
Thoracic spinal pain stemming from a lesion in a specified muscle caused by strain of that muscle beyond its normal physiological limits.

Clinical Features
Thoracic spinal pain, with or without referred pain, associated with tenderness in the affected muscle and aggravated by either passive stretching or resisted contraction of that muscle.

Diagnostic Criteria
The following criteria must all be satisfied.

1. The affected muscle must be specified.
2. There is a history of activities consistent with the affected muscle having been strained.
3. The muscle is tender to palpation.
4. a) Aggravation of the pain by any clinical test that can be shown to selectively stress the affected muscle, or
   b) Selective infiltration of the affected muscle with local anesthetic completely relieves the patient's pain.

Pathology
Rupture of muscle fibers, usually near their myotendinous junction, that elicits an inflammatory repair response.

Code
333.X1oS   Trauma
333.X7fS   Dysfunctional

Thoracic Trigger Point Syndrome (X-13)

Definition
Thoracic spinal pain stemming from a trigger point or trigger points in one or more of the muscles of the thoracic spine.

Clinical Features
Thoracic spinal pain, with or without referred pain, associated with a trigger point in one or more muscles of the vertebral column.

Diagnostic Criteria
The following criteria must all be satisfied.

71. A trigger point must be present in a muscle, consisting of a palpable, tender, firm, fusiform nodule or band orientated in the direction of the affected muscle's fibers
2. The muscle must be specified.
3. Palpation of the trigger point reproduces the patient's pain and/or referred pain.
4. Elimination of the trigger point relieves the patient's pain. Elimination may be achieved by stretching the affected muscle, dry needling the trigger point, or infiltrating it with local anesthetic.

Pathology
Unknown. Trigger points are believed to represent areas of contracted muscle that have failed to relax as a result of failure of calcium ions to sequestrate. Pain arises as a result of the accumulation of algogenic metabolites.

Remarks
For the diagnosis to be accorded, the diagnostic criteria for a trigger point must be fulfilled. Simple tenderness in a muscle without a palpable band does not satisfy the criteria, whereupon an alternative diagnosis should be accorded, such as muscle sprain, if the criteria for that condition are fulfilled, or spinal pain of unknown or uncertain origin.

Code
332.X1aS   Trauma
332.X6aS   Degeneration
332.X7hS   Dysfunctional

References
Simons, D.G., Myofascial pain syndromes: Where are we? Where are we going? Arch. Phys. Med. Rehab., 69 (1988) 207–212.

Travell, J.G. and Simons, D.G., Myofascial Pain and Dysfunction. The Trigger Point Manual. Williams & Wilkins, Baltimore, 1983.

Thoracic Muscle Spasm (X-14)

Definition
Thoracic spinal pain resulting from sustained or repeated involuntary activity of the thoracic spinal muscles.

Clinical Features
Thoracic spinal pain for which there is no other underlying cause, associated with demonstrable sustained muscle activity.

Diagnostic Features
None.

Pathology
Unknown. Presumably sustained muscle activity prevents adequate wash-out of algogenic chemicals produced by the sustained metabolic activity of the muscle.

Remarks
While there are beliefs in a pain–muscle spasm–pain cycle, clinical tests or conventional electromyography have not been shown to demonstrate reliably the presence of sustained muscle activity in such situations. The strongest evidence for repeated involuntary muscle spasm stems from sleep-EMG studies conducted on patients with low-back pain, but although it is associated with back pain, a causal relationship between this type of muscle activity and back pain has not been established.

Code
332.X1bS   Trauma
332.X2iS   Infection
332.X4*S   Neoplasm
332.X6bS   Degenerative
332.X7iS   Dysfunctional
332.X8fS   Unknown

References

Fischer, A.A. and Chang, C.H., Electromyographic evidence of paraspinal muscle spasm during sleep in patients with low back pain, Clin. J. Pain, 1 (1985) 147–154.

Garrett, W., Anderson, G., Richardson, W., et al., Muscle: future directions. In: (Eds.), New Perspectives on Low Back Pain, American Academy of Orthopaedic Surgeons, Park Ridge, Ill., 1989, pp. 373-379.

Garrett, W., Bradley, W., Byrd, S., et al., Muscle: basic science perspectives. In: J.W. Frymoyer and S.L. Gordon (Eds.), New Perspectives on Low Back Pain, American Academy of Orthopaedic Surgeons, Park Ridge, Ill., 1989, pp. 335-372.

Roland, M.O., A critical review of the evidence for a pain-spasm-pain cycle in spinal disorders, Clin. Biomech., 1 (1986) 102–109.

Thoracic Segmental Dysfunction (X-15)

Definition
Thoracic spinal pain ostensibly due to excessive strains imposed on the restraining elements of a single spinal motion segment.

Clinical Features
Thoracic spinal pain, with or without referred pain, that can be aggravated by selectively stressing a particular spinal segment.

Diagnostic Criteria
All the following criteria should be satisfied.

1. The affected segment must be specified.
2. The patient's pain is aggravated by clinical tests that selectively stress the affected segment.
3. Stressing adjacent segments does not reproduce the patient's pain.

Pathology
Unknown. Presumably involves excessive strain imposed by activities of daily living on structures such as the ligaments, joints, or intervertebral disk of the affected segment.

Remarks
This diagnosis is offered as a partial distinction from spinal pain of unknown origin, insofar as the source of the patient's pain can at least be narrowed to a particular offending segment. Further investigation of a patient accorded this diagnosis might result in the patient's condition being ascribed a more definitive diagnosis such as discogenic pain or zygapophysial joint pain, but the diagnosis of segmental dysfunction could be applied if facilities for undertaking the appropriate investigations are not available, if the physician or patient does not wish to pursue such investigations, or if the pain arises from multiple sites in the same segment.

For this diagnosis to be sustained it is critical that the clinical tests used be shown to be able to stress selectively the segment in question and to have acceptable interobserver reliability.

Code
333.X1pS/C   Trauma
333.X7dS/C   Dysfunctional

Radicular Pain Attributable to a Prolapsed Thoracic Disk (X-16)

Code
303.X1aR   Trauma
303.X6bR   Degenerative
203.X1cR   Trauma
203.X6bR (arm)   Degenerative

E. LOCAL SYNDROMES OF THE UPPER LIMBS AND RELATIVELY GENERALIZED SYNDROMES OF THE UPPER AND LOWER LIMBS

GROUP XI: PAIN IN THE SHOULDER, ARM, AND HAND

Tumors of the Brachial Plexus (XI-1)

Definition
Progressive aching, burning pain with paresthesias and sensory and motor impairment in the distribution of a branch or branches of the brachial plexus due to tumor.

Site
Shoulder and upper limb.

System
Nervous system.

Tumors
Benign tumors: schwannoma, neurofibroma. Malignant tumors: malignant schwannoma and fibrosarcoma, metastatic neoplasm or direct invasion from other lesion, neuroblastoma, ganglioneuroma (secondary neoplasia of peripheral nerves occurs frequently in lymphoma, leukemia, multiple myeloma). Breast, lung and thyroid neoplasia frequently involve the brachial plexus.

Main Features
Incidence: the specific tumors of peripheral nerve are extremely rare. *Sex Ratio:* there is no sex predilection. *Age of Onset:* young adulthood. They are more common with von Recklinghausen's disease. *Pain Quality:* the pain tends to be constant, gradual in onset, aching, and burning, and associated with paresthesias in the distribution of the pain, progressive wasting of muscles depending upon what groups are involved, and sensory loss. *Intensity:* severe.

Associated Symptoms
The pain is generally not affected by activity. There is associated sensory loss and muscle wasting depending upon the area of the brachial plexus involved. Pain relief is often not adequate, even with significant narcotics.

Signs and Laboratory Findings
The laboratory findings are those of the underlying disease. Signs are loss of reflexes, sensation, and muscle strength in the distribution of the involved portion of the plexus. There may be a local mass. The diagnosis is usually made promptly by X-ray or by CT scan. Electromyographic studies validate the location of the lesion, and there may be a palpable mass in the supraclavicular space.

Usual Course
These tumors are relentlessly progressive unless treated.

Social and Physical Disability
Those related to the loss of function.

Summary of Essential Features
The tumors are associated with slowly progressive pain and paresthesias, and subsequently severe sensory loss and motor loss. The diagnostic criteria are the increasing aching, burning pain, its distribution in the brachial plexus, the associated paresthesias, motor and sensory loss, and the presence of a mass by palpation and on X-ray or CT scan.

Diagnostic Criteria
1. Burning pain of increasing severity referred to the upper extremity. Occasional superimposed lancinating pain in the same distribution.
2. Subsequent progressive motor and sensory loss and autonomic dysfunction.
3. CT scan may show tumor involvement of the brachial plexus.

Differential Diagnosis
Includes all those lesions above, the scalenus anticus syndrome, and abnormalities of the first thoracic rib or the presence of a cervical rib.

Code
102.X4b
202.X4b

Chemical Irritation of the Brachial Plexus (XI-2)

Definition
Continuous burning pain occasionally accompanied by severe paroxysms, in the distribution of the brachial plexus or one of its branches, with sensory-motion deficits due to effects of local injection of chemical irritants.

Site
Upper limb.

System
Nervous system.

Main Features
Prevalence: injections in the shoulder area with any noxious agent are extremely rare. However, the pain syndromes from these injections are quite well defined. *Incidence:* the pain begins almost immediately with the injection and is continuous. *Pain Quality:* it is usually burning in character, superficial, and unaffected by activity. Occasional paroxysms may occur. It frequently persists even after neurological loss has resolved and is not necessarily associated with paresthesias or sensory loss. There are no differences between noxious agents as to time pattern, occurrence, character, intensity, or duration.

Signs and Laboratory Findings
The signs are of brachial plexus injury. Atrophy, sensory loss, and paresthesias occur in the appropriate area depending upon the portion of the plexus injured. There are no specific laboratory findings.

Usual Course
Pain is generally acute with the injection and gradually improves. Most disappear within a few weeks. Those that persist continue unabated permanently.

Complications
The complications are those of brachial plexus injury.

Pathology
The pathology is a combination of intraneural and extraneural scarring with focal demyelinization.

Summary of Essential Features
These are those of brachial plexus injury. The diagnosis can only be made by history of injection.

Diagnostic Criteria
1. History of injection of chemical irritant.
2. Burning pain with occasional superimposed paroxysms referred to the upper extremity.
3. Pain syndrome stabilizes or actually improves after days to weeks.

Differential Diagnosis
This includes all of the muscular and bony compressions, anomalies, and tumors previously described.

Code
102.X5
202.X5

Traumatic Avulsion of the Brachial Plexus (XI-3)

Definition
Pain, most often burning or crushing with super-added paroxysms, following avulsion lesions of the brachial plexus.

Site
Felt almost invariably in the forearm and hand irrespective of the roots avulsed. Occasionally, in avulsion of C5 root only, pain may be felt in shoulder.

System
Nerve roots torn from the spinal cord.

Main Features
Prevalence: some 90% of the patients with avulsion of one or more nerve roots suffer pain at some time. Virtually all patients with avulsion of all five roots suffer severe pain for some months at least. *Age of Onset:* vast majority of patients with this lesion are young men between the ages of 18 and 25 suffering from motorcycle accidents. The older the patient the more likely he is to suffer pain from the avulsion lesions. *Pain Quality:* the pain is characteristically described as burning or crushing, as if the hand were being crushed in a vise or were on fire. The pain is constant and is a permanent background to the patient's life, and in a high proportion of patients (in one series, 90%), there were periodic paroxysms or shots of pain lasting for a few seconds and of agonizing intensity. These paroxysms stop the patient in his tracks and may cause him to cry out and grip his arm and turn away. *Time Pattern:* frequency varies between a few an hour, a few a day, or a few a week. In a few patients they can be very frequent, with as many as 20 or 30 in an hour. There is no set pattern to the paroxysms, and the patient has no warning of their arrival. The constant pain may also be described as severe pins and needles and electric shocks, but it is most often burning or crushing. In some patients there is a gradual increase in the intensity of the pain over a period of days, building up to a very high level of pain lasting a day or more and then gradually subsiding over the next few days. In these patients the pain is particularly unpleasant and interferes seriously with their lives.

Associated Symptoms
Aggravating factors: cold weather, extremes of temperature, emotional stress, and intercurrent illness all aggravate the pain. The pain is almost invariably relieved by distraction involving absorbing work or hobbies. The pain is at its worst when the patient has nothing with which to occupy his mind. Patients often grip the anesthetic and paralyzed arm or hit the shoulder to try and

relieve the pain. Drugs are singularly unhelpful and a full range of analgesics is usually tried, but very few patients respond significantly. Alcohol helps, probably by relaxing the patient and promoting sleep. A number of patients have found that smoking cannabis can markedly reduce the pain, but if so it interferes with their concentration, and very few indeed are regular cannabis smokers.

Signs
Paralysis and anesthetic loss in the territory of the avulsed nerve root, i.e., avulsion C5–T1—a totally paralyzed and insensitive arm. Most patients ask their doctors about amputation as a means of relieving the pain, and it has to be made clear to them the pain is central and amputation has no effect at all. In fact, there is a good likelihood of adding stump pain to their existing pain. Avulsion of T1 is associated with a Horner's sign, drooping of the eyelid and constriction of the pupil.

Myelography often shows evidence of meningoceles or root avulsion. Electrophysiological tests may well show the presence of sensory action potentials in anesthetic, areas indicating that the lesion must be proximal to the posterior root ganglion. A flare response to intradermal histamine is occasionally useful, particularly in C5 lesions, again indicating preganglionic lesions.

Usual Course
Two-thirds of patients come to terms with their pain or say the pain is improved within three years of onset. If the pain is still severe at three years after onset, it is likely to last for the rest of their lives, and in these patients the pain steadily gets worse as they get older.

Complications
Rarely, trophic lesions of the anesthetic arm, e.g., burns or infections, or severe depression may occasionally follow prolonged pain, but it is remarkable how these young men manage to come to terms with their disability.

Social and Physical Disability
The major disability is the paralysis of the arm and the effect this has on work, hobbies, and sport. Pain itself can interfere with ability to work and can cut the patient off from normal social life.

Pathology
Avulsion is associated with spontaneous firing of deafferented nerve cells in the spinal cord at the level of the injury and may in time cause abnormal firing at higher levels of the central nervous system.

Summary of Essential Features and Diagnostic Criteria
The pain in avulsion lesions of the brachial plexus is almost invariably described as severe burning and crushing pain, constant, and very often with paroxysms of sharp, shooting pains that last seconds and vary in frequency from several times an hour to several times a week. So characteristic is the pain of an avulsion lesion that it is virtually diagnostic of an avulsion of one or more roots. Traction lesions of the brachial plexus that involve the nerve roots distal to the posterior root ganglion are seldom if ever associated with pain. Sometimes in regeneration spontaneously, or after nerve grafts for rupture of nerve roots distal to the intervertebral foramen, a causalgic type of pain develops, but this is highly characteristic of causalgia and cannot be confused with avulsion or deafferentation pain.

Code
203.X1c

Reference
Wynn Parry, C.B., Pain in avulsion lesions of the brachial plexus, Pain, 9 (1980) 41–53.

Postradiation Pain of the Brachial Plexus (XI-4)

Code
203.X5

Painful Arms and Moving Fingers (XI-5)

See XXXI-9, Painful Legs and Moving Toes.

Code
202.X8

Reference
Verhagen, W.I.M., Horstink, M.W.I.M., and Notermans, S.L.H., Painful arm and moving fingers, J. Neurol. Neurosurg. Psychiatry, 48 (1985) 384–398.

Brachial Neuritis (Brachial Neuropathy, Neuralgic Amyotrophy, Parsonage-Turner Syndrome) (XI-6)

Definition
Severe pain in shoulder and arm with progression to weakness and atrophy and, less frequently, numbness and paresthesias.

Site
Shoulder and upper limb.

System
Peripheral nervous system (brachial plexus).

Main Features
Severe sharp or burning nonlocalized pain in the entire upper extremity; this is usually unilateral but may be bilateral. It involves the proximal more frequently than the distal muscles.

Signs and Laboratory Findings
Diffuse weakness in nonroot and nondermatomal pattern with a patchy pattern of hypoesthesia. Laboratory tests of the spinal neuraxis are negative, but diffuse electromyographic abnormalities appear in the affected extremity with sparing of cervical paravertebral muscles.

Usual Course
Recovery is slow and may last one year or longer.

Summary of Essential Features
Onset of severe unilateral (or rarely bilateral) pain followed by weakness, atrophy, and hypoesthesia with slow recovery. The diagnosis is confirmed by positive electrodiagnostic testing and negative studies of the cervical neuraxis.

Differential Diagnosis
Avulsion of the brachial plexus; thoracic outlet syndrome.

Code
202.X8a

Bicipital Tendinitis (XI-7)

Definition
Severe pain with acute onset due to inflammation of the long head of biceps tendon.

Site
Interior shoulder.

System
Musculoskeletal system.

Main Features
Severe pain, usually with acute onset in the anterior shoulder, following trauma or excessive exertion. It may radiate down the entire arm and is usually self-limited, but there may be recurrent episodes.

Aggravating Factors
Movement of shoulder and elbow.

Signs
Tendon palpation in the shoulder bicipital groove is painful. Pain is reproduced by resisted supination of the flexed forearm (Jergason's sign).

Usual Course
Occurs primarily after repeated use or heavy strain on tendon. It may become chronic.

Relief
Nonsteroidal anti-inflammatory agents; local steroid injection.

Complications
Frozen shoulder (adhesive capsulitis).

Pathology
Inflammation of the tendon sheath.

Essential Features
Acute pain in the anterior shoulder, aggravated by forced supination of the flexed forearm.

Differential Diagnosis
Subacromial bursitis, calcific tendinitis, rotator cuff tear.

Code
231.X3

Subacromial Bursitis (Subdeltoid Bursitis, Supraspinatus Tendinitis) (XI-8)

Definition
Aching pain in the shoulder due to inflammation of subacromial bursa.

Site
Shoulder and upper arm.

System
Musculoskeletal system.

Main Features
Age of Onset: common over 30 years of age. *Pain Quality:* the condition presents with aching pain in the deltoid muscle and upper arm above the elbow aggravated by using the arm above the horizontal level (painful abduction). The pain is aggravated by sleeping on the affected shoulder. It is usually precipitated by repeated or minor trauma.

Signs
Tenderness over the insertion of supraspinatus tendon. Painful arc of abduction, and internal rotation.

Radiologic Finding
High riding humeral head on X-ray when chronic attenuation of bursa occurs.

Usual Course
Recurrent acute episodes may produce chronic pain.

Relief
Nonsteroidal anti-inflammatory agents, local steroid injection, ultrasound, deep heat, physiotherapy.

Complications
Frozen shoulder (adhesive capsulitis).

Pathology
Chronic inflammation of bursa; tendon.

Essential Features
Aching pain in shoulder with inflammation of the subacromial bursa and exacerbation on movement as well as tenderness over the insertion of the supraspinatus tendon.

Differential Diagnosis
Calcific tendinitis, rotator cuff tear.

Code
238.X3

Rotator Cuff Tear—Partial or Complete (XI-9)

Definition
Acute severe aching pain due to traumatic rupture of supraspinatus tendon.

Site
Shoulder and upper arm.

System
Musculoskeletal system.

Main Features
Acute severe aching pain in the shoulder following trauma, usually a fall on the outstretched arm. Abduction is extremely painful or impossible. The patient is unable to sleep on the affected side.

Signs
A partial tear is distinguished from a complete tear by subacromial injection of local anesthetic; partial tears will resume normal passive range of motion. The arm may drop to the side if passively abducted to 90° ("drop arm sign") if there is a complete tear.

Radiologic Finding
High riding humeral head on X-ray.

Complications
Frozen shoulder.

Essential Features
Acute severe pain due to trauma at the supraspinatus tendon.

Differential Diagnosis
Calcific tendinitis, subacromial bursitis.

Code
231.X1a

Adhesive Capsulitis and Frozen Shoulder (XI-10)

Code
232.X2   Infective
232.X3b   Inflammatory
232.X7   Dysfunctional

Lateral Epicondylitis (Tennis Elbow) (XI-11)

Definition
Pain in the lateral epicondylar region of the elbow due to strain or partial tear of the extensor tendon of the wrist.

System
Musculoskeletal system.

Main Features
Acute, subacute, or chronic pain of the elbow during grasping and supination of the wrist. *Age of Onset:* most common between 40 and 60 years of age. *Pain Quality:* pain radiates down the lateral forearm or to the upper arm.

Aggravating Factors
Repeated trauma.

Relief
Relieved by local steroid injection and physiotherapy.

Signs
Tenderness of the wrist extensor tendon about 5 cm distal to the epicondyle. Resisted wrist dorsiflexion reproduces pain.

Usual Course
Usually self limiting; several months duration.

Laboratory and Radiologic Findings
Negative.

Pathology
Strain or partial tear of tendon at tendoperiosteal junction.

Essential Features
Pain at the lateral epicondyle, worse on movement, aggravated by overuse.

Differential Diagnosis
Nerve entrapment, cervical root impingement, carpal tunnel syndrome.

Code
235.X1a

Medial Epicondylitis (Golfer's Elbow) (XI-12)

Definition
Pain in the medial epicondylar region of the elbow.

Main Features
As for tennis elbow (XI-11) but much less common.

Aggravating Factors
As for tennis elbow.

Signs
Tenderness over the tendon insertion of the medial epicondyle.

Laboratory and Radiologic Findings
Negative.

Usual Course
As for tennis elbow.

Pathology
As for tennis elbow.

Differential Diagnosis
As for tennis elbow.

Code
235.X1b

DeQuervain's Tenosynovitis (XI-13)

Definition
Severe aching and shooting pain due to stenosing tenosynovitis of abductor pollicis longus or extensor pollicis brevis.

Site
Wrist.

System
Musculoskeletal system.

Main Features
Sudden onset of severe aching or shooting pains. There may be localized swelling and/or redness.

Aggravating Factors
Aggravated by pinch, grasping, or repetitive thumb and wrist movements.

Signs
Occasional tendon swelling; tenderness over the tendon in the anatomical snuff box area. Finkelstein's sign reproduces the pain; the patient's thumb is folded into a fist and then the wrist is deviated to the ulnar side.

Usual Course
May be single self-limited episode or recurrent and chronic.

Relief
Relief from local splinting or local steroid injection.

Pathology
Inflammatory lesion of tendon sheath usually secondary to repetitive motion or direct trauma.

Essential Features
Severe aching and shooting pain in the radial portion of the wrist related to movement.

Differential Diagnosis
Arthritis of the wrist, scaphoid injury.

Code
233.X3

Osteoarthritis of the Hands (XI-14)

Definition
Chronic aching pain in the fingers with degenerative changes of distal and proximal phalangeal joints of the hands.

System
Musculoskeletal system.

Main Features
The illness occurs mainly in women over 45 years of age. The pain is chronic and aching in the fingers and aggravated by use and relieved by rest. There may be mild morning stiffness for less than half an hour and subjective reduction of grip strength, worse with trauma to nodes.

Signs

Bony enlargements of the distal interphalangeal joints are called Heberden's nodes, and those of the proximal interphalangeal joints are called Bouchard's nodes. The fingers may be stiff and lose some degree of full flexion. Grip strength is usually normal when measured.

Radiologic Finding

Narrowing of joint spaces, sclerosis, and bony osteophytosis.

Relief

Analgesics, soaking in hot fluids.

Code

238.X6b

Cubital Tunnel Syndrome (XI-15)

Definition

Entrapment of the ulnar nerve in a fibro-osseous tunnel formed by a groove (trochlear groove) between the olecranon process and medial epicondyle of the humerus. The groove is converted to a tunnel by a myofascial covering, and the etiology of the entrapment is multiple.

Site

Elbow, forearm, and fingers (fourth and fifth).

System

Peripheral nervous system (ulnar nerve).

Main Features

Gradual onset of pain, numbness, and paresthesias in the distribution of the ulnar nerve, sometimes followed by weakness and atrophy in the same distribution; often seen in conjunction with a carpal tunnel syndrome ("double crush phenomenon").

Signs and Laboratory Findings

Tinel's sign at the elbow. The ulnar nerve is frequently thickened and adherent. On electrodiagnostic testing there is slowing of conduction in the ulnar nerve across the elbow, accompanied by denervation of those intrinsic muscles of the hand innervated by the ulnar nerve.

Usual Course

The course may be stable or slowly progressive; if the latter, surgery is necessary, either decompression or transposition of the nerve.

Summary of Essential Features and Diagnostic Criteria

A gradual onset of pain, paresthesias, and, at times, motor findings in the distribution of the ulnar nerve. Tinel's sign is found. The diagnosis is confirmed by slowing of conduction across the elbow and often by denervation of those intrinsic muscles of the hand innervated by the ulnar nerve.

Differential Diagnosis

Thoracic outlet syndrome, carpal tunnel syndrome.

Code

202.X6c

Carpal Tunnel Syndrome (XI-16)

Definition

Stinging, burning, or aching pain in the hand, often nocturnal, due to entrapment of the median nerve in the carpal tunnel.

Site

One hand (sometimes bilateral), in the fingers, often including the fifth digit, often spreading into the forearm and occasionally higher; not usually well localized.

System

Peripheral nervous system.

Main Features

Prevalence: very common. *Age of Onset:* usually fourth to fifth decades. *Sex Ratio:* female to male 5:1. *Quality:* pins and needles, stinging, often aching, occasionally burning. *Time pattern:* usually nocturnal, typically awakening the patient several times and then subsiding in a few minutes; aching pain is often more constant. *Intensity:* may be severe briefly.

Associated Symptom

Aggravated by handwork such as knitting.

Signs and Laboratory Findings

Clinical examination often normal, but one may find decreased pin-prick sensation on the tips of digits I–III, a positive Tinel's or Phalen's sign, or rarely, weakness and/or atrophy of the thenar muscles (abductor pollicis brevis); nerve conduction studies showing delayed sensory and motor conduction across the carpal tunnel are diagnostic.

Usual Course

Very slow progression for years.

Social and Physical Disability

May impair ability to do handwork.

Pathology

Compression of median nerve in wrist between the carpal bones and the transverse carpal ligament (flexor retinaculum); focal demyelination of nerve fibers, axonal shrinkage and axonal degeneration.

Summary of Essential Features and Diagnostic Criteria

Episodic paresthetic nocturnal pain in the hand with electrophysiological evidence of delayed conduction in the median nerve across the wrist.

Code

204.X6

Pain of Psychological Origin in the Shoulder and Arm (XI-17)

Code

233.X7b   Tension: arm
21X.X9a   Delusional: arm
21X.X9b   Conversion: arm
21X.X9d   Associated with depression

Crush Injury of Upper Limbs (XI-18)

Code

231.X1b

Pain in a Limb or Limbs, Not Otherwise Specified (XI-19)

Code

2XX.XXz   Upper limb or limbs
6XX.XXz   Lower limb or limbs

GROUP XII: VASCULAR DISEASE OF THE LIMBS

Raynaud's Disease (XII-1)

Definition

Episodic attacks of aching, burning pain associated with vasoconstriction of the arteries of the extremities in response to cold or emotional stimuli.

Site

Predominantly in the hands, unilateral initially, later bilateral. Rarely lower limbs and exposed areas of face.

System

Cardiovascular system.

Main Features

Prevalence: Raynaud's phenomena can occur in 5% of normal females as secondary to connective tissue disease. Raynaud's disease is uncommon, with a female to male ratio of 5:1. *Onset:* most common between puberty and age 40. Exacerbations during emotional stress and possibly at time of menses. *Start:* evoked by cold, nervousness, and other stimuli which vary among patients. A typical attack occurs in three phases. Initially the digits become ashen white, then they turn blue as the capillaries dilate and fill with slowly flowing deoxygenated blood. Finally the arterioles relax and the attack comes to an end with a flushing of the diseased parts. *Pain Quality:* initially the pain is deep and aching and varies from mild to severe, changing to severe burning dysesthesias in the phase of reactive hyperemia. *Time Pattern:* recurring irregularly with changes in environmental temperature and emotional status. *Intensity:* variable from mild to severe depending upon the temperature and other stimuli. *Duration:* minutes to hours. Sometimes may last days if painful ischemia skin ulcers develop.

Associated Symptoms and Signs

Numbness or hypoesthesia are present. Progressive spasm of the vessels leads to atrophy of the tip, giving the finger a tapered appearance. The nail becomes brittle and paronychia is common. Advanced cases may develop focal areas of necrosis at the fingertip, occasionally preceded by cutaneous calcification. These areas are extremely painful and tender to palpation. Anxiety and other signs of sympathetic overactivity such as increased sweating in the limbs and piloerection develop.

Relief

Temporary relief from sympathetic block, and occasional prolonged relief from sympathectomy in the early phases. Calcium channel blocking agents may help.

Pathology

The cause of "cold sensitivity" is unknown. Abnormalities in sympathetic activity have not been proven. However, local application of cold is necessary to elicit the response of Raynaud's syndrome, and the threshold for triggering the response is lowered by any factor that increases sympathetic outflow or circulating catecholamines.

Essential Features

Color changes of digits, excited by cold or emotions, involving both upper extremities and absence of specific organic disease.

Differential Diagnosis

Raynaud's disease, which has no other known cause, and Raynaud's phenomenon, which is a response occurring in other illnesses, should be distinguished. The following other diseases should be recognized:

- collagen-vascular diseases: scleroderma, rheumatoid arteritis, systemic lupus erythematosis, dermatomyositis, periarteritis nodosa;
- other vascular diseases: thromboangiitis obliterans, thrombotic or embolic occlusion, arteriosclerosis obliterans, syphilitic arteritis;
- trauma: vibration (air-hammer disease, etc.), percussion (digital pianist, typist, etc.), palmar (hypothenar hammer syndrome);
- neurovascular syndromes: thoracic outlet syndromes, spondylitis, causalgia;
- central and peripheral nervous disorders (rarely): syringomyelia, poliomyelitis, ruptured cervical disk, progressive muscular atrophy;
- cold injury: frostbite, nonfreezing cold injury, (pernio, immersion foot), cold sensitivity syndrome;
- lack of suspension stability of blood: cold agglutinins, cryoglobulinemia, cryofibrinogenemia, polycythemia vera;
- intoxication: ergot, arsenic, heavy metals (lead), nicotine, and tobacco.

Code

024.X7a   Face
224.X7a   Arms
624.X7b   Legs

Raynaud's Phenomenon (XII-2)

Definition

Attacks like those of Raynaud's disease but related to one or more other disease processes.

Usual Course

In accordance with the underlying disease.

Pathology

Systemic and vascular diseases such as collagen disease, arteriosclerosis obliterans, nerve injuries, and occupational trauma—for example in chain saw operators, pianists, and pneumatic hammer operators—may all contribute to the development of Raynaud's phenomenon.

Code

024.X7c   Face

224.X7c   Arms
624.X7c   Legs

Frostbite and Cold Injury (XII-3)

Definition

Severe burning pain in digits or exposed areas of face due to cold injury.

Site

Periphery of limbs (digits) and exposed areas of face.

System

Cardiovascular system.

Main Features

Prevalence: increased incidence in elderly patients with arterial disease and in young men with hazardous exposure to cold environment, e.g., soldiers, mountaineers. *Start:* frostbite commences with an initial vasospastic phase with pallor and numbness, followed by cyanosis. Rubor only returns on rewarming. Signs and severity vary steadily with degree of cold exposure, see below. *Pain Quality:* at time of exposure, numbness and tingling of digits and severe aching pain occur. After a few days, severe burning or stinging pain, particularly after exposure to warmth. Then pain becomes a deep aching or throbbing which may persist for many weeks. *Time Pattern:* single episode after cold exposure or recurring episodes if there is a predisposition to cold injury. *Intensity:* mild initially, then severe after a few days if limb warmed. *Duration:* usually two to three weeks to eight weeks, but pain can become chronic.

Associated Symptoms

In chronic stages: sometimes hyperesthesia and increased sweating, increased sensitivity to cold, numbness, aching, paresthesias, and dysesthesias.

Signs and Usual Course

First degree frostbite: edema, erythema, and hypoesthesia lasting two to three weeks followed by superficial desquamation. *Second degree frostbite:* vesicles and blisters in superficial skin layers. In two to three weeks vesicles dry and leave thickened epithelium (in absence of infection). *Third degree frostbite:* involves full skin thickness. Hard black scar develops and separates in about eight weeks. *Fourth degree frostbite:* results in deep tissue necrosis down to bone and requires amputation of the affected area.

Complications

Infections leading to cellulitis, tetanus, and gas gangrene are unlikely unless contamination occurs after rewarming; amputation may be required for gangrenous extremities after fourth degree injury; persistent cold sensitivity; paresthesias; hyperhidrosis and burning pain which may be prevented or relieved by sympathetic block or denervation.

Social and Physical Disability
Restriction of use of limbs due to cold sensitivity, hyperhidrosis, and pain.

Pathology
On initial exposure to cold, intense vasoconstriction occurs in extremity areas and results in reduced microcirculation flow with sludging of red cells; eventually flow ceases at the onset of freezing. Frozen tissue is bloodless, hard, cold, and pale. As tissues thaw, vasodilation occurs and flow is resumed; however, interstitial edema restricts flow, and white emboli dislodge from injured vessel walls and mix with platelets to form thrombi at venular bifurcations, and this obstructive process extends through to precapillary arterioles so that within one hour most of these microvascular channels are occluded.

Tissue necrosis is attributed to mechanical effects of microvascular occlusion, to extracellular ice crystals, and to cellular dehydration.

Essential Features
Exposure to cold below 0°C followed by tissue injury a variable period after exposure.

Differential Diagnosis
Erythema pernio (chilblains), trench foot, immersion foot, cold sensitivity, cold agglutinin syndrome, cryoproteinemia. Persistent pain and hyperhidrosis following frostbite may simulate causalgia.

Code
222.X1a	Arms
622.X1a	Legs

Erythema Pernio (Chilblains) (XII-4)

Definition
Pain and itching in areas of extremities following exposure to cold and wet environment above 0°C and associated with pigmented or purpuric skin lesions.

Site
Digits and limbs, especially lower limbs.

Main Features
Similar to first degree frostbite except that women are more susceptible (especially those with "sensitivity to cold"). At time of exposure numbness and tingling of digits may occur. Redness and itching of the skin is a feature, together with excessive sweating. The pain is often mild but may be associated with intense itching and with burning sensations. Pernio tends to be seasonal in occurrence, associated with cold exposure. The pain is always aggravated by warmth.

Associated Symptom
Blebs filled with clear or bloody fluid may form, and pigmented or purpuric lesions may develop.

Differential Diagnosis
Erythema nodosum, erythema induratum, Raynaud's disease, and acrocyanosis.

N.B. Acrocyanosis is painless.

Code
225.XI	Arms
625.XI	Legs

Acrocyanosis (XII-5)

Definition
Persistent blueness and coldness of hands and feet, sometimes with aching pain.

Site
Hands and feet, especially digits.

System
Vascular system.

Main Features
Blueness and coldness, more common in women, sometimes aching pain, often not.

Associated Features
Often chilblains. Trophic changes, ulceration, and gangrene do not occur. Symptoms are more marked in cold periods. Commences in late childhood and seems to have a hereditary background.

Code
222.X1b	Arms
622.X1b	Legs

References
Juergens, J.L., et. al., Peripheral Vascular Diseases, 5th ed., W.B. Saunders, Philadelphia, 1980.

Livedo Reticularis (XII-6)

Definition
Common, possibly vasospastic disorder in women under the age of 40; associated with persistent aching in the skin of the arms and itching of circular and reticular lesions which have a mottled cyanotic appearance.

Site
Upper or lower limbs.

Main Features
Occurring in women, the more severe form (cutis marmorata) is associated with persistent aching in the skin of the arm. Itching circular and reticular lesions with a mottled cyanotic appearance are evident.

Differential Diagnosis
Pernio, other skin changes.

Code

222.68a	Arms
622.68c	Legs

Volkmann's Ischemic Contracture (XII-7)

Code
222.X5

GROUP XIII: COLLAGEN DISEASE OF THE LIMBS

Scleroderma (XIII-1)

Definition
Intermittent vasospasm often with soreness, stiffness, or swelling of peripheral joints of the fingers and toes due to collagen disease of the skin, particularly affecting the limbs.

Main Features
Incidence: 3–5 new cases per million per annum. *Sex Ratio:* male to female 1:3. *Age of Onset:* from young adult life onward. *Pain:* is not a great problem in most cases. However, pain can occur intermittently with soreness and pain of Raynaud's phenomenon, especially aching pain in episodes ranging from mild to severe and changing to burning dysesthesias in the phase of reactive hyperemia. Numbness or hypoesthesias are present also.

Associated Symptoms and Signs
Stiffness and swelling of peripheral joints of the fingers and toes. A tight skin which may or may not be thickened. Skin temperature is often lowered, and the underlying tissues seem firm. Fingers although swollen and stiff can be moved with difficulty. The skin appears pale and waxen, skin temperature is lowered in the affected parts, and although pulses are palpable at the wrist, there is usually complete arterial obstruction in the digits. Microstomia and multiple telangiectasia may be observed over the face and hands.

Essential Features
Evidence of scleroderma with Raynaud's phenomenon.

Differential Diagnosis
See Raynaud's Disease (XII-1) and Raynaud's Phenomenon (XII-2).

Code

226.X5	Arms
626.X5	Legs

Ergotism (XIII-2)

Definition
Burning pain in the extremities, identical to Raynaud's phenomenon, associated also with systemic symptoms attributable to excessive ergot intake.

Site
Fingers and toes especially; viscera are occasionally involved also.

Main Features
Occurs in patients taking excess ergotamine tartrate or others (rarely) who have eaten rye or wheat contaminated by ergot. Uncommon in general. Presents with burning pain in the extremities identical to Raynaud's phenomenon.

Three stages can be seen in the changes in the circulation: (1) a stage of cyanosis or pallor from which recovery is rapid; (2) a stage of deep purple coloration in which blanching cannot be effected by pressure and from which recovery may be slow or may not occur; and (3) a stage of necrosis.

Severe cases of ergot intoxication are however sporadic. Symptoms can consist of dizziness, frontal headache, angina pectoris, Raynaud's phenomenon, coldness of the extremities, and pain. Both neurologic and vascular symptoms may produce the feeling of intense heat and cold, burning pains, known in the past as St. Anthony's fire.

Associated Symptom

Headaches, dizziness, nausea and vomiting, visual disturbances, angina pectoris, mono- or hemiplegia. May result in gangrene.

Usual Course

On discontinuation of ergot administration, pulses and signs of ischemia return to normal in 1 to 3 days. In stages 2 and 3, more vigorous therapy is needed with anticoagulant and vascular dilatation agents.

Complications

Gangrene. In some cases residual anesthesia of the skin or paralysis of the extremities may persist.

Pathology

Ergot intoxication results in constriction of the arteries. Because of the vasoconstriction, the endothelium of the vessels suffers, stasis occurs in the capillaries, and thrombosis follows. After thrombosis gangrene is inevitable. Actual intoxication is not necessary for diminution of arterial pulses. The chronic use of therapeutic doses leads to lowered foot systolic blood pressure. The degree of tolerance to the vasoconstrictive effects varies widely.

Summary of Essential Features and Diagnostic Criteria

Color changes of digits, burning pain as described, evidence of excessive ingestion of ergotamine.

Differential Diagnosis

See Raynaud's Disease (XII-1).

Code

281.X6   Arms
681.X5   Legs

References

Juergens, J.L., et al., Peripheral Vascular Diseases, 5th ed., W.B. Saunders, Philadelphia, 1980.

Dukes, M.N.G. (Ed.), Meyler's Side Effects of Drugs, 9th ed., Excerpta Medica, Amsterdam, 1980.

Goodman, L.S. and Gilman, A., The Pharmacological Basis of Therapeutics, 7th ed., Macmillan, New York, 1985.

GROUP XIV: VASODILATING FUNCTIONAL DISEASE OF THE LIMBS

Erythromelalgia (XIV-1)

Definition

Episodic burning pain in the extremities accompanied by bright red discoloration in response to increased environmental temperature.

Site

Extremities of the limbs, but almost always the feet rather than the hands.

System

Vascular system.

Main Features

Primary form rare and more often bilateral than the secondary type, which is related to the frequency of the conditions. Men in the middle-age group are more often involved, but women and children may also be affected. Characterized by severe, burning pain and red discoloration. The skin temperature is often raised, the skin flushed with venous engorgement, and the surface hyperesthetic. Attacks of severe burning pain last from a few minutes to many hours.

Associated Symptoms

Arteriosclerosis, hypertension, peripheral neuritis, cold injury, polycythemia, disseminated sclerosis, infections, hemiplegia, gout, or chronic heavy metal poisoning may be present. Ulcers or gangrene rare in primary type.

Signs and Laboratory Findings

Diagnosed by reproducing symptoms after raising skin temperature to 31–36°C. Relief from cooling. Skin cyanotic or deeply red in response to rise of temperature.

Pathology

Cause of most cases unknown. Secondary erythromelalgia may result from disorders listed above.

Differential Diagnosis

Burning pain which comes in attacks and affects the foot-sole or palm of the hand, closely related to objective increased local skin temperature. Reduction of pain by elevating or cooling the affected extremity.

Code

224.X8d   Hands   *Note:* add code for secondary
624.X8d   Feet   case according to etiology.

References

Juergens, J.L., et al., Peripheral Vascular Diseases, 5th ed., W.B. Saunders, Philadelphia, 1980.

Kappert, A., Lehrbuch und Atlas der Angiologie, 1st ed., Verlag Hans Huber, Bern, 1981.

Fitzpatrick, T.B., et al., Dermatology in General Medicine: Textbook and Atlas, 2nd ed., McGraw-Hill, New York, 1977.

Thromboangiitis Obliterans (XIV-2)

Definition
Pain in the fingers or hands or small digits of the feet, usually in males who smoke; associated with ulceration of fingertips and margins of nails; related initially to segmental inflammation of walls of medium and small arteries and veins.

Site
Fingers and hands, more often toes and feet, rarely the calf.

System
Cardiovascular system.

Main Features
Prevalence: a rare disease with a possible preponderance in Jews. Close association with smoking. *Sex Ratio:* males more than females—ratio above 9:1. *Age of Onset:* usual age of onset between 30 and 40 years. *Pain Quality, Time Pattern, Intensity:* usual onset is sharp pain in fingers or hands or more often in the foot or calf. There may be episodes of intermittent claudication in the hands or legs or constant burning in the tips of the digits (rest pain). *Intensity:* may be unbearable, often aggravated by elevation.

Associated Symptoms
Tenderness in superficial arteries, veins or nerves in affected area. Cold extremities (upper and lower), dysesthesias, and muscle weakness.

Signs
Coldness and sensitivity to cold, sensations of numbness, paresthesias, sometimes superficial thrombophlebitis. Ulceration of fingertips and margins of nails, gangrene of digits which may be wet gangrene if there is venous obstruction; edema present if there is venous obstruction. Absent ulnar or tibial artery pulsation and positive Allen test in cases affecting the arms (see Thoracic Outlet Syndrome [VII-4] for Allen test). Abnormal color of skin of digits: pale if elevated, red when first dependent, then blue. Cyclic color changes may occur in response to cold (Raynaud's phenomenon).

Laboratory Finding
Thermogram shows differences in temperature of digits. Skin plethysmography shows reduced blood flow in one or more digits, indicating local arterial disease. Tobacco sensitivity may be demonstrated. Vigorous muscle contraction of the digit may result in sufficient pressure to overcome intravascular pressure with cessation of blood flow as measured by plethysmogram. Doppler test may be helpful.

Usual Course
Gradual progression from age 30 for many decades. Favorably influenced if smoking ceases.

Complications
Gangrene and infection of digits. Osteoporosis of bones of extremities.

Pathology
Ulnar, palmar, and digital arteries affected early with segmental inflammation initially. Arteries are contracted and hard and lumens occluded by adherent mass. Arteries and veins bound together by inflammatory tissue. Acute stage: granulation tissue in all layers of affected arteries (pan-arteritis) and usually a thrombus in vessel lumen. Subacute stage: thrombus recanalized. Chronic stage: sclerotic thrombus, dense fibrous tissue encloses arteries, veins, and nerves.

Summary of Essential Features and Diagnostic Criteria
Organic arterial disease of one or more digits, almost always in a male under 40 with a history of migrating superficial thrombophlebitis.

Differential Diagnosis
Arteriosclerosis (larger vessels and more widespread), periarteritis nodosa (veins not involved), giant cell arteritis (mainly branches of carotid), thoracic outlet syndrome.

Code
224.X3c   Arms
624.X3b   Legs

References
Juergens, J. L., et al., Peripheral Vascular Diseases, 5th ed., W.B. Saunders, Philadelphia, 1980.

Rutherford, R.B., Vascular Surgery, W.B. Saunders,, Philadelphia, 1977.

Haimovici, M., Vascular Surgery: Principles and Techniques, McGraw-Hill, New York, 1976.

Chronic Venous Insufficiency (XIV-3)

Definition
Dull, aching pain in limbs, especially legs, characterized by abnormally dilated or tortuous veins.

Site
Limbs, usually the legs; especially the distal portions. Found equally on right or left sides. Bilateral in 7%.

Main Features

Prevalence: about 15% of adult population, severe in only 1%. *Sex Ratio:* more common in women. Prevalence increases with age, and there may be a hereditary predisposition. *Pain Quality:* dull, aching pain, usually associated with varicosities. Additional pain often due to thrombosis and/or thrombophlebitis acutely.

Associated Symptoms

Feelings of heaviness, numbness of the skin. Previous thrombophlebitis in a vein of the extremity, orthostasis with edema, developing during the day and disappearing during the night when the patient lies flat. After edema has been present for some time, areas of brown pigmentation (hemosiderin and melanin) may appear. Eczema is a common feature. After longer periods there is a tendency toward the development of subcutaneous fibrosis with induration and swelling.

Signs and Laboratory Findings

Edema, dilated superficial veins, varicosities, corona phlebectatica, hyper- and de-pigmentation, induration, open or healed ulcus cruris. In obscure or borderline cases phlebography is required.

Usual Course

Chronic, but dependent on stage of insufficiency and reaction on causal therapy.

Relief

Relief, even of ulcer pains, occurs gradually as a result of recumbency and more quickly if the extremity is elevated (relief after 5–30 minutes). Causal therapy for ulcers and dermatitis is indicated.

Complications

Ulceration. Neuritis of n. saphena longus is occasionally seen as a complication of chronic venous insufficiency.

Social and Physical Disability

Dependent on degree of insufficiency.

Pathology

Chronic venous insufficiency is the late consequence of extensive damage of the deep veins by thrombosis, in a given case, thrombophlebitis. The aching pain is associated with edema largely of the subcutaneous tissues. The more epicritic pain of ulcers and indurative cellulitis is usually due to secondary inflammation rather than congestion.

Etiology

Hereditary factors, blockage by thrombosis or other disease (rarely carcinoma).

Essential Features

Signs of venous insufficiency. Deep venous thrombosis in history.

Code

222.X4	Arms: neoplasm
222.X6	Arms
622.X4	Legs: neoplasm
622.X6	Legs

References

Juergens, J.L., et al., Peripheral Vascular Diseases, 5th ed., W.B. Saunders, Philadelphia, 1980.

Widmer, L.K., Peripheral Venous Disorders, Hans Huber Publishers, Bern, 1978.

Haimovici, M., Vascular Surgery: Principles and Techniques, McGraw-Hill, New York, 1976.

Rutherford, R.B., Vascular Surgery, W.B. Saunders, Philadelphia, 1977.

GROUP XV: ARTERIAL INSUFFICIENCY IN THE LIMBS

Intermittent Claudication (XV-1) and Rest Pain (XV-2)

Definition

Intermittent cramping pain in a muscular area produced by exercise and relieved by rest (XV-1), or constant pain in an extremity associated with hypoesthesia and/or dysesthesia and areas of skin ulceration or gangrene (XV-2).

Site

Intermittent claudication (pain after exercise) is almost always confined to the lower limbs. Pain from arterial insufficiency arising at rest may occur in lower limbs or upper limbs and may be related to gravity.

System

Cardiovascular system.

Main Features

Sex Ratio: males affected earlier than females. *Age of Onset:* over 30, increasing in later middle age and decreasing in the aged. *Pain Quality:* the intermittent pain is cramping and severe and arises, usually, after fixed and consistent amounts of exercise. Severe ischemia will result in rest pain and night pain. The pain is relieved by the dependent position, which initially causes the limb to flush red and then become cyanotic. Elevation of the limb causes blanching and increased pain.

Associated Symptoms

Hypothyroidism or myxedema, diabetes mellitus, hypercholesteremia, hyperlipidemia, xanthomatosis, and long-standing heavy smoking may be found. Occlusion leads to ulceration gangrene, etc.

Associated hypertensive ischemia ulceration: In patients with hypertension of long duration, ulceration of skin results from insufficiency of small arteries or arterioles. More common in women of age 45–70 years. Lesions usually in skin of legs but sometimes in the upper limbs.

Signs

A systolic murmur may be heard over the abdominal aorta or iliac arteries. Pain is relieved by the dependent position which initially causes the limb to flush red and then become cyanotic. Elevation of the limb causes blanching and increased pain. Absent or diminished pulses, reduced skin temperature, and coldness of the limb are characteristic.

Laboratory Finding

Arteriography demonstrates the level of arterial obstruction or obstructions.

Usual Course

May gradually progress so that the patient can walk less far. Sudden progression indicates acute occlusion of main or collateral arteries.

Relief

Relief may be provided by sympathectomy for rest pain; claudication is less often relieved by this technique.

Complications

Ulceration, gangrene.

Pathology

Claudication intermittens is a symptom that always indicates an inadequate supply of arterial blood to contracting muscle. Atherosclerosis is usually the underlying condition.

Etiology

May be due to (a) arteriosclerosis, characterized by local deposition of fat under and within the intima of arteries, most commonly the aorta, coronary, cerebral arteries; (b) arteriosclerosis obliterans, an obstructive late stage of atherosclerosis characterized by partial or complete occlusion of arteries by atheromata, often with superimposed thrombosis: more common in men, involves large vessels such as aorta and arteries of lower limb; or (c) Monckeberg's medial calcification and sclerosis, much more common in men, patients usually over 50 years of age. Changes confined to muscular media of medium-sized arteries, e.g., radial or ulnar, leading to nodularities around the artery. Only rarely leads to obstruction of arteries. Intermittent claudication and rest pain are more benign with this type of arterial disease than with others.

Essential Features

Exercise-induced pain which passes off very quickly by rest. Signs of arterial or arteriolar insufficiency.

Differential Diagnosis

Neurogenic claudication intermittens. Arterial or arteriolar vascular insufficiency by other conditions like entrapment syndromes, arteriospastic or arteritic conditions.

Code

224.X8c	Intermittent claudication: arms
624.X8c	Intermittent claudication: legs
222.X8b	Rest pain: arms
622.X8b	Rest pain: legs

References

Silva, D.A. and Widmer, L.K., Peripheral Venous Disorders, Hans Huber, Bern, 1978.

Juergens, J.L., et al., Peripheral Vascular Diseases, 5th ed., W.B. Saunders, Philadelphia, 1980.

Gangrene Due to Arterial Insufficiency (XV-3)

Code

222.X8d	Arms
622.X8d	Legs

GROUP XVI: PAIN OF PSYCHOLOGICAL ORIGIN IN THE LOWER LIMBS (XVI-1)

General Descriptions
See section I-16.

Pain of psychological origin in the limbs is rarely considered to be due to muscle tension. Delusional or conversion pain in these (and other) locations may be more common on the left. Recurrent or chronic limb pain due to inappropriate use of muscle groups whether or not for psychological reasons may be quite common.

Code

633.X7c	Tension: legs
61X.X9d	Delusional: legs
61X.X9e	Conversion: legs
61X.X9f	With depression: legs

References

Merskey, H. and Watson, G.D., The lateralization of pain, Pain, 7 (1979) 271–280.

Hall, W. and Clarke, I.M.C., Pain and laterality in a British pain clinic sample, Pain, 14 (1982) 63–66.

F. VISCERAL AND OTHER SYNDROMES OF THE TRUNK APART FROM SPINAL AND RADICULAR PAIN

GROUP XVII: VISCERAL AND OTHER CHEST PAIN

Acute Herpes Zoster (XVII-1)

Code
303.X2d

Postherpetic Neuralgia (XVII-2)

Code
303.X2e

The syndromes of herpes zoster and postherpetic neuralgia are similar in all regions and are normally unilateral and limited to one or two dermatomal segments. For a general description of them see II-4 and II-5.

Postinfectious and Segmental Peripheral Neuralgia (XVII-3)

Definition
Paroxysmal pain in the distribution of an intercostal nerve commonly associated with cutaneous tenderness in the affected dermatome.

Site
In the distribution of spinal nerve roots or trunks (if segmental neuralgia); in the distribution of the intercostal nerves; or in the distribution of the posterior primary division of the nerve trunk (if peripheral neuralgia).

System
Peripheral nervous system.

Main Features
Pain Quality: sharp or burning pain, usually intermittent, often precipitated by lateral movements of trunk or vertebral column. Associated with tenderness at points of exit of the nerve from a deep to a more superficial plane, e.g., at mid-axillary or parasternal lines. Post-traumatic intercostal neuralgia often has continuous pain with exacerbation.

Etiology
Neuralgic pains may be due to postinfectious radiculitis, osteoarthritic spurs, other spinal lesions, trauma, toxic and metabolic lesions, etc. In acute cases they are most often precipitated by upper respiratory infection or trauma. In chronic cases bad body mechanics, lordosis or scoliosis, trauma, and arthritis are the most common causes. Primary neuralgia occurs rarely.

Differential Diagnosis
From neuralgias attributable to specific causes, or described above.

Code
306.X2	Postinfectious
306.X8	Unknown
306.X1 or 303.X1a	Post-traumatic

Angina Pectoris (XVII-4)

Definition
Pain, usually constricting, and a heavy feeling in the chest, related to ischemia of the myocardium without myocardial necrosis.

Site
Pain classically is in the precordium, although radiation to the arms and hands is common, particularly to the medial aspect of the left arm. Pain may also radiate up into the sides of the neck or jaw or into the back or epigastrium.

System
Cardiovascular system.

Main Features
Prevalence: common in middle and older age groups, males more than females. *Pain Quality:* the pain tends to be dull, crushing, or constricting and heavy. It is frequently precipitated by stress, either physical or psychological. It usually lasts a few minutes but can be prolonged or intermittent, lasting hours or occasionally longer.

Associated Symptoms
As noted, pain is aggravated by stress and relieved promptly by rest or nitroglycerin. Frequently patients also experience breathlessness, sweating, nausea, and belching.

Signs and Laboratory Findings
Frequently there are no objective findings but patients

may at the time demonstrate a tachycardia, a mitral regurgitant murmur of papillary muscle dysfunction, an S3 or S4, and reversed splitting of the second heart sound. Laboratory testing may show characteristic electrocardiographic changes, most commonly ST segment depression. Between pains, a stress electrocardiogram may show ST depression with exercise. Coronary angiography may show typical atherosclerotic narrowing of the coronary arteries.

Usual Course
Anginal pain typically is brief and intermittent, brought on by exertion or stress and relieved by rest and nitroglycerin. It may remain stable over many years, or may become "atypical" or accelerate to "preinfarction (or "unstable") angina."

Complications
Arrhythmia and myocardial infarction may occur.

Social and Physical Disability
If angina is brought on by little extra stress, there is serious reduction in the work capacity. If the patient is particularly fearful, angina can cause interruption of normal psychological function as well. The big concern is usually fear of progression to sudden death or myocardial infarction, though limitation of activity level may also be a serious threat.

Pathology
A list of risk factors predisposing individuals to atherosclerotic heart disease continues to develop but includes age, sex, hypertension, smoking, family history, hyperlipidemia, obesity, sedentary life-style, diabetes, etc. Superimposed on atherosclerotic coronary artery narrowing, such factors as increased cardiac oxygen demand, decreased flow related to coronary artery spasm, or arrhythmias may be contributory.

Summary of Essential Features and Diagnostic Criteria
Crushing retrosternal chest pain brought on by stress (physical or psychological) and relieved by rest and nitroglycerin, with ST depression on ECG but no evidence of infarction on sequential ECGs and cardiac enzymes.

Code
324.X6
224.X6   If mostly in the arms

Myocardial Infarction (XVII-5)

Definition
Pain, usually crushing, from myocardial necrosis secondary to ischemia.

Site
Retrosternal area with radiation to arms, neck, jaw, epigastrium.

System
Cardiovascular system.

Main Features
Prevalence: common in middle and older age groups, especially males. *Pain Quality:* the pain is dull, central, retrosternal, and heavy or crushing. Usually it is very severe and lasts several hours or until relieved by morphine. It may diminish slowly over a day or two.

Associated Symptoms
Breathlessness, sweating, nausea and vomiting, apprehension, and lightheadedness are common.

Signs and Laboratory Findings
Physical examination may be normal but may show hypertension, S3 or S4 gallop rhythm, and papillary muscle dysfunction with a mitral regurgitant murmur, as well as signs of forward or backward cardiac failure.

Laboratory abnormalities include elevation of cardiac enzymes such as CPK, LDH, and SGOT, classical sequential ECG changes (ST elevation and the development of Q waves), and abnormal radionuclide heart scan.

Usual Course
In patients surviving myocardial infarction the severe pain tends to diminish and disappear over several hours to a day or two. Often the patient is then pain free, although recurrent pain may represent angina or reinfarction.

Complications
Sudden cardiac death, arrhythmias, congestive heart failure, cardiogenic shock, post–myocardial infarction syndrome, pericarditis, septal perforation, valve cusp rupture, mural thrombus and embolism, myocardial aneurysm, deep vein thrombosis, and pulmonary embolism.

Social and Physical Disability
Myocardial infarction is a major cause of death and disability. Recovery frequently takes several months, and physical and psychological complications may prolong recovery and affect not only the patient but family members, friends, and employers. The significance of the heart as the source of life makes interpretation of this type of pain particularly threatening.

Pathology
The main pathogenic process is atherosclerosis of the coronary arteries. Other factors such as coronary artery spasm or arrhythmias, or decreased blood volume, or decreased total peripheral resistance may also be significant as "last straws." The risk factors mentioned with

angina—sex, age, hypertension, smoking, Type A personality, etc.—are important predisposing factors.

Differential Diagnosis
Angina pectoris, dissecting aneurysm, pulmonary embolism, esophageal spasm, hiatus hernia, and pericarditis.

Summary of Essential Features and Diagnostic Criteria
Crushing retrosternal chest pain with myocardial necrosis as evidenced by ECG and enzyme changes.

Code
321.X6
221.X6   If in the arms

Pericarditis (XVII-6)

Definition
Pain, often sharp, arising from inflammation of the pericardium.

Site
The pain is classically in the precordium but may radiate through to the midthorax posteriorly or follow the pattern of angina, or to the superior border of the trapezius muscles.

System
Cardiovascular system.

Main Features
Most cases are acute, and this is particularly true of pericarditis causing pain. Pain may be severe and pleuritic. It may be aggravated by swallowing. It may be steady, crushing substernal pain. It may occasionally be synchronous with the heartbeat.

Associated Symptoms
Weight loss, fatigue, and fever are common especially in chronic cases.

Signs and Laboratory Findings
Leaning forward may reduce the pain. The hallmark sign is a triphasic pericardial friction rub. If there is a significant effusion, heart sounds may be decreased and a paradoxical pulse may be elicited.

Laboratory signs include a "water bottle" configuration on chest X-ray if there is an effusion, as well as changes in fluoroscopy, echocardiography, or angiography. Even without an effusion the electrocardiogram may show typical changes, ST elevation, or inverted T waves.

Usual Course
The course varies depending on the etiology and may range from being acute to chronic.

Complications
May interfere with cardiac output.

Social and Physical Disabilities
Probably only significant in chronic cases where weight loss and generalized debility are part of the syndrome.

Etiology
A wide range of etiologies can cause pericarditis and its subsequent pain. The most treatable causes are infections, collagen, vascular, and drug-induced effects. Postmyocardial injury is also an important etiology.

Summary of Essential Features and Diagnostic Criteria
Sharp retrosternal pain aggravated by breathing and relieved by leaning forward, with auscultation revealing a friction rub, ECG showing ST elevation or T wave inversion, and echocardiogram showing an echo-free pericardial space.

Differential Diagnosis
Angina, myocardial infarction, pulmonary embolism, hiatus hernia, and esophageal spasm, etc.

Code
323.X2   Known infection
323.X3   Unknown infective cause
323.X1   Trauma
323.X4   Neoplasm
323.X5   Toxic

If the pain (although resulting from pericarditis) assumes a spinal thoracic pattern, code according to X-7.1 with suffix letters.

Aneurysm of the Aorta (XVII-7)

Definition
Pain from an abnormal widening of the aorta.

Site
Central chest pain which may radiate to the mid-scapular region.

System
Vascular system.

Main Features
Deep, diffuse, aching central chest pain is associated with large aneurysms. If dissection occurs, sudden and severe pain occurs, maximal at onset.

Associated Symptoms
Acute congestive heart failure may develop.

Signs and Laboratory Findings

A discrepancy may develop between pulses or blood pressures in the two arms. A new aortic regurgitant murmur may develop. A neurological impairment may develop. Chest X-ray may show widening of the superior mediastinum. Aortography may demonstrate a false lumen.

Usual Course

If there is a large aortic aneurysm, there can be chronic dull, central chest aching. If dissection occurs, an acute medical and surgical emergency has developed.

Complications

Chronic complications include pain and emboli. Acute complications include acute aortic valvular incompetence, occlusion of major vessels, hypotension, and death.

Social and Physical Disability

The main problems with aortic aneurysms are life and death considerations.

Pathology

"True" aneurysms involve all three layers—intima, media, and adventitia. "False" aneurysms involve disruption of the inner and medial segments so that the wall of the aneurysm consists only of adventitia and/or perivascular clot.

In the past, syphilis was the main cause. Cystic medial necrosis is a major cause of dissection. Arteriosclerosis is a major cause. Occasionally Marfan's syndrome is the cause. Hypertension is important and so is trauma.

Summary of Essential Features and Diagnostic Criteria

A rare cause of chronic chest pain with a wide superior mediastinum on chest X-ray. A dramatic cause of excruciating acute pain with importance because of medical and surgical therapies available.

Differential Diagnosis

Angina, pulmonary diseases, and thoracic disk disease.

Code

322.X6   Chronic aneurysm

If the pain assumes a thoracic spinal pattern (although of visceral origin), code according to X-7.2 as 322.X6a.

Diseases of the Diaphragm (XVII-8)

Definition

Pain from the diaphragm related to irritation of the diaphragmatic nerves by a disease process above the diaphragm, in the diaphragm (rare), or below the diaphragm.

Site

Diaphragmatic pain is deep and difficult to localize. Noxious stimulation may affect phrenic nerve sensory fibers C3, C4, and C5 and therefore is often felt at the shoulder tips and along the upper border of the trapezius muscle, or it may affect the intercostal nerves T6, T7, T8, and T9 with radiation of pain into the anterior chest, the upper abdomen, and the corresponding region of the back.

System

The system is musculoskeletal, cardiac, pulmonary, or intestinal depending upon the disease.

Main Features

The pain is deep, dull, poorly localized, and non-specific if it involves only the central chest and upper abdomen and upper back, but becomes better identified if there is shoulder tip radiation as well.

Associated Symptoms

These symptoms depend most on the underlying pathology, so that if there is pulmonary pathology, respiratory symptoms may be prominent. Likewise, if the basic disease is gastrointestinal or subphrenic, gastrointestinal complaints are most likely associated. Hiccoughs may be present.

Signs and Laboratory Findings

Frequently there are no physical findings, but if there are, the most classic would be elevation of a hemidiaphragm. Laboratory testing might show elevation of the diaphragm on chest X-ray, abnormal movement of the diaphragm on fluoroscopy, a pleural effusion on chest X-ray, an echo-free space on abdominal ultrasound, a space between liver and heart on radio-nuclide imaging, or a space beneath the diaphragm on CT scan or nuclear magnetic resonance scanning.

Usual Course

There is usually a specific therapy once the etiology is determined, but a considerable time may elapse before a conclusive diagnosis is reached.

Complications

Depend on the underlying cause.

Social and Physical Disability

These relate partly to the underlying disease process and partly to the vagueness of understanding of the cause of pain. This latter can be extremely frustrating to doctor and patient alike.

Etiology

Although a wide range of causes can cause disease affecting the diaphragm, the most important are infections and neoplasms.

Summary of Essential Features and Diagnostic Criteria

Abdominal pain in epigastrium with radiation to central chest, posterior midthorax and shoulder tip(s), with evidence of space-occupying lesions above or below the diaphragm.

Differential Diagnosis

Involves a wide range of cardiac, pulmonary, musculoskeletal, and gastrointestinal uses.

Code

423.X2   Infection: chest or pulmonary source
423.X4   Neoplasm: chest or pulmonary source
433.X2   Musculoskeletal
453.X2   Infection: gastrointestinal source
453.X4a   Neoplasm: gastrointestinal source
453.X6   Cholelithiasis

Carcinoma of Esophagus (XVII-9)

Definition

Pain due to malignant disease of the esophagus resulting from malignant transformation of either the squamous epithelium of the upper esophagus or the mucosa of the lower esophagus.

Site

Retrosternal pain, extending sometimes to the back.

System

Gastrointestinal system.

Main Features

This is a relatively uncommon tumor in the Western World but has localized areas of high incidence, especially in Iraq and Iran among the Kurds. Pain is not usually a prominent feature. The presenting symptom is usually dysphagia without pain, which usually occurs only when the cancer extends beyond the esophagus. At that point dysphagia and retrosternal pain may become continuous and radiate through the back.

Associated Symptoms

Dysphagia is the major symptom; others include regurgitation and recurrent pneumonia.

Signs and Laboratory Findings

Evidence of weight loss and cervical lymphadenopathy, particularly deep to the sternomastoid. Chest X-ray may show a dilated esophagus; barium swallow, a narrowing of the esophageal lumen; iron-deficiency anemia.

Usual Course

Unless the tumor is removed, the patient will become obstructed.

Complications

Esophageal obstruction, erosion into a bronchus, bronchoesophageal stricture, erosion into aorta with catastrophic hemorrhage.

Social and Physical Disability

If the tumor is inoperable and the patient cannot eat, a plastic tube can be passed through the tumor or a feeding jejunostomy performed.

Pathology

Chronic ingestion of carcinogens in certain areas of the world, e.g., Kurdistan and Lake Victoria, East Africa. Smoking—chronic disorders of esophagus, e.g., achalasia, Barrett's esophagus.

Summary of Essential Features and Diagnostic Criteria

Presents with dysphagia with pain as a late feature. Diagnosed by barium swallow and esophagoscopy with biopsy or cytology.

Differential Diagnosis

Benign stricture, achalasia.

Code

353.X4

Slipping Rib Syndrome (XVII-10)

(also known as Clicking Rib Syndrome and Rib Tip Syndrome)

Definition

Chronic pain at the costal margin which may mimic visceral pain.

Site

Eighth, ninth, or tenth rib cartilages, one or more rib cartilages being involved. The condition may be bilateral.

Main Features

Prevalence: fairly common. *Age of Onset:* 15–60 years. *Sex Ratio:* more common in females (3F:1M). *Quality:* a constant dull ache or a sharp stabbing pain which may itself be followed by a dull ache. *Time Pattern:* the pain may last from several hours to many weeks, and some patients have constant pain.

Aggravating Factors

Movement, especially lateral flexion and rotation of the trunk. Rising from a sitting position in an armchair is often a particularly painful stimulus.

Signs

Manipulation of the affected rib and its costal cartilage will exactly reproduce the presenting pain.

Usual Course
Some cases may resolve spontaneously, but most patients have symptoms permanently.

Relief
Restriction of movement may give relief.

Complications
Depression and anxiety. Patients may be misdiagnosed and undergo unnecessary investigations and even inappropriate surgical procedures.

Social and Physical Disability
Physical activities are often restricted by pain or fear of provoking an exacerbation.

Pathology
No specific histological changes identified. Cause of pain is presumed to be irritation of intercostal nerve by adjacent hypermobile rib cartilage.

Summary of Essential Features and Diagnostic Criteria
A fairly common condition which should be considered in any patient complaining of upper abdominal pain. The diagnosis is clinical and should be made only when the patient's symptoms are exactly reproduced by manipulation of the appropriate rib or ribs. An intercostal nerve block with local anesthetic may produce confirmatory evidence where the clinical findings are equivocal.

Treatment
Reassure patient—this may be sufficient for some patients who do not have severe pain. If severe pain persists, then the offending costal cartilage should be excised.

Differential Diagnosis
Biliary tract pathology, duodenal and gastric ulceration.

Code
333.X6

References
Copeland, G.P., Machin, D.G., and Shennan, J.M., Surgical treatment of the slipping rib syndrome, Br. J. Surg., 71 (1984) 522–523.

Holmes, J.F., Slipping rib cartilage, Am. J. Surg., 54 (1941) 326–338.

Postmastectomy Pain Syndrome: Chronic Nonmalignant (XVII-11)

Definition
Chronic pain commencing immediately or soon after mastectomy or removal of a lump, affecting the anterior thorax, axilla, and/or medial upper arm.

Site
Anterior thorax, axilla, medial upper arm; usually one side only.

System
Peripheral nervous system.

Main Features
Prevalence: infrequent. *Age of Onset:* any age. *Sex:* females. *Pain Quality:* often burning, intensified by touch or clothing. *Time Pattern:* constant; unremitting to analgesic. *Intensity:* moderate to severe. *Duration:* years.

Associated Symptoms
The patient may be unable to tolerate a prosthesis, clothing, or touch.

Signs
Increased response to touch; hyperesthesia and allodynia to skin stroking or skin traction. Reduction in appreciation of pinprick, cold, and touch related to the incision and upper arm.

Usual Course
May remain intractable to physical measures. Commonly responds to amitriptyline. May also respond to ointments based on capsaicin.

Complications
Can be compounded by emotional stress, recurrence of disease.

Social and Physical Disability
Impairment of social, occupational, and sexual activities.

Pathology
None known.

Summary of Essential Findings and Diagnostic Criteria
Pain commencing postoperatively, usually immediately, at the site of the mastectomy, without objective evidence of local abnormality.

Allodynia over widespread areas of the chest or arm, or both; sensory loss over anterior chest or arm, or both.

Differential Diagnosis
Herpes zoster, local infection, radiation necrosis in ribs, recurrent neoplasm.

Code
303.X9

Late Postmastectomy Pain or Regional Carcinoma (XVII-12)

Definition
Shooting, jabbing, or burning pain commencing more than three years after the initial treatment for cancer of the breast and due to local metastases.

Site
Spine, thorax at site of cancer, arms.

Main Features
Prevalence: fairly common. *Age:* 35 and upward. *Sex Ratio:* most common in females. *Pain Quality:* varies according to etiology. With skeletal secondary deposits, pain is increased with movement. Shooting or jabbing pain occurs with brachial plexus lesion, usually spontaneously, sometimes with paresthesias. Burning, shooting, and numb feelings are found with brachial plexus damage from radiation. *Intensity:* moderate to severe. *Duration:* less than 12 months, due to short life expectancy.

Associated Symptoms
Weakness and reduced range of movement of the ipsilateral limb.

Signs
Ipsilateral Horner's syndrome; lower brachial plexus signs, e.g., anesthesia, muscle weakness, and wasting; chest wall or axillary or supraclavicular recurrent disease. Bony tenderness to percussion.

Usual Course
With skeletal secondaries and brachial plexus damage, the course is usually progressive deterioration. However, with radiation damage to the brachial plexus, the course is more protracted, with onset more than five years after treatment and long survival.

Complications
Patients with skeletal, visceral, and brachial plexus damage have a short survival of less than one year. Radiation damage is a progressive disorder with disability and long survival.

Social and Physical Disability
Moderate impairment of social and occupational activity, with depression related to chronic illness.

Pathology
Local skin, subcutaneous, skeletal, or visceral metastatic disease; with recurrent disease there is local lymphatic spread, and extradural and brachial plexus involvement. Radiation damage to the brachial plexus is more common in patients who have received repeated or excessive doses of radiation, and in such patients, telangiectasia may be present in the skin with pigmentation and signs of radiation arthritis.

Diagnostic Criteria
Pain arising more than three years after mastectomy for cancer, at the above sites. Objective evidence of recurrent disease.

Differential Diagnosis
Herpes zoster; pleurisy related to infection; and second tumor, e.g., Pancoast's tumor with brachial plexus involvement.

Code
307.X4

Post-thoracotomy Pain Syndrome (XVII-13)

Definition
Pain that recurs or persists along a thoracotomy scar at least two months following the surgical procedure.

Site
Chest wall.

Systems
Skeletal and nervous systems.

Main Features
Pain following thoracotomy is characterized by an aching sensation in the distribution of the incision. It usually resolves in the two months following the surgery. Pain that persists beyond this time or recurs may have a burning dysesthetic component. There may also be a pleuritic component to the pain. Movements of the ipsilateral shoulder make the pain worse.

Associated Symptoms
If the thoracotomy was done for tumor resection and there was evidence of pleural or chest wall involvement at the time of surgery, it is likely that the pain is due to tumor recurrence in the thoracotomy scar.

Signs and Laboratory Findings
There is usually tenderness, sensory loss, and absence of sweating along the thoracotomy scar. Auscultation of the chest may reveal decreased breath sounds due to underlying lung consolidation or a malignant pleural effusion. A specific trigger point with dramatic pain relief following local anesthetic injection suggests that the pain is benign in nature and due to the formation of a traumatic neuroma. A CT scan through the chest is the diagnostic procedure of choice to establish the presence or absence of recurrent tumor.

Usual Course

If the pain is due to traumatic neuromata, it usually declines in months to years and can be relieved by antidepressant-type medications and anticonvulsants. If the pain is due to tumor recurrence, some relief may be obtained by an intercostal nerve block or radiation therapy.

Complications

Immobility of the upper extremity because of exacerbation of the pain may result in a frozen shoulder. Aggressive physiotherapy is necessary to prevent this complication.

Pathology

For benign disease, the pathology is that of neuroma formation. If there is an underlying malignancy, there is tumor infiltration of the intercostal neurovascular bundle.

Summary of Essential Features and Diagnostic Criteria

Persistent or recurrent pain in the distribution of the thoracotomy scar in patients with lung cancer is commonly associated with tumor recurrence. CT scan of the chest is the diagnostic procedure of choice to demonstrate this recurrence.

Differential Diagnosis

Epidural disease and tumor in the perivertebral region can also produce intercostal pain if there is recurrent disease following thoracotomy.

Code

303.X1d	Neuroma
333.X4a	Metastasis

Internal Mammary Artery Syndrome (XVII-14)

Definition

Burning anterior chest pain commencing immediately or soon after coronary artery bypass surgery in which the internal mammary artery has been used for grafting.

Site

Anterior thorax, usually left side and occasionally bilaterally (always at the site of the graft).

System

Peripheral nervous system.

Main Features

Burning pain across a well-circumscribed area defined by the sternum medially, the intercostal junction at T2 or T3 superiorly, the intercostal junction at T5 or T6 inferiorly, and approximately the nipple line laterally. It is most frequently associated with sharp, spontaneous pains radiating to the chest, axilla, or neck. The pain may be mild, moderate, or intense.

Associated Symptoms

The patients usually do not tolerate contact with clothing or the water of the shower. Occasionally the pain is confused with angina.

Signs and Laboratory Findings

While the area is anesthetic or hypoesthetic, most patients present with troublesome allodynia and also severe tenderness on palpation of the sternum and the costosternal junctions at the site of the harvesting of the graft. Most patients will continue to demonstrate slow healing at the site of the median sternotomy. An active bone scan may be found up to 4 years after surgery due to compromise of the sternal blood supply as a result of harvesting the internal mammary artery.

Usual Course

Without treatment the pain may decrease in intensity during the first year post surgery, may remain the same, or may become intractable. Thoracic sympathetic ganglia blocks may significantly reduce pain, allodynia, and bone tenderness but only temporarily.

Complications

Pain can be compounded by emotional stress and suspicion of recurrence of heart disease.

Social and Physical Disability

Depending on the degree of discomfort, impairment ranges from negligible to serious.

Pathology

Trauma or resection of the anterior intercostal nerve.

Diagnostic Criteria

Burning pain, numbness, hyperesthesia and deep bone tenderness are almost all simultaneously present at the area of harvesting of the graft.

Relief

The application of TENS/desensitization may be very beneficial within the first few months after surgery. A combination of TENS and tricyclic medication should be tried subject to consideration of the effects of tricyclic antidepressants on the underlying heart disease. Patients may benefit from reassurance that this pain does not arise from recurrent heart disease.

Differential Diagnosis

Ischemic heart pain, costochondritis, hyperesthesia from the scar.

Code

303.X1f

Reference
Mailis, A., Chan, J., Basinski, A., Feindel, C., Vanderlinden, G., Taylor, A., Flock, D. and Evans, D., Chest wall pain after aorto-coronary bypass surgery using internal mammary artery graft: a new pain syndrome? Heart Lung, 18 (1989) 553–558.

Tietze's Syndrome — Costo-Chondritis (XVII-15)

Code
332.X6

Fractured Ribs or Sternum (XVII-16)

Code
335.X1

Xiphoidalgia Syndrome (XVII-17)

Code
494.X8

Reference
Bonica, J.J., The Management of Pain, Vol. 2, Lea & Febiger, Philadelphia, 1990, pp. 1129–1130.

Carcinoma of the Lung or Pleura (XVII-18)

Code
323.X4a

GROUP XVIII: CHEST PAIN OF PSYCHOLOGICAL ORIGIN

Muscle Tension Pain (XVIII-1)

Definition
Virtually continuous pain in the thorax, due to sustained muscle contraction and related to emotional causes.

Site
Either symmetrical, more often in the posterior thoracic region, or precordial.

System
Central nervous system (psychological and social).

Main Features
Tension pain is rare in the posterior thoracic region compared with tension headache (perhaps one-tenth or less of the frequency of the latter). Precordial pain is more common, often associated with tachycardia or a fear of heart disease. The exact prevalence is unknown. The other features of these pains are the same as for muscle tension pain in general (III-1, 2). See also I-16.

Code
333.X7h

Delusional Pain (XVIII-2)

See the general description of delusional pain (I-16). Perhaps more frequent in the precordial region.

Code
31X.X9d

Conversion Pain (XVIII-3)

See the description of conversion pain in general (I-16). Most frequent in precordium; may be associated with tachycardia and fear or conviction of heart disease being present. Often mimics angina, but without adequate evidence of organic disease.

Differential Diagnosis
As for conversion pain in general and angina pectoris.

Code
31X.X9e

With Depression (XVIII-4)

See I-16 for general description.

Code
31X.X9f

GROUP XIX: CHEST PAIN REFERRED FROM ABDOMEN OR GASTROINTESTINAL TRACT

Subphrenic Abscess (XIX-1)

Definition
Pain, often referred to the shoulder, from a collection of pus under the diaphragm.

Site
Upper abdominal pain and tenderness along the costal margins. Shoulder pain may be present.

System
Gastrointestinal.

Main Features
Deep, dull and often poorly localized pain in epigastrium with tenderness beneath the rib margin. Shoulder tip pain often occurs also. Often follows intra-abdominal surgery, especially with perforated viscus. May follow closed blunt trauma.

Associated Symptoms
Fever, malaise, weight loss, hiccoughs.

Signs and Laboratory Findings
These may be vague. The patient may be febrile and cachectic. There may be a pleural effusion or lack of diaphragmatic movement. There may be tenderness to percussion or to palpation of the upper abdomen. White blood cell count and erythrocyte sedimentation rate may be elevated. Chest X-ray may show pleural effusion or elevated hemi-diaphragm. Abdominal ultrasound or CT scan may reveal the collection of pus.

Usual Course
Treatment with antibiotics with or without surgery usually leads to resolution. There may be a prolonged phase of prediagnosis.

Complications
Prolonged fever and weight loss. May lead to death. Chronic pain. Septic shock.

Social and Physical Disability
May lead to usual effects both of chronic sepsis and chronic pain.

Etiology
Most common organisms are *E. coli*, non–group A streptococci, staphylococci, Klebsiella-enterobacter, and anaerobes.

Differential Diagnosis
A wide range of upper gastrointestinal diseases.

Summary of Essential Features and Diagnostic Criteria
Chronic illness often after abdominal surgery with fever and abdominal pain, often with shoulder tip radiation.

Code
353.X2   Thorax
453.X2a   Abdomen

Herniated Abdominal Organs (XIX-2)

Definition
Pain related to the protrusion of an abdominal organ through the normal containing walls of the abdomen.

Site
Pain can be related either to the organ herniating or the walls of the orifice. For hiatus hernias the main pain is epigastric.

System
Gastrointestinal system.

Main Features
Burning epigastric pain (or retrosternal pain, or both), often following eating or lying recumbent.

Associated Symptoms
The patient may also complain of chest pain similar to angina, right upper quadrant abdominal pain similar to that in cholelithiasis, epigastric pain like that in peptic ulcer disease, abdominal bloating and air swallowing.

Signs and Laboratory Findings
There are usually no physical findings. Radiographic techniques will show evidence of abdominal viscera in places they are not supposed to be, such as gastric mucosa above the diaphragm or colon above the diaphragm.

Usual Course
Pain typically is intermittent and aggravated by certain foods, aspirin, alcohol, bending over or straining, abdominal pressure or tight clothing, and carbonated beverages. Likewise, more esophageal reflux may occur with caffeine or nicotine, which relax the lower esophageal sphincter.

Complications
Pain and gastrointestinal upset.

Social and Physical Disability

May lead to chronic complaint, usually not too severe.

Etiology

Traumatic and congenital or degenerative weaknesses in the diaphragm are of key etiologic significance, although the exact cause is often obscure.

Summary of Essential Features and Diagnostic Criteria

Epigastric discomfort and esophageal reflux are key symptoms, with radiographic or endoscopic evidence of extra-abdominal organs.

Differential Diagnosis

Angina, cholelithiasis, acid-pepsin disease without hernias, and pancreatitis, etc.

Code

355.X6   Thoracic pain
455.X6   Abdominal pain

Esophageal Motility Disorders (XIX-3)

Definition

Attacks of severe pain, usually retrosternal and midline, due to a diffuse disorder of the esophageal musculature with severe attacks of spasm and/or failure of relaxation of the cardiac sphincter.

Site

Pain is usually well localized to the midline behind the sternum, between the epigastrium and the suprasternal notch.

System

Gastrointestinal system.

Main Features

Prevalence: uncommon. *Sex Ratio:* males and females equally affected. *Age of Onset:* occurs in young adults and middle aged. *Pain Quality:* sudden onset of pain, usually sharp and stabbing, spasmodic and severe, at times excruciating, lasting from 30 seconds to a few minutes, and leaving a residue of retrosternal soreness. The bouts are usually infrequent. Air swallowing and belching are common, and the pain is aggravated by swallowing.

Associated Symptoms

Dysphagia occurs in patients with achalasia of the lower esophageal sphincter. There is a sensation of the food sticking in the lower part of the esophagus. With the aid of gravity, the weight of the food causes the sphincter to open when the patient rises from the chair, and the sticking sensation disappears. Relieving factors include smooth muscle dilatation agents such as glyceryl trinitrate or amyl nitrite, which may relieve the pain.

Signs and Laboratory Findings

Patients usually point out their pain with one finger. Gastroscopy, barium swallow, cine-esophagoscopy or esophageal manometry may show evidence of increased or asynchronous esophageal motility. A barium swallow may show disordered esophageal contractions with or without 'spasm' or esophageal dilatation. The cardiac sphincter may remain closed until a large amount of barium fills the esophagus, when it will suddenly open. In patients with prolonged achalasia the esophagus may contain foreign material, which is undigested food. Esophageal manometry will show disordered motility with a lack of normal peristalsis and occasional high-pressure contractions or 'spasm.' In patients with achalasia the cardiac sphincter will fail to relax normally following swallowing, although sphincter pressure is normal. Special pressure devices in the esophagus for 24 to 48 hours may pick up very high pressure contractions, which may be related to the pain.

Usual Course

Pain tends to be severe and episodic. It may vary from very occasional to cyclic or be continuous throughout the day. Anxiety and eating may aggravate it. Most patients with motility disorders run a benign course with occasional attacks of pain. Occasionally the symptoms progress to the point where the patient has to undergo active therapy. In contrast, patients with achalasia usually progress to the point where they require definitive treatment.

Complications

If the pain is severe, it may lead to anorexia and weight loss. Vomiting may be a problem. Patients with achalasia can develop aspiration pneumonia from retained esophageal contents. The incidence of esophageal cancer in those patients is slightly increased.

Social and Physical Disability

Severe pain may restrict normal activities and be socially disabling.

Pathology

This is mainly a physiologic rather than a pathologic problem. Stress may be an important contributing factor. There is frequently a positive family history.

Summary of Essential Features and Diagnostic Criteria

This syndrome consists of short attacks of acute severe retrosternal pain which may be relieved by nitrites, with or without dysphagia. The diagnosis is made with a combination of barium swallow appearances and disordered esophageal motility and normal mucosal appearances on esophagoscopy.

Differential Diagnosis
Pericarditis, pulmonary embolism, angina pectoris, dissecting aneurysm, tertiary esophageal contractions in the elderly, and carcinoma of the esophagus.

Code
356.X7

Esophagitis (XIX-4)

Definition
Pain due to inflammation of the esophageal mucosa.

Site
Retrosternal or epigastric pain, depending on the etiology, e.g., upper esophagus, monilial; lower esophagus, acid reflux.

Main Features
Prevalence: common, especially in middle aged and obese. *Sex Ratio:* more common in women. *Pain Quality:* burning retrosternal pain, especially at night if lying flat, or on bending over. *Time Pattern:* may last minutes or hours.

Associated Symptoms
Aggravated by very hot or cold drinks, acidic drinks, alcohol, or strong coffee. Relieved by antacids or food.

Signs and Laboratory Findings
No physical findings. There may be iron-deficiency anemia and positive occult blood tests.

Usual Course
Chronic, intermittent, rarely constant.

Complications
Chronic occult GI bleeding, stricture of lower esophagus.

Social and Physical Disability
Unable to tolerate certain foods, unable to sleep flat in bed.

Pathology
Peptic: Dysfunction of cardiac sphincter results in intermittent regurgitation of gastric acid contents into lower esophagus when intragastric or intra-abdominal pressure is increased and aided by gravity. *Monilial:* Commonly secondary to immunosuppression and corticosteroids.

Summary of Essential Features and Diagnostic Criteria
Burning retrosternal pain from esophageal inflammation.

Code
355.X2   Monilial
355.X3a   Peptic

Reflux Esophagitis with Peptic Ulceration (XIX-5)

Definition
Retrosternal burning chest pain due to acid reflux causing inflammation and ulceration.

Site
Typically retrosternal midline pain radiating from behind the xiphisternum up as far as the neck.

System
Gastrointestinal system (esophageal mucosa).

Main Features
Prevalence: common in young adults and middle age group, starting in third decade. *Sex Ratio:* more common in females, especially in the obese or during pregnancy. *Time Pattern:* bouts of pain occur often after postural changes such as bending over or lying down. They also may be associated with a sour taste or waterbrash. *Intensity:* attacks are usually mild, except with ulceration, where they are very severe and last minutes to hours. With ulceration, pain may be continuous.

Associated Symptoms
Sour taste, waterbrash.

Aggravating Factors
Certain postures such as bending over, sitting in a slumped position, or lying down; very hot or cold drinks; acidic drinks. Relieved by antacids.

Signs and Laboratory Findings
The only abnormal findings are appearances of esophagitis (reddening or hemorrhagia mucosa) or of actual ulceration on esophagoscopy. Esophageal motility studies may show a decrease in cardiac sphincter pressure, a pH probe may detect acid reflux, and the pain may be reproduced by the infusion of 0.1 N hydrochloric acid proximal to the cardiac sphincter.

Usual Course
In the majority of patients the symptoms persist intermittently for years. In pregnant women they usually disappear after childbirth, except in the obese patients.

Pathology
Changes in the lower esophageal mucosa may vary from the mildest changes with blunting of the rete papillae to severe hemorrhage inflammation with ulceration and loss of mucosa.

Complications

Patients with ulceration may develop a stricture in the region of the ulcer which can cause dysphagia. Rarely a malignancy may develop in the area of chronic esophagitis.

Summary of Essential Features and Diagnostic Criteria

Esophagitis with nonmalignant ulceration presents with retrosternal pain especially on bending or lying down, or on drinking very hot or cold fluids or eating acidic foods. The diagnosis is made on the history, esophagoscopy, and esophageal motility studies.

Differential Diagnosis

Monilial esophagitis, herpetic esophagitis, foreign body in wall of esophagus, Crohn's disease.

Code
355.X3b

Gastric Ulcer with Chest Pain (XIX-6)

Code
355.X3c

Duodenal Ulcer with Chest Pain (XIX-7)

Code
355.X3d

Thoracic Visceral Disease with Pain Referred to Abdomen (XIX-8)

See Pericarditis (XVII-4) and Diaphragmatic Hernia (XIX-2).

GROUP XX: ABDOMINAL PAIN OF NEUROLOGICAL ORIGIN

Acute Herpes Zoster (XX-1)

Code
403.X2d

Postherpetic Neuralgia (XX-2)

Code
403.X2b

Segmental or Intercostal Neuralgia (XX-3)

See description of these conditions in thoracic section. Characteristics as for thoracic pain of similar etiology.

Differential Diagnosis

Also includes entrapment in rectus sheath or operative scars. Post-traumatic pain often has continuous ache with paroxysmal exacerbations.

Code
406.X2   Postinfectious
406.X8   Unknown
406.X1 or 403.X1   Post-traumatic

Twelfth Rib Syndrome (XX-4)

Definition

Chronic pain in the loin, sometimes with acute exacerbations and radiation to the groin.

Site

Eleventh or twelfth rib, or both.

Systems

Skeletal and nervous systems.

Main Features

A fairly common condition that seems to occur more often in women than men (4:1). Patients usually develop the problem between the ages of 20 and 40 years. There is not usually any history of trauma, but it may start during a pregnancy. The pain may take the form of a sharp pain or a dull ache, or a combination of the two (the initial lancinating pain being followed by a prolonged period of aching pain). Patients are rarely free from pain, although the intensity varies from time to time. An attack of severe pain can be bad enough to mimic ureteric colic. The sharp pains usually last for several hours, and the subsequent dull ache subsides over a couple of days.

Aggravating Factors
Certain movements, involving alternating flexion and extension of the spine, e.g., using a vacuum cleaner.

Relief
Flexion of the spine (i.e., sitting forward).

Signs
Tenderness of the affected ribs. Manipulation of the ribs should *exactly* reproduce the patient's syndrome.

Laboratory Findings
None diagnostic but a chest X-ray, intravenous urogram, and spinal X-rays will help to exclude other causes of loin pain.

Usual Course
Pain continues indefinitely.

Complications
Depression.

Social and Physical Disability
Quality of life moderately or severely impaired. Patients usually limit physical activities lest they provoke an acute attack.

Pathology
No histological abnormality identified in ribs. It is assumed that the cause is irritation of an intercostal nerve by the offending rib.

Summary of Essential Features and Diagnostic Criteria
Loin pain, either intermittent or continuous and sometimes with radiation to the groin. Frequently misdiagnosed as pain of renal origin. Diagnosis is clinical and depends upon exactly reproducing the patient's pain by palpation of the rib. Confirmatory evidence can often be obtained by using local anesthetic to block the appropriate intercostal nerve, but a negative test would not necessarily exclude the syndrome.

Treatment
Reassure the patient of the benign nature of the condition. Excise as much of the shaft of the rib as possible.

Differential Diagnosis
Renal or ureteric pathology, spinal problems, pulmonary pathology.

Code
433.X6a

Reference
Machin, D.G. and Shennan, J.M., Twelfth rib syndrome: a differential diagnosis of loin pain, Br. Med. J., 287 (1983) 586.

Abdominal Cutaneous Nerve Entrapment Syndrome (XX-5)

Definition
Segmental pain in the abdominal wall due to cutaneous nerve entrapment in its muscular layers, commonly at the outer border of the rectus sheath or by involvement in postoperative scar tissue.

Site
Unilateral in the abdomen, usually confined to a single dermatome.

System
Peripheral nervous system.

Main Features
Initially there is abdominal wall pain, which is sharp and burning but intermittent. Later the patients typically complain of a constant dull ache, with an additional sharp, stabbing pain in the anterolateral subcostal region on twisting, coughing, or straining. The aching pain is worse when sitting and easier when standing or walking. In women, pressure of tight garments on the abdomen can aggravate the pain.

With nerve entrapment in the rectus sheath the pain occurs, or is made worse, when the abdominal wall is tensed, for example if the patient is asked to raise the head and neck off the examining couch. The diagnosis is frequently missed when the abdomen is relaxed, as it is for conventional examination. The diagnosis may also be supported by the response of pain on localized pressure of the fingertip, pencil head, or similar object over the tender area.

The measures in examination assist in determining which thoracic nerve is trapped and may require injection.

Relief
Relief is obtained immediately by injection of local anesthetic into the trigger zone.

Differential Diagnosis
Serious intra-abdominal pathology, such as acute appendicitis, is normally not so prolonged over weeks or months. The pain of appendicitis is present even when the abdomen is relaxed and usually is associated with other well-known physical signs. Entrapment neuropathy may require distinction from other causes of segmental pain (see intercostal neuralgia). Pain of psychological origin, especially in young women, is another diagnostic alternative.

Code
433.X6b

GROUP XXI: ABDOMINAL PAIN OF VISCERAL ORIGIN

Cardiac Failure (XXI-1)

Definition
Dull aching pain from congestive failure.

Site
Pain from congestive heart failure is usually epigastric or in the right upper abdominal quadrant.

System
Gastrointestinal system. Pain is thought to be related to distension of the hepatic capsule. Bowel ischemia may also be a factor.

Main Features
Dull aching pain in association with a tender enlarged liver and other signs of congestive heart failure.

Associated Symptoms
Dyspnea, increased abdominal girth, ankle edema, decreased exercise tolerance.

Signs and Laboratory Findings
Physical findings of congestive heart failure may include crackles on auscultation, elevated jugular venous pressure, hepatomegaly, and occasionally a pulsatile liver, ascites, and edema. An S3 and S4 gallop may be heard. Chest X-ray may show cardiomegaly and pulmonary edema. LDH, bilirubin, and SGOT may be elevated secondary to hepatic congestion.

Usual Course
This is variable depending on the treatability of the congestive failure. The pain may settle promptly with good medical management.

Complications
Long term this may result in "cardiac cirrhosis."

Social and Physical Disability
If prolonged, it may be part of a disability secondary to heart failure.

Pathology
Passive congestion of the liver is the pathological finding. The primary pathology is usually coronary artery disease.

Essential Factors
Dull aching right upper quadrant and epigastric pain with a large tender liver and elevated liver enzymes in association with other findings of heart failure.

Differential Diagnosis
Hepatitis and diseases of the gallbladder.

Code
452.X6

Gallbladder Disease (XXI-2)

Definition
Pain due to an inflammatory disorder of the gallbladder usually associated with gallstones.

Site
Right upper quadrant, but also epigastrium and other parts of the abdomen.

System
Gastrointestinal; gallbladder and bile duct.

Main Features
Prevalence: common, especially in middle age, except in ethnic minorities with high prevalence when younger age groups are also often affected (e.g., some North American Indians). *Sex Ratio:* much more common in women. *Pain Quality:* pain associated with passage of stone into the cystic duct is a severe colic, short lived with associated sweating.

Associated Symptoms
Anorexia, nausea and vomiting, jaundice, dark urine, pale stool. Relieved with antispasmodics or opiates. Dyspepsia with fatty foods.

Signs and Laboratory Findings
Tenderness in right upper quadrant. Neutrophil leucocytosis; hyperbilirubinemia; elevation in serum transaminases and alkaline phosphatase. Evidence also from ultrasound and cholecystograms.

Usual Course
Resolves within two or three days unless stone impacts in common bile duct, causing obstructive jaundice.

Complications
Obstructive jaundice, mucocele of the gallbladder, empyema of gallbladder with or without rupture.

Pathology
Gallstones may be cholesterol from lithogenic bile, pigment secondary to chronic hemolysis, or mixed.

Summary of Essential Features and Diagnostic Criteria
Acute right upper quadrant pain, dyspepsia to fatty foods. Diagnosis by ultrasound or cholecystogram.

Differential Diagnosis
Hepatitis, renal colic, hepatic flexure syndrome.

Code
456.X6

Post-cholecystectomy Syndrome (XXI-3)

Definition
Right upper quadrant pain in patients following chole-cystectomy.

Site
Right upper quadrant.

System
Gastrointestinal (external biliary tree).

Main Features
Prevalence: this pain is a common occurrence soon after the gallbladder has been removed, often with a short initial pain-free period. *Sex Ratio:* it is more common in females. *Pain Quality:* the pain is similar to "gall-bladder" pain, may be colicky in nature, daily, but not at night, may be dull or very intense lasting all day, and may continue for months or years.

Associated Symptoms
Nausea, occasionally vomiting. Aggravated by eating.

Signs and Laboratory Findings
Tenderness in right upper quadrant in region of the scar. No abnormal laboratory tests.

Usual Course
Chronic, unrelenting.

Complications
Risk of analgesic addiction or further unnecessary surgery.

Social and Physical Disability
Those of chronic pain and addiction.

Summary of Essential Features and Diagnostic Criteria
Right upper quadrant pain in a patient following chole-cystectomy with no obvious cause. Endoscopic retro-grade cholangiography often reproduces the pain.

Differential Diagnosis
Retained bile duct stone, hepatic flexure syndrome.

Code
457.X1

Chronic Gastric Ulcer (XXI-4)

Definition
Attacks of periodic upper abdominal pain due to ulceration of the gastric mucosa.

Site
Pain is generally rather diffuse over the central upper abdomen. It may radiate in any direction and occasionally through to the back.

System
Gastrointestinal system.

Main Features
Sex Ratio: males and females are about equally affected, although in some areas it is more common in females, e.g., Australia. *Age of Onset:* can occur at any age, but most common in the middle-aged and the elderly. *Time Pattern:* sudden onset of pain after meals from within one-half to two hours. Pain may be aggravated by eating, relieved by fasting or antacids. At first may be periodic and infrequent, every two to three months lasting for a few days.

Associated Symptoms
Anorexia and mild weight loss, often nausea, but vomiting is rare and associated with a prepyloric ulcer.

Signs and Laboratory Findings
May be anemic. Patient shows site of pain by pointing to diffuse area of upper abdomen with hand. Tender on palpation in that area. The diagnosis is made on endoscopy or barium meal (upper gastrointestinal series). Mild iron-deficiency anemia, or elevation of ESR, or both may be found on blood examination.

Usual Course
Periodic pain becomes more frequent and perhaps severe and for longer duration until pain-free periods may disappear. Pain commonly responds to regular antacid and anticholinergic therapy and particularly to H2 receptor antagonists, but there is a high incidence of relapse.

Complications
Gastric ulcers may bleed, usually chronically, presenting with iron-deficiency anemia but occasionally acutely presenting with hematemesis and melena; chronic ulceration leads to scarring so that prepyloric ulcers may cause obstruction with vomiting. Peptic ulcers may perforate, though usually insidiously, resulting in erosion into adjacent structures such as the pancreas. This causes localized but rarely generalized pancreatitis, or acute perforation with resulting acute peritonitis.

Social and Physical Disability
Recurrent or chronic pain will restrict normal activities and reduce productivity at work.

Pathology
Chronic ulceration with transmural inflammation results in localized fibrosis and cicatrization.

Summary of Essential Features and Diagnostic Criteria
Chronic gastric ulcer is a syndrome of periodic diffuse postprandial upper abdominal pain relieved by antacids. The diagnosis is made by endoscopy or barium contrast radiology.

Code
455.X3a

Chronic Duodenal Ulcer (XXI-5)

Definition
Attacks of periodic epigastric pain due to ulceration of the first part of the duodenal mucosa.

Site
Pain is classically localized to a spot high in the epigastrium, either central or under the right costal margin, and commonly radiates through to the back.

System
Gastrointestinal.

Main Features
Occurs at any age but commonly in young and middle-aged adults and is still more common in men. However, the incidence is less than 2:1, males to females. Commonly occurs when the patient is fasting, especially at night, and is relieved by eating or antacids. Periodic pain, which commonly lasts from a few days to two or three weeks, with pain-free periods lasting for months.

Associated Symptoms
Weight loss uncommon; patients may actually gain weight. Dyspepsia and often nausea occur, but vomiting is uncommon.

Signs and Laboratory Findings
Patient often points to site of pain, which is also tender, with one finger. The diagnosis is made on endoscopy or barium meal (upper gastrointestinal series). Mild iron-deficiency anemia and elevated ESR may occur. Rarely hypercalcemia is discovered in association with hyperparathyroidism.

Usual Course
Attacks of periodic pain may become more frequent and for longer duration. Pain commonly responds to appropriate doses of antacids and healing is promoted by H2 receptor antagonists. But there is a high incidence of relapse, which can be considerably prevented by maintenance doses.

Complications
Duodenal ulcers may acutely bleed or perforate.

Social and Physical Disability
Restriction of normal activities and reduction of productivity at work.

Pathology
Chronic ulceration with transmural inflammation resulting in localized fibrosis and cicatrization.

Summary of Essential Features and Diagnostic Criteria
Chronic duodenal ulcer is a syndrome of periodic, highly localized, upper epigastric pain relieved by antacids. The diagnosis is made by endoscopy or barium contrast radiology.

Code
455.X3b

Carcinoma of the Stomach (XXI-6)

Definition
Constant upper abdominal pain due to neoplasm of the stomach.

Site
Anywhere in the upper abdomen.

System
Gastrointestinal system.

Main Features
Uncommon, occurring predominantly in middle-aged and elderly patients but can occur in the third decade of life. There may be a past history of a gastric ulcer or partial gastrectomy 15 years or more previously. Pain varies from a dull discomfort to an ulcer-like pain, which is not relieved by antacids, to a constant dull pain.

Associated Symptoms
Anorexia and weight loss early in the disease, together with fatigue. The patient may present with acute gastrointestinal bleeding, hematemesis and/or melena, or signs of anemia, e.g., fatigue, shortness of breath on exertion, and even angina and swelling of the ankles. Later, symptoms of obstruction either at the pylorus, with gastric distension and forceful vomiting, or at the cardia, with dysphagia and regurgitation, may occur.

Signs and Laboratory Findings
Physical findings include those of obvious weight loss of cachexia, a palpable mass in the epigastrium, and an enlarged liver. Laboratory findings are mainly of anemia, which may be microcytic due to chronic blood loss, normocytic due to chronic disease, or macrocytic due to

achlorhydria and even to underlying pernicious anemia. Occult blood is commonly present in the stool. Hypoproteinemia is found, at times associated with a protein-losing enteropathy. Liver chemistry tests, especially alkaline phosphatase, will be abnormal in patients with hepatic metastases.

Usual Course
If the patient presents early in the course of the disease the tumor may be resectable, although the chance of recurrence in the local lymph glands is high.

Complications
There may be obstruction at the cardia or pylorus, or metastases in the liver or in more distant organs such as the lungs or bone, resulting in bone pain.

Social and Physical Disability
Inoperable patients continue with anorexia and weight loss, become cachectic and totally incapacitated.

Pathology
The tumor is usually an adenocarcinoma. It may present as an ulcerating lesion or with diffuse infiltration of the stomach wall (linitis plastica).

Summary of Essential Features and Diagnostic Criteria
Indefinite onset of anorexia, weight loss, and fatigue in an elderly patient with vague upper abdominal discomfort developing into constant upper abdominal pain associated with anemia. The overall prognosis depends on the stage of the tumor at the time of diagnosis, early resectable tumors having an excellent prognosis.

Differential Diagnosis
Gastric ulcer.

Code
453.X4c

Carcinoma of the Pancreas (XXI-7)

Definition
Chronic constant abdominal pain or discomfort due to neoplasia anywhere within the pancreatic gland.

Site
Central or paraumbilical or upper abdominal over the surface markings of the pancreas.

System
Gastrointestinal system.

Main Features
Uncommon, occurring predominantly in older patients, i.e., average age 65 years, but can occur in third decade of life. Pain can vary from a dull discomfort to, in the later stages, an excruciating severe pain boring through to the back, which is difficult to relieve with analgesics.

Associated Symptoms
Generalized symptoms of fatigue, anorexia, weight loss, fever, and depression occur early in the course of the disease. The patient may present with a sudden onset of diabetes mellitus late in life, without a family history, or with recurrent venous thromboses. Later symptoms include jaundice with pale stools and dark urine, pruritus, nausea, and vomiting.

Signs and Laboratory Findings
Evidence of recent weight loss and eventually cachexia are common. Jaundice and a central or lower epigastric hard mass are late findings, and a palpable spleen tip is uncommon. Laboratory findings usually show normochromic normocytic anemia with or without thrombocytosis, elevated fasting or two-hour postprandial blood glucose. Later, an elevated alkaline phosphatase and serum conjugated bilirubin may occur and the serum amylase may be slightly elevated.

Usual Course
Only a minority of patients, from 20 to 40%, are operable at the time of diagnosis. Only about 20% of those (i.e., 5 to 10% overall) have a potentially curative resection with a four-year survival of about 40%, or 4% of the whole.

Complications
These include diabetes mellitus, obstructive jaundice, portal vein thrombosis, and small or large intestinal obstruction.

Social and Physical Disability
The symptom complex with weight loss and generalized weakness is eventually totally incapacitating.

Pathology
The tumor is usually adenocarcinoma.

Summary of Essential Features and Diagnostic Criteria
Indefinite onset of anorexia, weight loss and fatigue in an elderly patient with vague central abdominal discomfort eventually turning to severe constant pain with or without obstructive jaundice. The overall prognosis even with modern imaging techniques is poor.

Differential Diagnosis
Malignancy in other organs, stricture or impacted stone in the common bile duct.

Code
453.X4b

Chronic Mesenteric Ischemia (XXI-8)

Definition
Intermittent central abdominal pain or discomfort related to ischemia of the large or small intestine.

Site
Central, periumbilical, occasionally radiating to the back.

System
Gastrointestinal system.

Main Features
Progressively severe abdominal pain precipitated by ingestion of a large meal. It may progress to almost constant pain and fear of eating.

Associated Symptoms
There may be symptoms suggestive of gastric or duodenal ulceration or intermittent incomplete small bowel obstruction.

Signs and Laboratory Findings
There may be evidence of generalized atherosclerosis as shown by absent femoral popliteal or pedal pulses, or the presence of an epigastric bruit. No specific laboratory findings are diagnostic. Weight loss is associated with a severe form of this disease. Arteriographic evaluation indicates severe stenosis or occlusion of all three mesenteric vessels, including the inferior mesenteric artery, the superior mesenteric artery, and the celiac axis. A meandering artery, indicating collateral blood flow to the colon, is a common finding.

Usual Course
Progressive weight loss and abdominal pain if untreated. Sudden and complete infarction of the small bowel may occur.

Social and Physical Disability
This unusual problem may be part of a picture of generalized atherosclerosis, in which case the patient may suffer from angina, cerebral vascular disease, or intermittent claudication.

Pathology
Patients with true mesenteric ischemia show severe narrowing of all three mesenteric vessels by atherosclerosis, which leads to inadequate blood flow to the gastrointestinal system. Atherosclerosis is usually isolated at the origin of these three vessels.

Summary of Essential Features and Diagnostic Criteria
Mesenteric ischemia may result in central abdominal pain, associated with ingestion of meals. When this becomes severe, weight loss results and sudden small bowel infarction may occur.

Differential Diagnosis
This rare disease is usually diagnosed by exclusion of other causes of intra-abdominal pathology.

Code
455.X5

Crohn's Disease (XXI-9)

Definition
Pain due to chronic granulomatous disease of the gastrointestinal tract.

Site
Principally distal ileum and colon; less commonly anus.

System
Gastrointestinal system, sometimes including liver. Other systemic involvement is principally skeletal muscle.

Main Features
Becoming increasingly common in young adults but can occur at any age; males and females affected equally; pain usually due to obstruction in the distal ileum with colicky central abdominal pain in bouts; or localized inflammation (abscess formation) may cause a constant severe pain. Both pains will persist until treated.

Associated Symptoms
Intestinal obstruction associated with distention, nausea and vomiting, alteration in bowel habit, constipation or diarrhea or both, aggravated by eating, relieved by "bowel rest." Localized inflammation associated with fever, anorexia, and malaise.

Signs and Laboratory Findings
Mass in right lower quadrant; central abdominal distension; increased bowel sounds.

Usual Course
The symptoms in patients with Crohn's disease will often settle with bowel rest (parenteral nutrition), with anti-inflammatory therapy, Salazopyrine, or Metronidazole with or without corticosteroids.

Complications
Strictures, fistulas.

Social and Physical Disability
A high proportion of patients with Crohn's disease require surgery.

Etiology
Unknown.

Essential Features

Pain due to a chronic inflammatory granulomatous condition of the GI tract resulting in narrowing of the ileum and inflammatory "skip" lesions of the colon.

Differential Diagnosis

Small intestine—benign strictures; large intestine—ulcerative colitis.

Code

456.X3a   Colicky pain
452.X3a   Sustained pain

Chronic Constipation (XXI-10)

Definition

Abdominal pain, usually dull, due to chronic alteration in bowel habit resulting in fewer bowel movements and diminished mean daily fecal output.

Site

Left lower quadrant and upper abdomen.

System

Gastrointestinal system.

Main Features

Common in any age group but becoming increasingly common in the elderly. More common in women during menstruation, pregnancy, and menopause. The pain is located over the cutaneous markings of the colon, most commonly in the left lower quadrant and upper abdomen over the transverse colon. The pain may vary from being constant and dull to sharp or very severe, but it never prevents sleep. It may last all day, every day, with exacerbations associated with eating; defecation may bring partial temporary relief.

Associated Symptoms

The pain may be aggravated by eating and relieved by defecation. However certain high-fiber foods such as vegetables and bulk laxatives failing to cause defecation increase the pain, as do bowel irritants. Stool softeners can relieve the pain.

Signs and Laboratory Findings

The abdomen may be chronically distended; colonic fecal contents are palpable as well as the colon itself, especially the descending and transverse colon, which can be tender. The rectum may be full of hard feces (rectal constipation) or empty, but with feces palpable in the sigmoid colon on bimanual examination (sigmoid constipation).

Usual Course

Unless the constipation is due to some correctable abnormality, such as carcinoma or a particularly poor diet, the course is usually chronic, i.e., continuous for years.

Complications

There is a suggestion on epidemiological and experimental grounds that chronic constipation predisposes to diverticular disease and carcinoma. Neither is proven in humans. Fecal impaction, particularly in the elderly, can lead to large bowel obstruction or spurious diarrhea.

Social and Physical Disability

Severe constipation, particularly in the elderly, can cause spurious diarrhea resulting in fecal incontinence.

Pathology

Chronic constipation is most closely related to diet. The Western world's highly refined low-fiber diet predisposes to small stool weights and constipation, which is little known in Third World countries. Rarer causes include disorders of colonic muscle such as congenital megacolon and Hirschprung's disease.

Summary of Essential Features and Diagnostic Criteria

Abdominal pain, usually dull, sometimes exacerbated by eating due to chronic constipation, which is largely a disorder of Western civilization and increases with age. The diagnosis is made from the history and physical examination.

Differential Diagnosis

Diverticular disease, carcinoma of the colon.

Code

453.X7a

Irritable Bowel Syndrome (XXI-11)

Definition

Chronic abdominal pain of no apparent cause associated with alteration of bowel habit.

Site

Anywhere over the cutaneous markings of the colon but maximal on the left lower quadrant over the descending colon.

System

Gastrointestinal system.

Main Features

Very common, maximum in second, third, and fourth

decades but onset at any age from first to eighth decade. More common in females, with ratio varying from 2:1 to 5:1. The pain varies from dull to very severe, often throughout the day with some fluctuations, but never wakes the patient at night. It occurs daily throughout the year and in some patients "never misses a day," often for many years. The pain is out of keeping with the patient's physical condition.

Associated Symptoms
Nausea and vomiting but not anorexia or weight loss. There is always an alteration in bowel habit, either morning diarrhea with five to six bowel actions followed by normal bowel action later in the day or chronic constipation. Pain aggravated by eating, occasionally by milk and smoking. It may be relieved by defecation, lactose-free diet, and stopping smoking.

Signs and Laboratory Findings
Tenderness over part of colon. Extremely tender on rectal examination and on sigmoidoscopy at rectosigmoid junction. Scars of previous surgery, e.g., appendectomy, cholecystectomy, and hysterectomy common. Majority of investigations negative. Barium enema shows colonic spasm; a small percentage are lactose intolerant.

Usual Course
Chronic, often lasts for many years.

Complications
May predispose to diverticular disease, secondary neuropsychiatric abnormalities.

Social and Physical Disability
The pain can be incapacitating and result in deterioration in performance, social relationships, etc.

Pathology
Disturbance of motility throughout GI tract from esophagus to anus. May be associated with increased sensitivity to GI hormones, e.g., cholecystokinin, and to prostaglandins (in the chronic diarrheal patients).

Essential Features
Usually there is a long history of constant abdominal pain and tenderness in young women; associated with alteration in bowel habit and no abnormal investigations.

Differential Diagnosis
Diverticular disease of the colon.

Code
453.X7b

Diverticular Disease of the Colon (XXI-12)

Definition
Pain, usually dull, arising in relation to multiple small sac-like projections from the lumen of the colon through the muscular wall and beyond the serosal surface.

Site
The pain is most commonly in the left lower abdominal quadrant, related to the sigmoid colon, spreading more widely if the disease involves the whole colon.

System
Gastrointestinal system.

Main Features
The pain is not a common symptom in this very common condition, which rarely presents before age 40, but becomes increasingly common with age. Males and females are equally affected. Pain may be dull and chronic, recurrent in nature, associated with constipation or acute severe pain in the left lower quadrant, associated with acute inflammation (acute diverticulosis), and lasting one to two weeks.

Associated Symptoms
Chronic constipation, acute or chronic abdominal distension, rectal bleeding (in diverticulitis). Aggravated by chronic constipation. Relieved by high cereal fiber diet (e.g., bran).

Signs and Laboratory Findings
Abdominal (colonic) distension. Palpable descending and sigmoid colons with or without tenderness. Barium enema shows multiple diverticuli.

Usual Course
Chronic disorder with constipation as the main problem. Acute attacks of diverticulitis occur infrequently. Patients rarely require operative intervention for subacute obstruction.

Complications
Acute diverticulitis, obstruction with or without spurious diarrhea, bleeding, peridiverticular abscess.

Social and Physical Disability
Chronic constipation and spurious diarrhea may lead to rectal incontinence. If surgery is needed, a permanent colostomy may be required.

Pathology
Hypertrophy of circular colonic muscle with penetration by sacs consisting of mucosa, connective tissue, and the serosal surface.

Summary of Essential Features and Diagnostic Criteria

A common chronic condition of the elderly resulting in constipation, colonic distension, and sometimes abdominal pain. The diagnosis is made by identification of diverticuli on barium enema.

Differential Diagnosis

Chronic constipation, carcinoma of the colon.

Code
454.X6

Carcinoma of the Colon (XXI-13)

Definition

Pain due to malignant neoplasm of the large bowel.

Site

Most commonly lower abdominal or perineal pain from a lesion of the rectosigmoid area. Then any part of the abdomen from involvement of the colon, including the cecum.

System

Gastrointestinal system.

Main Features

One of the most common cancers in the developed countries, in contrast to developing countries. It is common in the middle aged and elderly. However it can occur rarely in young adults and children. The sex ratio is equal. The illness presents commonly with an alteration in bowel habit or with iron-deficiency anemia. There are several possible mechanisms of pain: the most common is due to obstruction with colon distension. Rarely pain is due to erosion through the colonic wall with peritoneal involvement. Pain is persistent and progressive until treated.

Signs and Laboratory Findings

A palpable abdominal mass or colonic distension or a palpable rectal mass. Positive fecal occult blood. Iron-deficiency anemia. Visualization by barium enema or endoscopy.

Usual Course

The pain is short lived once the diagnosis is made, and it disappears with surgical removal of tumor, but pain may result later from metastases.

Complications

Acute or chronic rectal bleeding. There may be obstruction with a change in bowel habit, rarely colonic perforation or fistula formation into another viscus such as the bladder.

Social and Physical Disability

Surgical treatment may involve a permanent colostomy.

Pathology

The pathology is that of adenocarcinoma, beginning in the mucosa or in an adenomatous polyp, and spreading through the muscular wall to the serosa and via the lymphatic system and later the mesenteric blood supply to metastases to the liver, lung, etc.

Summary of Essential Features and Diagnostic Criteria

One of the most common cancers in the Western world, manifesting either as iron deficiency anemia, rectal bleeding, or an alteration in bowel habit, sometimes with abdominal or perineal pain. Diagnosed by endoscopy or barium enema.

Differential Diagnosis

Benign polyps and strictures, diverticular disease, ischemia colitis.

Code
452.X4

Gastritis and Duodenitis (XXI-14)

Code
45X.X2c

Dyspepsia and Other Dysfunctional Disorders in Stomach with Pain (XXI-15)

Code
45X.X7c or 45X.X8

Radiation Enterocolitis (XXI-16)

Code
453.X5

Ulcerative Colitis and Other Chronic Colitis and Other Ulcer (XXI-17)

Code
453.X8a

Post–Gastric Surgery Syndrome, Dumping (XXI-18)

Code
454.X1a

Chronic Pancreatitis (XXI-19)

Code
453.XXd

Recurrent Abdominal Pain in Children (XXI-20)

Definition
Recurrent abdominal pain is a syndrome consisting of paroxysmal episodes of unexplained abdominal pain in children.

Site
Abdomen.

System
Probably gastrointestinal system in most cases.

Main Features
Very common, affecting 10% of children, increasing from age 4. Pain usually lasts less than one hour and is self limiting. The child is healthy between bouts of pain.

Associated Symptoms
May be associated with nausea, vomiting, pallor, limb pains, and headache.

Signs
The pain is often periumbilical but can be anywhere in abdomen. If pain always occurs at a site other then periumbilical the possibility of other organ system pathology (e.g., genito-urinary) arises.

Laboratory Findings
Blood count, urinalysis, ESR normal.

Usual Course
Variable; in more severe cases the condition is chronic over many years.

Social and Physical Disability
Usually only during pain episodes. Disability depends on the reaction of the family, child, and doctor.

Relief
Fiber supplement, behavior management if clearly of behavioral origin.

Pathology
None.

Diagnostic Criteria
Paroxysmal abdominal pain interfering with normal activities occurring at least three times over at least three months.

No organic findings.

Code
456.X7

References
Apley J., The child with abdominal pains, 2nd ed., Blackwell Scientific, London, 1975.

Feldman, W., McGrath, P., Hodgson, C., Ritter, H. and Shipman, R., The use of dietary fibre in the management of simple childhood idiopathic recurrent abdominal pain: results in a prospective double blind randomized controlled trial, Am. J. Dis. Child., 139 (1985) 1216-1218.

McGrath, P. and Feldman, W., Clinical approach to recurrent abdominal pain in children, Dev. Behav. Pediatr., 7 (1986) 56-61.

Carcinoma of the Liver or Biliary System (XXI-21)

Code
453.X4

Carcinoma of the Kidney (Grawitz Carcinoma) (XXI-22)

Code
453.X4

GROUP XXII: ABDOMINAL PAIN SYNDROMES OF GENERALIZED DISEASES

Familial Mediterranean Fever (FMF) (XXII-1)

Definition
Disease of unknown cause predominant in those of Mediterranean stock, notably Sephardic Jews, Armenians, and Arabs. Classic features are periodic acute self-limiting febrile episodes with peritonitis, pleuritis, synovitis, and/or erythema resembling erysipelas.

Site
Abdomen or chest.

System
Peritoneal and pleural cavity.

Main Features
Prevalence: unknown. *Sex Ratio:* affects either sex. *Age of Onset:* attacks usually appear before age 20. Hereditary; transmitted as a single genetic characteristic with autosomal recessive inheritance. *Onset:* abdominal pain (peritoneal) most frequent presenting feature, varies in severity from mild abdominal discomfort with mild pyrexia to board-like rigidity, absent peristalsis and vomiting. *Time Pattern:* attacks settle within 48 hours, leaving no residual signs. Pleural attacks resemble peritoneal ones but are less common and usually precede or follow abdominal pain. Chest wall tenderness may be marked during attack, and transient pleural effusion may occur. Attacks occur with varying frequency.

Associated Symptoms
Erysipelas-like erythema over the cutaneous aspects of thighs, legs, or dorsa of feet. Arthralgias or acute arthritis involving mainly large joints such as knees or ankles. Attacks typically accompanied by fever and sometimes myalgia. Precipitants such as exercise, emotional stress, menstruation, fatty food, and cold exposure have been implicated. Relief obtained only from strong analgesics, though colchicine may diminish frequency of attacks.

Laboratory Findings
Hemocytosis may occur. Pleural fluid contains polymorphs but is sterile.

Complications
Amyloidosis is the commonest cause of death and is chiefly nephropathic. Its occurrence is highly variable depending on race and geography. When it does occur death is usually before age 40.

Social and Physical Disability
Interruption of work when severe. No physical disability if amyloidosis does not supervene.

Pathology
Unknown.

Treatment
Colchicine is effective.

Diagnostic Criteria
Periodic attacks of peritonitis (rarely pleuritis) occurring in people chiefly of Mediterranean stock. Self-limiting and associated with fever, leucocytosis, and occasional rash. Arthralgic amyloidosis may supervene and lead to death in renal failure. Sporadic cases in people of other races have been described.

Differential Diagnosis
Other causes of peritonitis, peptic ulcer, porphyria.

Code
434.X0b or 334.X0b

Abdominal Migraine (XXII-2)

Definition
Characterized by recurrent attacks of abdominal pain, and/or vomiting occurring in association with typical migraine or as a replacement or migraine equivalent.

System
Unknown; vasospasm in the autonomic diencephalic centers has been postulated.

Site
Abdomen.

Main Features
Prevalence: unknown; but uncommon in contrast to common or classical migraine. *Sex Ratio:* males more than females. *Age of Onset:* most common in children between 2 and 11; occurs in young adults. *Aura:* prodromal symptoms may occur such as listlessness, mood disturbance, yawning or, rarely, typical aura of common migraine. *Pain:* may be anywhere in abdomen but usually epigastric or periumbilical; a diffuse burning or aching increasing in severity lasting several hours but terminated by sleep; frequently associated with nausea

and vomiting and is commonly replaced by vomiting alone. *Frequency:* more common in childhood as "bilious" attacks. Attacks occur often during episodes of stress, frustration, or personal conflict.

Signs
Skin may show vasodilation; nonspecific fever has been recorded.

Laboratory Findings
EEG during attack may show mild generalized dysrhythmia, with high-voltage slow waves, thought to indicate cerebral hypoxia; transient leucocytosis may occur at height of attack.

Course
Tends to become less frequent with age and usually disappears when personal conflicts resolve.

Complications
None.

Social and Physical Disabilities
Reduced work performance in some.

Pathology
Unknown.

Summary of Essential Features and Diagnostic Criteria
Recurrent attacks of vomiting and/or abdominal pain occurring either as a migraine equivalent or associated with a migraine attack; more frequent in childhood and often associated with stress or personal conflict.

Differential Diagnosis
Gallstones; peptic ulcer, porphyria, irritable gut syndrome, etc.

Code
404.X7a

Porphyria — Hepatic Porphyrias

A group of disorders characterized by increased formation of porphyrins and/or porphyrin precursors in the liver. The principal clinical manifestations are photosensitivity and neurological lesions, which result in abdominal pain, peripheral neuropathy, and mental disturbance.

Within this group three diseases are recognized: (1) intermittent acute porphyria (IAP); (2) hereditary coproporphyria (HCP.); and (3) variegate porphyria (VP).

Intermittent Acute Porphyria (IAP) (XXII-3)

Definition
Inherited disturbance of porphyrin metabolism not associated with photosensitivity, with attacks of abdominal pain as a constant feature, and sometimes variable hypertension, peripheral and central neuropathy (mainly motor), or psychosis.

Site
Abdomen, either generalized or localized.

System
Autonomic peripheral or central nervous system.

Main Features
Prevalence: exact incidence unknown. *Sex Ratio:* females to males 3:2. *Age of Onset:* after puberty. *Inheritance:* transmitted by a single autosomal-dominant gene with variable penetrance; positive family history commonly obtained. *Manifestations:* colicky abdominal pain, moderate or severe, generalized or localized is usually the first and most prominent syndrome. Constipation, abdominal distension, and profuse vomiting common; attacks are intermittent, lasting several days to several months with periods of remission during which symptoms are slight or absent. Attacks may be precipitated by (a) a wide variety of drugs, hormones; or (b) metabolic and nutritional factors (dieting, low carbohydrate intake).

Associated Symptoms
Neurological symptoms and signs are variable but may include peripheral neuritis (motor), autonomic, brain stem, cranial nerve, and cerebral dysfunction. Hypertension is frequent.

Signs
The abdomen is soft, tenderness is marked, and rebound tenderness is absent. Abdominal distension, slight fever, and leucocytosis may occur.

Laboratory Findings
X-rays often show areas of intestinal distension proximal to areas of spasm. Hyponatremia may be severe. Porphobilinogen and delta-aminolevulinic acid (ALA) in urine.

Usual Course
Severe cases may terminate in death from respiratory failure or from azotemia. Many, however, are clinically mild or latent and may exhibit only minor or vague complaints.

Social and Physical Disabilities
Pain often results in frequent admissions to hospital. Great caution needed when administering any drug.

Pathogenesis

The primary genetic defect is a generalized deficiency of enzyme uroporphyrinogen I synthetase acting in the pathway of heme synthesis, predominantly in the liver. This leads to depression of ALA synthetase activity and overproduction of ALA and porphobilinogen.

Essential Features

Acute intermittent abdominal colic without photosensitivity, with or without neuropsychiatric associated symptoms and hypertension, and typical urinary findings (q.v.).

Diagnostic Criteria

Intermittent abdominal pain with excess porphobilinogen and/or ALA in urine.

Differential Diagnosis

Peptic ulcer, gallstones, appendicitis, diverticulitis, irritable colon, lead poisoning, etc.

Code

404.X5a

Hereditary Coproporphyria (HCP) (XXII-4)

Definition

An inherited disturbance of porphyrin metabolism characterized by attacks of abdominal pain, occasional photosensitivity, neurological and mental disturbance (see Intermittent Acute Porphyria [IAP] [XXII-3]).

Site

Abdomen (see IAP).

System

Autonomic nervous system.

Main Features

Very rare; only a few families described; autosomal dominant; both sexes affected; often clinically silent (see IAP). Similar but milder disturbance; acute attacks often precipitated by drugs.

Associated Features

As in IAP but photosensitivity occurs, though uncommonly.

Usual Course

As in IAP but milder.

Pathology

Due to probable partial block in conversion of coproporphyrin III to protoporphyrinogen IX. Coproporphyrinogen oxidase activity decreased, probably mainly in liver.

Code

404.X5b

Variegate Porphyria (VP) (XXII-5)

(South African Genetic Porphyria or Protocoproporphyria Hereditaria)

Definition

A rare hereditary disorder of porphyria metabolism characterized by acute attacks of abdominal pain, neuropsychiatric manifestations, and photocutaneous lesions.

Site

Abdomen, diffuse or localized.

System

Autonomic nervous system.

Main Features

Prevalence: unknown. Sporadic families reported throughout the world. First reported in Dutch descendants in South Africa where incidence is 3 in 1000 Afrikaners. Autosomal dominant in either sex. *Onset:* usually in third decade, with cutaneous photosensitivity being initial feature. Attacks of abdominal pain, identical to those described in IAP (see XXII-3). *Frequency:* variable. Provoked by a variety of drugs, particularly barbiturates and sulfonamide, hormones, anesthetics, ethanol.

Signs

See IAP.

Laboratory Findings

Excretion of large amounts of protoporphyrin and coproporphyrin in feces. Urinary porphyrin precursors only modestly increased or normal, except during acute attack. Dehydration may lead to azotemia, and hyponatremia is common.

Usual Course

Variable; not as severe as IAP. Permanent neuropathic change can occur.

Pathology

Partial enzyme block between protoporphyrinogen and heme is postulated. No major anatomic abnormalities at autopsy.

Diagnostic Criteria

Intermittent acute abdominal pain with prominent cutaneous photosensitivity and often neuropsychiatric manifestations.

Differential Diagnosis

See IAP.

Code

404.X5c

GROUP XXIII: ABDOMINAL PAIN OF PSYCHOLOGICAL ORIGIN

Muscle Tension Pain (XXIII-I)

Rare. See general description (I-16.1 and III-1, III-2).

Code
433.X7c

Delusional or Hallucinatory Pain (XXIII-2)

See general description (I-16.2).

Code
41X.X9d

Conversion Pain (XXIII-3)

See general description (I-16.3).

Abdominal pain of psychological origin occurs as the Couvade syndrome in men during their wives' pregnancies. This may be manifest as pains of discomfort, or at the time of labor, very rarely in developed societies, as an episode of pains resembling contractions.

Code
41X.X9e

Reference
Trethowan, W.H. and Conlon, M.F., The Couvade syndrome, Br.. J. Psychiatry, 111, 470 (1965) 57–66.

Associated with Depression (XXIII-4)

Rare in some cultures, common in others.

Code
41X.X9f

Reference
Magni, G., Rossi, M.R., Rigatti-Luchini, S. and Merskey, H., Chronic abdominal pain and depression: epidemiologic findings in the United States Hispanic Health and Nutrition Examination Survey, Pain, 49 (1992) 77–85.

Abdominal Pain—Visceral Pain Referred to the Abdomen

Pericarditis: see XVII-6.

Diaphragmatic Hernia: see XIX-2.

Aneurysm of the Aorta: see XVII-7.

Disease of the Diaphragm: see XVII-8.

GROUP XXIV: DISEASES OF THE BLADDER, UTERUS, OVARIES, AND ADNEXA

Mittelschmerz (XXIV-1)

Definition
Mittelschmerz, also called midcycle pain, occurs as recurrent pain episodes at the time of ovulation.

System
Female internal genital organs; in an ovary, a tube, or the uterus.

Site
Either unilateral or bilateral in the lower abdomen. May be felt always in the same iliac fossa, or alternately on one side or the other, or in the whole lower abdomen.

Main Features
Prevalence: Mittelschmerz is the complaint of 1 to 3% of patients in a gynecological outpatient clinic. It is mostly found in young women, between 20 and 30 years of age. *Symptoms:* usually presents as a recurrent pain around the time of ovulation. It may last from a few hours to 1 or 2 days, sometimes up to 4 days. The severe form is infrequent. It presents around the date of ovulation as a severe pain in an iliac fossa, lasting some 20 to 30 minutes and then gradually fading away. It may be accompanied by symptoms and signs of intraperitoneal bleeding: anemia, abdominal meteorism, diaphragmatic and/or shoulder pain, and fainting. *Time Course:* the severe form recurs only rarely; it may be followed by the

recurrent less severe form. The less severe form may last for several years.

Associated Symptoms
Increase of cervical mucorrhea; sometimes accompanied by midmenstrual bleeding.

Signs
In the less severe form, there are no signs, or only tenderness on bimanual palpation, especially in the corresponding iliac fossa. When the severe form is accompanied by intraperitoneal bleeding, there are signs of acute anemia, or rebound tenderness on palpation of the abdomen.

Complications
None in the less severe forms. In the severe forms there may be massive intraperitoneal hemorrhage; as in these cases an operation is necessary, this may be followed by postoperative adhesions around the ovary or the adnexa.

Pathology
No definite pathology known; pathophysiology remains to be elucidated. Possible causes include maturation of the follicle or ovulation itself or contractions of the tubal wall in a case of hydrosalpinx, or an increase in the basal tone of the myometrial contractions around the time of ovulation. It may also be due, although rarely, to a focus of endometriosis.

Treatment
If the pain is mild in the less severe form: analgesics. The pain episode may be prevented by cyclic estroprogestogens. In more severe forms with intraperitoneal bleeding, a laparotomy may be necessary.

Diagnostic Criteria and Differential Diagnosis
The essential feature is recurrence at the time of ovulation. It may be useful to confirm the coincidence with the periovulatory period by means of the basal body temperature, which will show a shift toward a premenstrual plateau. Severe cases with right-sided location may erroneously be taken for appendicitis. Appendicitis frequently starts with a pain in the periumbilical region, and it gives rise to nausea or vomiting, muscle guarding, and a slight fever. When accompanied by intraperitoneal hemorrhage, the time of occurrence will differentiate severe Mittelschmerz from ectopic pregnancy or rupture of a corpus luteum cyst, but blood transfusion and laparotomy will be indicated in both cases.

Code
765.X7a

Reference
Renaer, M., Midcycle pain. In: M. Renaer (Ed.), Chronic Pelvic Pain, Springer Verlag, Berlin, 1981, pp. 65–68.

Secondary Dysmenorrhea (XXIV-2)

Definition
Dysmenorrhea is called secondary if a structural anomaly is found that is probably responsible for the pain or when the pain seems to have a psychological origin.

System
Genital system.

Site
Pelvis. The pain is more often unilateral than in the primary variety, especially when the causal condition is unilateral, as for example in some cases of endometriosis.

Main Features
These resemble primary dysmenorrhea, but the pain often lasts longer, e.g., as in endometriosis.

Main Causes
The main causes of secondary dysmenorrhea are: endometriosis, adenomyosis, submucous fibroids, and various causes of obstructive dysmenorrhea, as described below.

ENDOMETRIOSIS is a condition caused by foci of ectopic endometrium, located in the pouch of Douglas, on the ovaries, or on the broad ligament, which undergo to a variable extent the influence of the sexual steroids secreted during the menstrual cycle. *Main Features:* up to 40% of the endometriotic lesions remain symptomless. The most frequent symptom is pain, which may present as dysmenorrhea or as premenstrual pain with menstrual exacerbation, or continuous pain with or without menstrual exacerbation. The menstrual pain may last the whole duration of the menstrual period and sometimes even one day after its end. For the other clinical features of endometriosis, refer to the section on Endometriosis (XXIV-4).

ADENOMYOSIS The presence of islands of endometrium deep in the uterine muscle wall is called adenomyosis or endometriosis interna. *Main Features:* clinical diagnosis is difficult, so diagnosis has generally to await microscopic examination of a hysterectomy specimen. The prevalence varies greatly, depending on the depth of penetration of endometrial tissue into the myometrium required by the pathologist in order to consider a case as adenomyosis. The prevalence is of the order of 3% to 8% of hysterectomies. Fifty percent of patients are in the fifth decade. The most common symptoms are menorrhagia or metrorrhagia and dysmenorrhea; but both symptoms, abnormal bleeding and menstrual pain, coincide in only 20% of cases. The dysmenorrhea is usually severe and may be incapacitating.

Associated Symptoms: adenomyosis frequently causes infertility. *Signs:* the uterus is either symmetrically or asymmetrically enlarged and firm, and there are generally no well-circumscribed nodules as in a polyfibromatous uterus. *Usual Course:* the uterine volume enlarges progressively over the years but rarely grows larger than a 14-week gestation. The pain and the abnormal bleeding disappear at menopause but, owing to the severity of symptoms, most patients have to undergo a hysterectomy before menopause. *Complications:* none. *Pathology:* adenomyosis is diagnosed only when endometrial glands are found at least one low-power microscopic field below the myoendometrial junction. The nests of endometrial tissue are generally surrounded by a proliferation of fibrous tissue. *Diagnostic Criteria:* differentiation from uterine fibroids may be difficult. In adenomyosis no nodules are found; the uterus varies in consistency, size, and tenderness on palpation during the menstrual cycle, size and tenderness increasing premenstrually. Hysterography performed with a water-soluble contrast medium may suggest adenomyosis if, in a patient with dysmenorrhea and menorrhagia, the uterine cavity has an irregular shape and if small diverticula are found either in the fundus or along the lateral borders.

FIBROIDS Fibroids are rarely responsible for pain or dysmenorrhea. They may cause colicky pains generally accompanied by menorrhagia when they are extruded out of the myometrium into the uterine cavity or pushed against or through the cervical isthmus. *Diagnostic Criteria:* if the uterine size is only slightly enlarged, hysterography may detect a submucous fibroid or a fibroid polyp. A circular or polycyclic filling defect is then found that generally deforms the uterine cavity, whereas a mucous polyp does not.

OBSTRUCTIVE DYSMENORRHEA Secondary dysmenorrhea is called obstructive when obstruction of the menstrual flow is due to an organic cause, either congenital or acquired. *Main Features:* the prevalence is difficult to evaluate. In congenital forms the pain mostly begins a few months after menarche, as it starts only when enough blood has been retained to distend the vagina or the uterus. When there is an atresia of the hymen, there is dysmenorrhea with cryptomenorrhea as the menstrual blood is retained in the vagina. If there is retention of fluid in one half of a double uterus, the menstrual pain will be unilateral.

Associated Symptoms: The asymmetrical varieties of double uteri are frequently accompanied by absence or hypotrophy of one kidney. The retained blood may distend the vagina and the uterus and give rise to a retrograde menstruation, which, after a few months, may cause implantation of menstrual debris, i.e., endometriosis. *Signs:* If there is atresia of the hymen, retention of

blood in the vagina will manifest itself by distention of the vagina with the hymen bulging at the introitus and the posterior wall of the vagina bulging into the rectum. Retention of blood in one half of a double uterus will cause an asymmetrical enlargement of the uterus. The distended blind half of a double vagina will bulge into the other half of the vagina. *Pathology:* Various congenital anomalies may cause secondary dysmenorrhea, e.g., atresia of the hymen, a rudimentary uterine horn, a double uterus one half of which does not communicate with the vagina, or a uterus duplex bicollis, one half of which opens into a blind half of a double vagina. Acquired forms may be due to adhesions in the cervical canal after amputation of the cervix or conization or electrocoagulation. Adhesions may also be situated in the lower part of the uterine cavity, for example, in an Asherman syndrome.

Diagnostic Criteria: Diagnosis must rely on history and clinical examination. An early unilateral dysmenorrhea, combined with the presence of an asymmetrical mass in the lower abdomen or in the vagina is suggestive of an asymmetric malfusion deformity. Vaginography after injection of an opaque medium into the blind vagina or hysterography through the accessible cervix may be used. Radiological exploration of the reno-ureteral tract is also indicated.

ACQUIRED FORMS Main Features:. the acquired forms are usually easy to diagnose. If dysmenorrhea or cryptomenorrhea appear after an amputation of the cervix or an electrocoagulation or a conization of the cervix, or after a curettage performed for retained products of conception, the diagnosis is easy and the condition may be cured with a dilatation of the cervix or with a curettage by means of a smooth curette in order to destroy the adhesions. A laparotomy will rarely be required to divide the adhesions under visual control.

DYSMENORRHEA OF PSYCHOLOGICAL ORIGIN The frequency of such dysmenorrhea has been exaggerated. The diagnosis of dysmenorrhea of psychological origin should be accepted only where no organic cause can be found and when psychopathologic evaluation reveals neurotic behavior or other psychopathological problems sufficient to account for the complaint.

Code

765.X6a	With endometriosis
765.X4	With adenomyosis or fibrosis
765.X0	With congenital obstruction
765.X6b	With acquired obstruction
765.X9a	Psychological, tension
765.X9b	Psychological, delusional
765.X9c	Psychological, conversion

Primary Dysmenorrhea (XXIV-3)

Note: Endometritis does not cause pain, either acute or chronic.

Definition

Dysmenorrhea, or painful menstruation, refers to episodes of pelvic pain whose duration is limited to the period of menstrual blood flow, or which start one or, at the earliest, two days before and stop one or, at the latest, two days after the blood flow. In primary dysmenorrhea there is no structural lesion.

System

Female internal genital organs; either the uterus or both adnexa or one adnexum.

Site

The pain is localized either in the whole lower abdomen nearly always symmetrically or in an iliac fossa. It may radiate towards the sacro-gluteal zone in the lower back, i.e., to the superior half of the sacrum and, laterally, to one or both gluteal regions. It sometimes radiates into the anterior and superior aspect of one or both thighs.

Main Features

There are two varieties of dysmenorrhea; primary or essential and secondary or symptomatic. If the pain has a lower abdominal location, which is usually symmetrical, and if no structural anomaly is found on clinical examination, the dysmenorrhea is termed primary. Cases with structural organic anomalies are classified as secondary (see XXIV-2).

Prevalence: between 5 and 10% of all girls in their late teens and early 20s suffer from severe, mostly primary, dysmenorrhea during the first hours of their periods. In one study, 72% of women aged 19 years had some dysmenorrhea. *Age of Onset:* primary dysmenorrhea mostly starts a few months after menarche and lasts for several years. *Pain Quality:* the pain is generally colicky; in about one-fourth of all cases the pain is continuous. *Intensity:* the pain may be mild. It is called severe (or second degree) if it seriously interferes with the patient's work. Third degree or incapacitating dysmenorrhea has an intensity that compels the patient to stay in bed. *Duration:* in most cases the pain starts a few hours or half a day before the beginning of the blood flow, and usually lasts less than one day.

Associated Features

With third degree primary dysmenorrhea there may be nausea, vomiting and/or diarrhea.

Usual Course

Primary dysmenorrhea may disappear spontaneously after a few years, but it mostly disappears in 8 cases out of 10 after the birth of the first baby.

Complications

None.

Social and Physical Disability

Third degree dysmenorrhea is the cause of periodic absence from work or school in many teenagers and young women.

Pathology

No definite pathology known.

Pathophysiology

Primary dysmenorrhea is found at the end of an ovulatory cycle; it has also been reported in women taking oral contraceptives. In some patients uterine contractions during dysmenorrheic episodes show well-coordinated contractions with extremely high intrauterine pressures, in others "dysrhythmic" contractions with high or low pressures, and in others an elevated intrauterine pressure between contractions. Several authors have found elevated prostaglandin concentrations in endometrium and menstrual fluid of patients with primary dysmenorrhea. Although the exact mechanism of primary dysmenorrhea is unknown, it is probable that in most cases the pain is due to hypertony of the uterine isthmus, i.e., failure of the normal menstrual relaxation with temporary obstruction of the flow of menstrual blood. This is combined with an increased production (or perhaps increased retention) of prostaglandins, which leads to increased, or dysrhythmic, myometrial contractions, sensitization of nerve terminals to prostaglandins, and ischemia of the uterine wall.

Treatment

Mild and moderate cases are best treated by analgesics. In severe cases the pain can be prevented by cyclic estro-progestogens, or the pain may, when it appears, be alleviated by prostaglandin inhibitors.

Differential Diagnosis

From conditions causing secondary dysmenorrhea, namely endometriosis, etc. Primary dysmenorrhea is characterized by the absence of any structural abnormality of the internal female genital organs. Recent observations have shown that in about 10% of cases with a negative clinical examination, laparoscopic visualization of the internal genitalia may detect endometriotic lesions, so that the diagnosis of primary dysmenorrhea is not as simple as previously thought.

Code

765.X7b

Reference

Andersch, B. and Milsom, I., An epidemiologic study of young women with dysmenorrhea, Am. J. Obstet. Gynecol., 144 (1982) 655–660.

Endometriosis (XXIV-4)

Definition
Lower abdominal pain due to foci of ectopic endometrium located outside the uterus (endometriosis externa of endometriosis).

System
Genital system.

Site
The pain may be located in one or in both iliac fossae or over the whole lower abdomen. It frequently radiates toward the sacro-gluteal region in the lower back.

Main Features
Prevalence: the frequency with which endometriosis is found depends on the circumstances in which it is sought. It was found in 15 and 20% of two different series of laparoscopies, but, on the other hand, it was found in 50% of a large series of laparotomies. Because many endometriotic lesions remain symptomless, the true incidence is difficult to determine. The ectopic foci are located either in the pouch of Douglas or on the ovaries or on the posterior leaf of the broad ligament and, less frequently, on the wall of rectum or sigmoid colon; rather seldom they infiltrate the bladder wall or the wall of the ureter. *Age of Onset:* It used to be thought that endometriosis usually develops in the late twenties or in the thirties, but since more laparoscopies have been performed on younger patients it has been found rather frequently in teenagers, especially those complaining of secondary dysmenorrhea and/or infertility. *Symptoms:* In some 30 to 40% of patients with endometriosis there are no complaints except perhaps infertility. The main symptom of endometriosis is pain; it may manifest itself as dysmenorrhea, as premenstrual pain with menstrual exacerbation, or as chronic pain. Lesions located in the pouch of Douglas may provoke firm adhesions between the anterior wall of the rectum and the posterior vaginal wall; this location may cause pain on defecation during menstruation. Foci located in the pouch of Douglas or a fixed uterine retroversion due to endometriotic adhesions frequently cause deep dyspareunia. Endometriotic foci that penetrate into or through the bladder wall may cause painful micturition with or without hematuria during menstruation.

Signs
On pelvic examination a fixed painful retroversion may be found, or tender, enlarged, adherent adnexa on one or both sides. Small, tender nodular lesions, which are frequently palpated either in a sacro-uterine ligament or on the posterior surface of the uterus, are almost pathognomonic of endometriosis.

Usual Course
The ectopic foci remain receptive in a variable degree to the ovarian steroids, and they will undergo the same histological changes as the "eutopic" endometrium. The ectopic tissue may grow on the surface of the peritoneum or it may become buried in a fibrous capsule. The encapsulated lesions are those most likely to become painful, whereas the superficial ones are usually painless. The pain may start as secondary dysmenorrhea; it may later become premenstrual as well as menstrual, or may become continuous. The pain due to endometriotic foci is usually alleviated by pregnancy. At menopause, the pain usually disappears.

Complications
Infertility is a frequent complication. Subocclusion or occlusion of the small or the large intestine is possible but infrequent. Rupture of an endometriotic cyst located in an ovary may cause an acute abdominal emergency due to irritation of the peritoneum by the old blood flowing from the ruptured cyst.

Pathogenesis
Retrograde menstruation, i.e., passage of menstrual blood and endometrial debris through the tubes toward the pelvic cavity, often occurs. This seems to be the pathogenetic mechanism in most cases of endometriosis. However, it does not explain all the possible locations of the foci. Tiny fragments of menstrual endometrium may be carried away by lymphatics and, more rarely, by veins of the endometrium.

Diagnostic Criteria
The history and the findings on clinical examination will frequently lead to the diagnosis. When any doubt remains, a therapeutic trial with cyclic estroprogestogens will alleviate the pain in 8 of 10 cases. Laparoscopic inspection of the pelvic cavity has been used rather frequently in recent years to verify the diagnosis and to evaluate the extent of the lesions. Acute pain episodes in the right iliac fossa due to endometriosis may be mistaken for appendicitis. Recurrent episodes of lower abdominal pain, tenderness, and a slight fever may erroneously be taken for recurrent pelvic inflammatory disease.

Treatment
Treatment of endometriosis will be hormonal or surgical or combined. It will vary depending on age of the patient, stage of the disease, and the main presenting problem—pain or infertility or both. Hormonal treatment consists of cyclic estroprogestogens or in the continuous daily administration of oral progestogens, for example, Lynestrenol or norethisterone acetate. The two last drugs produce a hypoestrogenic amenorrhea. During recent years excellent results have been obtained by the continuous oral administration of Danazol, a strong anti-

gonadotropin and mild androgenic drug. Surgical treatment will, depending on the indication and the stage of the disease, consist of conservative surgery preferably by microsurgical techniques, or semiradical or radical surgery, i.e., total hysterectomy and bilateral salpingo-oophorectomy.

Code
764.X6

References
Varangot, J., Giraud, J.R. and Bignon-Schnizer, J., Pathologie, clinique et pathologie de l'endométriose génitale, Bull. Fed. Soc. Gynec. Obstet. Fr., 17 (1965) 239–292.

Chalmers, J.A., Endometriosis, Butterworth, London, 1975.

Posterior Parametritis (XXIV-5)

Definition
Pain with low grade infection of parametrial tissues, especially the posterior parametrium. Synonyms: pelvic lymphangitis, chronic parametrial cellulitis.

System
Uterine cervix and parametrial tissues.

Main Features
Site: Lower abdomen, sometimes the back also. *Prevalence:* Because histological proof of the diagnosis is usually missing, the prevalence is unknown, but the condition is seen infrequently. It may be found soon after a delivery, especially if the cervix has been torn and infected. *Symptoms:* The patient complains of lower abdominal pain with or without low backache, and deep dyspareunia. There is usually no fever. The pain may occur during the premenstrual period and disappear during menstruation, or it may be continuous, with premenstrual exacerbation.

Signs
A more or less severely torn cervix is found and either an acute or a chronic cervicitis. One or both utero-sacral ligaments are tender on palpation.

Pathology
Posterior parametritis on chronic cervicitis is believed to be due to extension of a cervical infection along the lymphatics of the parametrium. Chronic cervicitis is not painful by itself.

Diagnostic Criteria and Treatment
Diagnosis of cervicitis depends on finding agglutinated leukocytes in the cervical mucus during the periovulatory period. The presence of an infected cervical canal and of a tender posterior parametrium and the absence of a history and of clinical findings suggestive of endometriosis make the diagnosis of posterior parametritis

plausible. In these circumstances treatment with broad-spectrum antibiotics and local heat is indicated. If the pain disappears, this confirms the diagnosis. If the pain and the parametrial tenderness persist, another cause of the pain should be looked for by laparoscopy.

Code
733.X2

Reference
Renaer, M., Chronic Pelvic Pain in Women, Springer Verlag, Berlin, 1981.

Tuberculous Salpingitis (XXIV-6)

Definition
Pelvic pain due to tuberculosis salpingitis.

Main Features
Prevalence: genital tuberculosis has become quite uncommon in most developed countries thanks to the gradual disappearance of pulmonary tuberculosis. It remains a problem in many less developed countries where pulmonary tuberculosis is still widely prevalent. *Symptoms:* The most frequent symptoms are sterility, pelvic pain, poor general condition, and menstrual disturbances. Genital tuberculosis presents under two forms, either the silent or the active form. In the silent forms there are no particular symptoms; there is no pain and no fever. In the active or advanced forms there are general symptoms and signs of the tuberculous process, meno- or metrorrhagias, sometimes amenorrhea. Pelvic pain may be present. In the active cases there is usually pyrexia, weight loss, and night sweats.

Signs
On pelvic examination a fixed retroversion with palpable tubo-ovarian masses may be found. Spontaneous pain and dysmenorrhea may be explained by a pyo- or hydro-salpinx or by a tuberculous pelvioperitonitis. Dyspareunia may be due to a fixed retroversion or to adherent adnexal masses.

Usual Course
The tuberculous process may become latent or may heal spontaneously. It may, on the other hand, evolve towards a pyosalpinx or an ovarian abscess or to a tuberculous pelvioperitonitis or a general peritonitis.

Diagnostic Criteria
In advanced cases general symptoms and signs of the tuberculous process, abdominal pain or discomfort, signs of a pelvic infection, together with a positive tuberculin test and bacteriological evidence of tuberculosis constitute the basis of the diagnosis. Tubercle bacilli may be cultured either from menstrual blood or from an endometrial biopsy, taken preferably in the premenstrual

phase. Silent cases are usually diagnosed by the presence of tubercular lesions in an endometrial biopsy taken during the evaluation of infertility cases.

Treatment

Treatment is essentially medical by means of a combined drug regimen with Rifamycin, isoniazid, and ethambutol. It should last for a minimum of 18 months to two years. Surgery will be resorted to only if pelvic masses persist or increase under medical treatment, if endometrial lesions persist, and if pain or other pelvic symptoms are not alleviated by drug therapy.

Code

763.X2

Reference

Schaefer, G., Female genital tuberculosis, Clin. Obstet. Gynecol., 19 (1976) 223–239.

Retroversion of the Uterus (XXIV-7)

Definition

Lower abdominal pain due to a retroverted uterus.

Main Features

Retroversion of the uterus is found in 15 to 20% of adult women, but only a small number of mobile retroversions cause symptoms. In a few cases it may give rise to intermittent pain with or without deep dyspareunia. The pain will be located either in the lower abdomen or in the sacro-gluteal region or in both sites. The pain usually is worse during the premenstrual period and mostly disappears or decreases after the first or second day of the period. It also decreases with horizontal rest. On pelvic examination the retroverted uterus is tender and frequently slightly enlarged and softer than normal.

Pathology

It has repeatedly been observed that the size of a painful retroverted uterus diminishes and that it becomes firmer after anterior reposition. If the pain disappears after correction of the retroversion and insertion of a pessary, it does so gradually during the two to three days following the reposition. These circumstances seem to indicate that circulatory disturbances, probably passive pelvic congestion, cause the pain.

Diagnostic Criteria

The uterus is said to be retroverted when the axis of the cervix is directed towards the symphysis pubis and the axis of the uterine corpus towards the excavation of the sacrum. A retroversion is either mobile or fixed. A retroversion is said to be fixed when adhesions bind the uterine corpus down in the pouch of Douglas. A mobile retroversion should be considered the cause of the pain only if no other causes of pain are found, such as endo-metriosis or posterior parametritis on a chronic cervicitis, and if the pain disappears after anterior reposition of the uterus. It is then maintained in its corrected position by inserting a vaginal pessary. If a patient with a fixed retroversion complains of some symptoms, it is usually impossible to prove which symptoms are due to the retroversion and which are not. Treatment must therefore be directed against the causal disorder, which may be either endometriosis or sequelae of acute pelvic inflammatory disease or of a pelvioperitonitis, or a tuberculous salpingitis.

Treatment

A mobile retroversion that causes no symptoms does not require any treatment. If the patient complains of pain, reposition of the uterus will be tried and a pessary inserted. If the pain disappears the pessary may be left in situ for 6 or 8 weeks. It is then removed and nothing more is necessary if the pain does not recur. If it does, operative correction of the retroversion may be undertaken.

If the retroversion is fixed, treatment must be directed against the causal condition and a suspension operation should be performed only when the retroversion itself is probably the cause of the complaint, as in some cases of dyspareunia, or when there are other reasons for surgical intervention, e.g., tubal surgery for infertility.

Code

765.X7c

Reference

Renaer, M., Pain in gynecologic practice. III. The symptomatology of uterine retroversion and, in particular, pain in uterine retroversion (Dutch), Verhand. Koninkl. Acad. voor Gen. van België, 17 (1955) 433–457.

Ovarian Pain (XXIV-8)

Definition

Lower abdominal pain due to an ovarian lesion.

RECURRENT PAINFUL FUNCTIONAL OVARIAN CYSTS
Main Features: lower abdominal pain due to recurrent painful functional cysts is sometimes, although rarely, seen in young women. It is called by some "painful ovarian dystrophy." *Diagnostic Criteria:* if the condition is very painful, laparoscopy may be indicated in order to ascertain the cause of the pain; the cystic fluid may then be aspirated and submitted to cytological examination. If the result of this examination is compatible with a functional cyst, it is recommended to treat it conservatively by means of oral contraceptives. There is a good chance that the cyst and the pain will disappear, whereas surgical exploration with wedge resection of the ovary is

likely to be followed by a recurrence of the cyst and of the painful episode.

Code
764.X7a

OVARIAN REMNANT SYNDROME Pain due to ovarian remnants following operation. *Main Features:* when a bilateral oophorectomy has been performed in conditions that make it difficult to be sure that all ovarian tissue is removed, e.g., when the ovaries were embedded in endometriotic scar tissue or were surrounded by dense adhesions, active rests of ovarian tissue may cause a painful condition called the ovarian remnant syndrome. *Diagnostic Criteria:* an ovarian remnant will be suspected when the patient presents evidence of estrogen secretion that persists after a short course of corticoids prescribed to suppress adrenal androstenedione secretion and its peripheral conversion to estrone. Treatment will consist of metecious excision of the residual ovarian tissue.

Code
764.X7b

References
Stone, S.C. and Schwartz, W.J., A syndrome characterized by recurrent symptomatic functional ovarian cysts in young women, Am. J. Obstet. Gynecol., 134 (1979) 310–314.

Symmonds, R.E. and Pettit, P.D.N., Ovarian remnant syndrome, Obstet. Gynecol., 54 (1979) 174–177.

Chronic Pelvic Pain Without Obvious Pathology (CPPWOP) (XXIV-9)

Definition
Chronic or recurrent pelvic pain that has apparently a gynecological origin but for which no definite lesion or cause is found.

System
Genital system.

Site
Lower abdomen.

Main Features
Chronic pelvic pain without obvious pathology is the name given recently to a syndrome that has been known and described for more than a century under many different names, some of them being: parametropathia spastica, pelvic congestion and fibrosis, pelipathia vegetativa, and pelvic sympathetic syndrome. *Prevalence:* this syndrome is rather uncommon. Until 20–30 years ago, it was considered rather common, but the diagnosis should be considered only under the following conditions: (1) if the patient's symptoms are not due to a gynecological cause; (2) if the pain has characteristics of a gynecological pain; and (3) if the syndrome is not due to one of the acknowledged causes of gynecological pain, which supposes that the patient underwent a laparoscopy.

It has become clear that formerly many chronic painful conditions have erroneously been classified under the above heading.

Associated Symptoms
The most important symptom is lower abdominal pain and, less frequently, low back pain. The lower abdominal pain may be felt either in the whole lower abdomen or in both iliac fossae, or in one fossa only. The low back pain may be felt over the whole width of the sacrogluteal zone or over a part of this zone. The pain is usually more severe for several days before menstruation, and its intensity decreases on the first or second day of the period. Deep dyspareunia is a frequent complaint.

Medical treatment is not well-defined and is therefore not usually successful in chronic cases. When a chronic pelvic pain syndrome has lasted for several months and has not been cured by medical treatment, it is useful to perform a laparoscopy in order to look for nonpalpable lesions, such as endometriosis or sequelae of chronic pelvic inflammatory disease, which might explain the pain. By definition, those lesions are not found in CPPWOP.

Signs
On abdominal examination tenderness at ovarian points may occur. Uterine tenderness may be found. On gynecological examination the uterus and adnexa may be tender; there is frequently tenderness of the posterior parametrium, and sometimes it is shortened. The vagina usually appears congested.

Pathology
Besides lower abdominal pain with or without sacrogluteal pain and the frequent complaint of deep dyspareunia, many patients have several complaints including one or more that are usually considered functional; these patients may therefore be called polysymptomatic. Most oligosymptomatic patients complain merely of spontaneous pelvic pain and deep dyspareunia. During the last decades various conditions have been suspected as possible causes. It has been thought that in a percentage of cases the syndrome is due to traumatic laceration of a sacrouterine ligament or of a posterior leaf of one or both broad ligaments. It seems, however, that the role of those tears is negligible.

There is good indirect evidence that circulatory factors may give rise to chronic or intermittent lower abdominal pain. There is uterine and pelvic phlebographic evidence for the presence of passive pelvic congestion in a percentage of cases with CPPWOP, but this passive pelvic congestion does not seem to be the sole factor that causes the pain. Pelvic varicosities are likely to be the major cause of the pain. Tenderness with or without shortening of the posterior parametrium is found in the majority of cases of CPPWOP; because pressure or traction exerted on the posterior parametrium usually reproduces the pain the patient feels either spontaneously or during intercourse, this condition seems to intervene in the pain mechanism in many cases. However, the morphological or functional basis of this tenderness remains to be elucidated. All those who studied the psychological characteristics of these patients found definite psychopathological anomalies or stress situations in most, although not all, of the patients examined.

It is probable that patients with CPPWOP constitute a heterogenous group made up of a spectrum of miscellaneous conditions. At one end, there are patients with very little peripheral noxious stimulation whose complaints will, to a large extent, have a psychological explanation. The other extreme is made up of persons with rather intense peripheral noxious stimulation: either pelvic circulatory disturbances or tenderness of the posterior parametrium and, less often, uterine cramps or a real tear in a sacro-uterine ligament, and little or no psychological factor. In between these extremes there are apparently a number of mixed cases with less pronounced peripheral noxious stimulation and one or more of the psycho-physiological mechanisms that may induce complaints and care-seeking behavior. Varicosities may be a major contributory physical factor.

Treatment
Even if one does not find a satisfactory explanation, the patient's complaints should be taken seriously. The doctor should try to obtain information concerning the patient's family and personal history, her marital life, and her general behavior. As said earlier, the diagnosis of CPPWOP cannot be made without the aid of laparoscopy; this may be useful in lessening the anxiety of the patient. CPPWOP is frequently associated with psychological problems or with a neurotic disorder, in which case treatment should attend to those conditions.

Some patients have been helped with cyclic estroprogestogens; others have had hypo-estrogenic amenorrhea induced by continuous administration of oral progestogens e.g., 5 mg of Lynestrenol daily or 5 mg of Norethisterone acetate daily during several months, but we think this of little value. Many gynecologists have performed, or still perform, a total hysterectomy for CPPWOP The low percentage of good long-term results has shown that

a total hysterectomy is not an effective treatment in this syndrome and that it should be performed only if the patient has been treated conservatively for several months or years, is oligosymptomatic, and does not present psychopathologic disturbances.

Code
763.X8
See also I-16.

References
Beard, R.W., Highman, J.H., Pearce, I. and Reginald, P.W., Diagnosis of pelvic varicosities in women with chronic pelvic pain, Lancet, ii (1984) 946–949.

Renaer, M., Jijs, P., Van Assche, A. and Vertommen, H., Chronic pelvic pain without obvious pathology: personal observations and a review of the problem, Eur. J Obstet. Gynecol. Reprod. Biol., 10 (1980) 415–453.

Taylor, H.C., Vascular congestion and hyperemia. I. Physiologic basis and history of the concept, Am. J. Obstet. Gynecol., 57 (1949) 211–230.

Taylor, H.C., Vascular congestion and hyperemia. II. The clinical aspects of the congestion-fibrosis syndrome, Am. J. Obstet. Gynecol., 57 (1949) 637–653.

Taylor, H.C., Vascular congestion and hyperemia. III. Etiology and therapy, Am. J. Obstet. Gynecol., 57 (1949) 654–668.

Pain from Urinary Tract (XXIV-10)

Code
763.XXb or 863.XX

Pain of Vaginismus or Dyspareunia (XXIV-11)

Code
864.X7

Carcinoma of the Bladder (XXIV-12)

Code
763.X4

GROUP XXV: PAIN IN THE RECTUM, PERINEUM, AND EXTERNAL GENITALIA

Neuralgia of Iliohypogastric, Ilio-Inguinal, or Genito-Femoral Nerves (XXV-I)

Testicular Pain

Definition
Burning or lancinating or other pain syndrome due to injury of the respective nerve, usually following surgical intervention in the hypogastric or inguinal region.

Site
Inguinal area and external genitalia.

System
Peripheral nervous system.

Main Features
The pain can occur immediately after the operation but not infrequently occurs after months or years. Sometimes there is no history of operation or trauma. The pain is burning or lancinating and radiates to the area supplied by the sensory nerve. For the iliohypogastric nerve the pain radiates to the midline above the pubis but also laterally to the hip region. For the ilio-inguinal and the genito-femoral nerve the pain radiates from the groin into the anterior part of the labia major (or the scrotum and the root of the penis) and on the inside or the anterior surfaces of the thigh, sometimes down to the knee.

Usually the pain is continuously present, but it can be intensified by forcible stretching of the hip joint, coughing, sneezing, sexual intercourse, or general tension in the abdominal muscles. The patient frequently adopts a posture that eases discomfort, with a slight flexure of the hip and a slight forward inclination of the trunk.

Signs
On examination the pain can be triggered in a narrowly circumscribed area of the operative scar. Usually, there is a tenderness along the course of the nerve from near the anterior superior iliac spine to the external genitalia; when the genito-femoral nerve is involved, the internal ring of the inguinal canal can be very painful. As a rule, cutaneous sensibility is more or less impaired in the region innervated by the affected nerve. Usually, there is an increased threshold for touch and prick sensation in combination with hyperalgesia; the hypoesthesia is some times best demonstrated with cold stimuli. In some cases scratching the skin induces less reddening or an absence of it on the affected side as compared to the intact side, indicating the degeneration of afferent C-fibers. Although motor impairment of abdominal muscles can be present, this is hard to evaluate because the motor tests usually exacerbate the pain. If the iliohypogastric nerve is damaged, the lower abdominal skin reflex may be absent. Typically, with involvement of the genital branch of the genito-femoral nerve in man, the cremaster reflex is absent on the affected side.

Usual Course
Without treatment, the pain may persist for several years without tendency to improvement. Surgical repair is the most effective treatment.

Pathology
If the nerve was sectioned during surgical intervention, histological examination may show a neuroma. If the nerve was ligated or entrapped by a tear, there is endoneural fibrosis.

Diagnostic Criteria
Typical pain radiation with sensory impairment and pain relief by local anesthetic.

Treatment
The pain can be relieved by injection of a local anesthetic proximally from the injury side; for the iliohypogastric and ilio-inguinal nerve the injection is done two finger-widths medially from the anterior superior iliac spine, where they leave the internal oblique muscle.

Diagnostic Criteria
1. Burning pain with occasional superimposed paroxysms in the distribution of the involved nerve.
2. Increased threshold to light touch and pinprick associated with hyperalgesia.
3. Reproduction of paroxysmal pain by tapping neuromata at the site of nerve injury.
4. Transient pain relief from proximal local anesthetic block.

Differential Diagnosis
Inguinal and femoral hernia; lymphadenopathy; periostitis of pubic tubercle.

Code
407.X7b
407.X1   Testicular pain

Rectal, Perineal, and Genital Pain of Psychological Origin (XXV-2)

About 10% of psychiatric patients with pain have rectal, perineal, or genital pain. This is usually mentioned as a secondary site of pain. Only about 2% report pain in these parts as the primary site. When that happens the rectal pain is usually associated with severe depressive or schizophrenic illness but may also be associated with conversion symptoms. It occurs in a few patients. For the general description, see I-16.

Conversion pain in these patients is usually accompanied by pains elsewhere. See also I-16.

Code
81X.X9d   Delusional
81X.X9e   Conversion
81X.X9f   Depressive

Pain of Hemorrhoids (XXV-3)

Code
853.X5

Proctalgia Fugax (XXV-4)

Definition
Severe brief episodic pain, seemingly arising in the rectum, occurring at irregular intervals.

Site
Localized in the anus.

System
Uncertain. Proctalgia fugax has been attributed to spasm of the sigmoid colon or levator ani. Others contend it is due to spasm of the pelvic floor.

Main Features
The pain is severe, episodic, and usually located in the midline somewhere above the anal sphincter. It does not radiate. The pain is sudden in onset, without warning, lasting from several seconds to 20 minutes. It may occur at any time of day, or may waken the sufferer from a deep sleep at night. Most sufferers have fewer than six single episodes per year.

Prevalence
The pain occurs in 14–19% of healthy subjects and is somewhat more common in women (17.7%) than in men (8.8%).

Precipitating Factors
A bowel movement, sexual activities, stress, heat, or cold may precipitate an attack.

Relieving Agents
The onset of action of most drugs is too slow to be of help. Heat and pressure to the perineum are sometimes helpful. Others assume the knee-chest position and then firmly pull the buttocks apart. There is no accepted method of preventing or treating this condition.

Complications
Nausea and sweating and/or fainting may occur during an attack.

Signs and Laboratory Findings
None unless fainting occurs.

Usual Course
The frequency of episodes tends to fall with age, and usually stops by the age of 70.

Social and Physical Disabilities
Between episodes of pain, the sufferer is completely well. Marital disharmony due to the fear of sexual intercourse precipitating an attack has been described.

Pathology or Other Contributing Factors
Proctalgia is thought by some to occur more commonly in sufferers from irritable bowel symptoms. Others report that patterns submitted to psychiatric assessment and personality tests were perfectionist, anxious, tense, and hypochondriacal.

Diagnostic Criteria
Episodic pain in the rectal area occurring in otherwise well subjects.

Differential Diagnosis
Ano-rectal disease, e.g., anal fissures, usually causes pain with each bowel movement and can be seen at anoscopy or sigmoidoscopy. Coccygodynia is accompanied by a tender coccyx. The pain of tabes is longlasting with tenesmus and radiation into the legs.

Code
856.X8

References
Douthwaite, A., Proctalgia fugax, Br. Med. J., 2 (1962) 164–165.

Thompson, W.G., Proctalgia fugax in patients with the irritable bowel, peptic ulcer or inflammatory bowel disease, Am. J. Gastroenterol., 79, 6 (1984) 450–452.

Harvey, R, Colonic modality in proctalgia fugax, Lancet, 2 (1979) 713–714.

Thiele, G., Coccygodynia and pain in the superior gluteal region and down the back of the thigh: causation by tonic spasm of the levator ani, coccygeus and pirifomis muscles and relief by massage of the muscles, JAMA, 109 (1937) 1271–1275.

Thompson, W.G. and Heaton, K., Proctalgia fugax, J. Roy. Coll. Phys. Lond., 14, 4 (1980) 247–248.

Mountifield, J.A., Proctalgia fugax: a cause of marital dysharmony, Can. Med. Assoc. J. (1986) 1269–1270.

Code
856.X8

Ulcer of Anus or Rectum (XXV-5)

Code
81X.XX

Injury of External Genitalia (XXV-6)

Code
832.X1

Carcinoma of the Prostate (XXV-7)

Code
862.X4

G. SPINAL PAIN, SECTION 3: SPINAL AND RADICULAR PAIN SYNDROMES OF THE LUMBAR, SACRAL, AND COCCYGEAL REGIONS

N.B. For explanatory material on this section and on section D, Spinal and Radicular Pain Syndromes of the Cervical and Thoracic Regions, see pp. 11-16 of the list of Topics and Codes.

GROUP XXVI: LUMBAR OR RADICULAR SPINAL PAIN SYNDROMES

In using this section, please refer back to the remarks upon Spinal and Radicular Pain Syndromes, pp. 11–16. Please note particularly the comments on coding at the top of sections IX and XXVI of the list of Topics and Codes, pp. 17 and 29.

Lumbar Spinal or Radicular Pain Attributable to a Fracture (XXVI-1)

Definition
Lumbar spinal pain occurring in a patient with a history of injury in whom radiography or other imaging studies demonstrate the presence of a fracture that can reasonably be interpreted as the cause of their pain.

Clinical Features
Lumbar spinal pain with or without referred pain.

Diagnostic Features
Radiographic or other imaging evidence of a fracture of one of the osseous elements of the lumbar vertebral column.

Schedule of Fractures
XXVI-1.1(S)(R)
       Fracture of a Vertebral Body
       Code 533.X1aS/C 633.X1aR
XXVI-1.2(S)
       Fracture of a Spinous Process
       Code 533.X1bS
XXVI-1.3(S)(R)
       Fracture of a Transverse Process
       Code 533.X1cS/C 633.X1cR
XXVI-1.4(S)(R)
       Fracture of a Superior Articular Process
       Code 533.X1dS/C 633.X1dR
XXVI-1.5(S)(R)
       Fracture of an Inferior Articular Process
       Code 533.X1eS/C 633.X1e
XXVI-1.6(S)(R)
       Fracture of a Lamina (pars interarticularis)
       Code 533.X1fS 633.X1fR

Lumbar Spinal or Radicular Pain Attributable to an Infection (XXVI-2)

Definition
Lumbar spinal pain occurring in a patient with clinical and/or other features of an infection, in whom the site of infection can be specified and which can reasonably be interpreted as the source of their pain.

Clinical Features
Lumbar spinal pain with or without referred pain, associated with pyrexia or other clinical features of infection.

Diagnostic Features
A presumptive diagnosis can be made on the basis of an elevated white cell count or other serological features of infection, together with imaging evidence of the presence of a site of infection in the lumbar vertebral column or its adnexa. Absolute confirmation relies on histological and/or bacteriological confirmation using material obtained by direct or needle biopsy.

Schedule of Sites of Infection
XXVI-2.1(S)(R)
       Infection of a Vertebral Body (osteomyelitis)
       Code 532.X2aS/C 632.X2aR
XXVI-2.2(S)(R)
       Septic Arthritis of a Zygapophyseal Joint
       Code 532.X2bS/C 632.X2bR
XXVI-2.3(S)(R)
       Infection of a Paravertebral Muscle
       (e.g., psoas abscess)
       Code 532.X2cS/C 632.X2cR
XXVI-2.4(S)(R)
       Infection of an Intervertebral Disk (diskitis)
       Code 532.X2dS/C 632.X2dR

XXVI-2.5(S)(R)
  Infection of a Surgical Fusion-Site
  Code 532.X2eS/C 632.X2eR
XXVI-2.6(S)(R)
  Infection of a Retroperitoneal Organ or Space
  Code 532.X2fS/C 632.X2fR
XXVI-2.7(S)(R)
  Infection of the Epidural Space (epidural abscess)
  Code 532.X2gS/C 632.X2gR
XXVI-2.8(S)(R)
  Infection of the Meninges (meningitis)
  Code 502.X2*S/C 602.X2cR
XXVI-2.9(S)(R)
  Acute Herpes Zoster
  Code 503.X2dS/C (low back)
  Code 603.X2dR (leg)
XXVI-2.10(S)(R)
  Postherpetic Neuralgia
  Code 503.X2bS/C (low back)
  Code 603.X2bR (leg)

Lumbar Spinal or Radicular Pain Attributable to a Neoplasm (XXVI-3)

Definition
Lumbar spinal pain associated with a neoplasm that can reasonably be interpreted as the source of the pain.

Clinical Features
Lumbar spinal pain with or without referred pain.

Diagnostic Features
A presumptive diagnosis may be made on the basis of imaging evidence of a neoplasm that directly or indirectly affects one or other of the tissues innervated by lumbar spinal nerves. Absolute confirmation relies on obtaining histological evidence by direct or needle biopsy.

Schedule of Neoplastic Diseases
XXVI-3.1(S)(R)
  Primary Tumor of a Vertebral Body
  Code 533.X4aS/C 633.X4aR
XXVI-3.2(S)(R)
  Primary Tumor of Any Part of a Vertebra Other than Its Body
  Code 533.X4bS/C 633.X4bR
XXVI-3.3(S)(R)
  Primary Tumor of a Zygapophysial Joint
  Code 533.X4cS/C 633.X4cR
XXVI-3.4(S)(R)
  Primary Tumor of a Paravertebral Muscle
  Code 533.X4dS/C 633.X4dR
XXVI-3.5(S)(R)
  Primary Tumor of Epidural Fat

  (e.g., lipoma)
  Code 533.X4eS/C 633.X4eR
XXVI-3.6(S)(R)
  Primary Tumor of Epidural Vessels
  (e.g., angioma)
  Code 533.X4fS/C 633.X4fR
XXVI-3.7(S)(R)
  Primary Tumor of Meninges
  (e.g., meningioma)
  Code 503.X4aS/C 603.X4aR
XXVI-3.8(S)(R)
  Primary Tumor of a Spinal Nerve
  (e.g., neurofibroma, schwannoma, neuroblastoma)
  Code 503.X4bS/C 603.X4bR
  Code 503.X4cS/C 603.X4cR
XXVI-3.9(S)(R)
  Primary Tumor of Spinal Cord (e.g., glioma)
  Code 533.X4gS/C 633.X4gR
XXVI-3.10(S)(R)
  Metastatic Tumor Affecting a Vertebra
  Code 533.X4hS/C 633.X4hR
XXVI-3.11(S)(R)
  Metastatic Tumor Affecting the Vertebral Canal
  Code 533.X4iS/C 633.X4iR
XXVI-3.12(S)(R)
  Other Infiltrating Neoplastic Disease of a Vertebra (e.g., lymphoma)
  Code 533.X4jS/C 633.X4jR

Lumbar Spinal or Radicular Pain Attributable to Metabolic Bone Disease (XXVI-4)

Definition
Lumbar spinal pain associated with a metabolic bone disease that can reasonably be interpreted as the source of the pain.

Clinical Features
Lumbar spinal pain with or without referred pain.

Diagnostic Features
Imaging or other evidence of metabolic bone disease affecting the lumbar vertebral column, confirmed by appropriate serological or biochemical investigations and/or histological evidence obtained by needle or other biopsy.

Schedule of Metabolic Bone Diseases
XXVI-4.1(S)(R)
  Osteoporosis of Age
  Code 532.X5aS/C 632.X5aR

XXVI-4.2(S)(R)
> Osteoporosis of Unknown Cause
> Code 532.X5bS/C   632.X5bR

XXVI-4.3(S)(R)
> Osteoporosis of Some Known Cause Other
> than Age
> Code 532.X5cS/C   632.X5cR

XXVI-4.4(S)(R)
> Hyperparathyroidism
> Code 532.X5dS/C   632.X5dR

XXVI-4.5(S)(R)
> Paget's Disease of Bone
> Code 532.X5eS/C   632.X5eR

XXVI-4.6(S)(R)
> Metabolic Disease of Bone Not Otherwise
> Classified
> Code 532.X5fS/C   632.X5fR

Lumbar Spinal or Radicular Pain Attributable to Arthritis (XXVI-5)

Definition
Lumbar spinal pain associated with arthritis that can reasonably be interpreted as the source of the pain.

Clinical Features
Lumbar spinal pain with or without referred pain.

Diagnostic Features
Imaging or other evidence of arthritis affecting the joints of the lumbar vertebral column.

Schedule of Arthritides
XXVI-5.1(S)(R)
> Rheumatoid Arthritis
> Code 534.X3aS/C   634.X3aR

XXVI-5.2(S)(R)
> Ankylosing Spondylitis
> Code 532.X8*S/C   632.X8*R

XXVI-5.3(S)(R)
> Osteoarthritis
> Code 538.X6aS/C   638.X6aR

XXVI-5.4(S)(R)
> Seronegative Spondyloarthropathy
> Not Otherwise Classified
> Code 532.X8bS/C   623.X8bR

Remarks
Osteoarthritis is included in this schedule with some hesitation because there is only a weak relation between pain and this condition as diagnosed radiologically.

The alternative classification to "lumbar spinal pain due to osteoarthrosis" should be "lumbar zygapophysial joint pain" if the criteria for this diagnosis are satisfied (see

XXVI-13) or "lumbar spinal pain of unknown or uncertain origin" (see XXVI-9).

Similarly, the condition of "spondylosis" is omitted from this schedule because there is no positive correlation between the radiographic presence of this condition and the presence of spinal pain. There is no evidence that this condition represents anything more than age-changes in the vertebral column.

References
Lawrence, J.S., Bremner, J.M. and Bier, F., Osteoarthrosis: prevalence in the population and relationship between symptoms and X-ray changes, Ann. Rheum. Dis. 25 (1966) 1–24.

Magora, A., and Schwartz, T.A., Relation between the low back pain syndrome and X-ray findings, Scand. J. Rehab. Med., 8 (1976) 115–125.

Lumbar Spinal or Radicular Pain Associated with a Congenital Vertebral Anomaly (XXVI-6)

Definition
Lumbar spinal pain associated with a congenital vertebral anomaly.

Clinical Features
Lumbar spinal pain with or without referred pain.

Diagnostic Features
Imaging evidence of a congenital vertebral anomaly affecting the lumbar vertebral column.

Remarks
There is no evidence that congenital anomalies per se cause pain. Although they may be associated with pain, the specificity of this association is unknown. This classification should be used only when the cause of pain cannot be otherwise specified, but should not be used to imply that the congenital anomaly is the actual source of pain.

Code
523.X0aS/C
623.X0aR

Pseudarthrosis of a Transitional Vertebra (XXVI-7)

Definition
Lumbar spinal or radicular pain stemming from a pseudarthrosis formed by a transitional vertebra.

Clinical Features

Lumbar, lumbosacral, or sacral spinal pain.

Diagnostic Criteria

The pseudarthrosis must be evident radiographically, and must be shown to be symptomatic by having the pain relieved upon selective anesthetization of the pseudarthrosis, provided that the local anesthetic injected does not spread to affect other structures that might constitute an alternative source of the patient's pain.

Pathology

Periostitis as a result of repeated contact between the two bones, progressing to sclerosis of the contact sites of the two bones.

Remarks

The majority of pseudarthroses between transitional vertebrae are asymptomatic. Consequently, the radiographic presence of a pseudarthrosis in a patient with spinal pain is insufficient grounds alone to justify the diagnosis. The pseudarthrosis must be shown to be symptomatic.

Reference

Jonsson, B., Stromqvist, B. and Egund, N. Anomalous lumbosacral articulations and low-back pain: evaluation and treatment, Spine, 14 (1989) 831–834.

Code

523.X0bS/C
623.X0bR

Pain Referred From Abdominal Viscera or Vessels and Perceived as Lumbar Spinal Pain (XXVI-8)

Definition

Lumbar spinal pain associated with disease of an abdominal viscus or vessel that reasonably can be interpreted as the source of pain.

Clinical Features

Lumbar spinal pain with or without referred pain, together with features of the disease affecting the viscus or vessel concerned.

Diagnostic Features

Reliable evidence of the primary disease affecting an abdominal viscus or vessel.

Schedule of Diseases

XXVI-8.1	Aortic Aneurysm (See also XVII-7) Code 522.X6	
XXVI-8.2	Gastric Ulcer (See also XXI-4) Code 555.X3a	
XXVI-8.3	Duodenal Ulcer (See also XXI-5) Code 555.3Xb	
XXVI-8.4	Mesenteric Ischemia (See also XXI-8) Code 555.X5	
XXVI-8.5	Pancreatitis (See also XXI-19) Code 553.XXf	
XXVI-8.6	Perforation of a Retroperitoneal Organ Code 552.X3	

Lumbar Spinal Pain of Unknown or Uncertain Origin (XXVI-9)

Definition

Lumbar spinal pain occurring in a patient who has not previously undergone surgery for that pain whose clinical features and associated features do not enable the cause and source of the pain to be determined, and whose cause or source cannot be or has not been determined by special investigations.

Clinical Features

Lumbar spinal pain with or without referred pain.

Diagnostic Features

Lumbar spinal pain for which no other cause has been found or can be attributed.

Pathology

Unspecified.

Remarks

This definition is intended to cover those complaints that for whatever reason currently defy conventional diagnosis. It does not encompass pain of psychological origin. It presupposes an organic basis for the pain but one that cannot be or has not been established reliably by clinical examination or special investigations, such as imaging techniques or diagnostic blocks.

This diagnosis may be used as a temporary diagnosis. Patients given this diagnosis could in due course be accorded a more definitive diagnosis once appropriate diagnostic techniques are devised or applied. In some instances, a more definitive diagnosis might be attainable using currently available techniques, but for logistic or ethical reasons these may not have been applied.

Upper Lumbar Spinal Pain of Unknown or Uncertain Origin (XXVI-9.1)

Definition

As for XXVI-9 but the pain is located in the upper lumbar region.

Clinical Features
Spinal pain located in the upper lumbar region.

Diagnostic Features
As for XXVI-9, save that the pain is located in the upper lumbar region.

Pathology
As for XXVI-9.

Remarks
As for XXVI-9.

Code
5XX.X8cS

Lower Lumbar Spinal Pain of Unknown or Uncertain Origin (XXVI-9.2)

Definition
As for XXVI-9 but the pain is located in the lower lumbar region.

Clinical Features
Spinal pain located in the lower lumbar region.

Diagnostic Features
As for XXVI-9, save that the pain is located in the lower lumbar region.

Pathology
As for XXVI-9.

Remarks
As for XXVI-9.

Code
5XX.X8dS

Lumbosacral Spinal Pain of Unknown or Uncertain Origin (XXVI-9.3)

Definition
As for XXVI-9 but the pain is located in the lumbosacral region.

Clinical Features
Spinal pain located in the lumbosacral region.

Diagnostic Features
As for XXVI-9, save that the pain is located in the lumbosacral region.

Pathology
As for XXVI-9.

Remarks
As for XXVI-9.

Code
5XX.X8eS

Lumbar Spinal or Radicular Pain after Failed Spinal Surgery (XXVI-10)

Definition
Lumbar spinal pain of unknown origin either persisting despite surgical intervention or appearing after surgical intervention for spinal pain originally in the same topographical location.

Clinical Features
Lumbar spinal pain occurring alone or in association with referred pain or radicular pain.

Diagnostic Criteria
As for lumbar spinal pain of unknown origin with the exception that the patient's history now includes an unsuccessful attempt at treating the pain in the same region by surgical means.

Pathology
Unknown.

Remarks
This diagnosis has been formulated as an entity distinct from lumbar spinal pain of unknown origin to accommodate beliefs that the failed attempt at surgical therapy complicates the patient's condition pathologically, psychologically, or both.

Conjectures may be raised as to the possible origin of this form of pain, such as neuroma formation, deafferentation, epidural scarring, etc, but until reliable diagnostic techniques are developed whereby these or similar conditions can be confirmed objectively, any attempt at diagnosis can only be presumptive.

The diagnosis does not apply if a patient presents with spinal pain that is not associated both topographically and temporally with the spinal surgery. In that case, the spinal pain should be accorded a separate diagnosis; the previous spinal pain treated surgically should be considered only as part of the patient's general medical history.

Code
533.X1gS/C
632.X1hR

Lumbar Discogenic Pain (XXVI-11)

Definition
Lumbar spinal pain, with or without referred pain, stemming from a lumbar intervertebral disk.

Clinical Features
Spinal pain perceived in the lumbar region, with or without referred pain to the lower limb girdle or lower limb.

Diagnostic Criteria
The patient's pain must be shown conclusively to stem from an intervertebral disk by demonstrating

either (1) that selective anesthetization of the putatively symptomatic intervertebral disk completely relieves the patient of the accustomed pain for a period consonant with the expected duration of action of the local anesthetic used;

or (2) that selective anesthetization of the putatively symptomatic intervertebral disk substantially relieves the patient of the accustomed pain for a period consonant with the expected duration of action of the local anesthetic used, save that whatever pain persists can be ascribed to some other coexisting source or cause;

or (3) provocation diskography of the putatively symptomatic disk reproduces the patient's accustomed pain, but provided that provocation of at least two adjacent intervertebral disks clearly does not reproduce the patient's pain, and provided that the pain cannot be ascribed to some other source innervated by the same segments that innervate the putatively symptomatic disk.

Pathology
Unknown, but presumably the pain arises as a result of chemical or mechanical irritation of the nerve endings in the outer anulus fibrosus, initiated by injury to the anulus, or as a result of excessive stresses imposed on the anulus by injury, deformity, or other disease within the affected segment or adjacent segments.

Remarks
Provocation diskography alone is insufficient to establish conclusively a diagnosis of discogenic pain because of the propensity for false-positive responses either because of apprehension on the part of the patient or because of the coexistence of a separate source of pain within the segment under investigation. If analgesic diskography is not performed or is possibly false-negative, criterion (3) must be explicitly satisfied. Otherwise, the diagnosis of "discogenic pain" cannot be sustained, whereupon an alternative classification must be used.

Code
533.X1iS	Trauma
533.X6aS	Degenerative
533.X7cS	Dysfunctional

References
Bernard, T.N., Lumbar discography followed by computed tomography: refining the diagnosis of low-back pain, Spine, 15 (1990) 690–707.

Bogduk, N., The lumbar disc and low back pain, Neurosurg. Clin. North Am., 2 (1991) 791–806.

Executive Committee of the North American Spine Society, Position statement on discography, Spine, 13 (1988) 1343.

Simmons, J.W., Aprill, C.N., Dwyer, A. P., and Brodsky, A.E., A reassessment of Holt's data on "the question of lumbar discography," Clin. Orthop., 237 (1988) 120–124.

Walsh, T.R., Weinstein, J.N., Spratt, K.F., et al., Lumbar discography in normal subjects, J. Bone Joint Surg., 72A (1990) 1081–1088.

Internal Disk Disruption (XXVI-12)

Definition
Lumbar spinal pain, with or without referred pain, stemming from an intervertebral disk, caused by internal disruption of the normal structural and biochemical integrity of the symptomatic disk.

Clinical Features
Lumbar spinal pain, with or without referred pain in the lower limb girdle or lower limb; aggravated by movements that stress the symptomatic disk.

Diagnostic Criteria
The diagnostic criteria for lumbar discogenic pain must be satisfied, and in addition, CT-diskography must demonstrate a grade 3 or greater grade of anular disruption as defined by the Dallas diskogram scale.

Pathology
The pathology of internal disk disruption is believed to be due to enzymatic degradation of the internal disk matrix. Initially, the degradation is restricted to the nucleus pulposus, but eventually it progresses in a centrifugal pattern along radial fissures into the anulus fibrosus. Biochemically the process involves activation of enzymes such as proteinases, cathepsin, and collagenase. Biophysically the process is characterized by denaturation and deaggregation of proteoglycans and diminished water-binding capacity of the nucleus pulposus.

The causes of disk degradation are still speculative but possibly involve disinhibition of proteolytic enzymes systems endogenous to the disk as a result of impaired nutrition to the disk or injuries to the vertebral endplate.

Pain arises as a result of chemical or mechanical stimulation of the nerve endings located in the outer third or outer half of the anulus fibrosus, and is aggravated by any movements that stress these portions of the anulus.

Code

533.X1tS	Trauma
533.X6bS	Degenerative
533.X7*S	Dysfunctional

References

Bernard, T.N., Lumbar discography followed by computed tomography: refining the diagnosis of low-back pain, Spine, 15 (1990) 690–707.

Bogduk, N., The lumbar disc and low back pain, Neurosurg. Clin. North Am., 2 (1991) 791–806.

Crock, H.V., Internal disc disruption: a challenge to disc prolapse 50 years on, Spine, 11 (1986) 650–653.

Vanharanta, H., Sachs, B.L., Spivey, M.A., et al., The relationship of pain provocation to lumbar disc deterioration as seen by CT/discography, Spine, 12 (1987) 295–298.

Lumbar Zygapophysial Joint Pain (XXVI-13)

Definition
Lumbar spinal pain, with or without referred pain, stemming from one or more of the lumbar zygapophysial joints.

Clinical Features
Lumbar spinal pain with or without referred pain.

Diagnostic Criteria
No criteria have been established whereby zygapophysial joint pain can be diagnosed on the basis of the patient's history or by conventional clinical examination. The condition can be diagnosed only by the use of diagnostic, intraarticular zygapophysial joint blocks. For the diagnosis to be declared, all of the following criteria must be satisfied.

1. The blocks must be radiologically controlled.
2. Arthrography must demonstrate that any injection has been made selectively into the target joint, and any material that is injected into the joint must not spill over into adjacent structures that might otherwise be the actual source of the patient's pain.
3. The patient's pain must be totally relieved following the injection of local anesthetic into the target joint.
4. A single positive response to the intraarticular injection of local anesthetic is insufficient for the diagnosis to be declared. The response must be validated by an appropriate control test that excludes false-positive responses on the part of the patient, such as:

- no relief of pain upon injection of a nonactive agent;
- no relief of pain following the injection of an active local anesthetic into a site other than the target joint; or
- a positive but differential response to local anesthetics of different durations of action injected into the target joint on separate occasions.

Local anesthetic blockade of the nerves supplying a target zygapophysial joint may be used as a screening procedure to determine in the first instance whether a particular joint might be the source of symptoms, but the definitive diagnosis may be made only upon selective, intraarticular injection of the putatively symptomatic joint.

Pathology
Still unknown. May be due to small fractures not evident on plain radiography or conventional computerized tomography, but possibly demonstrated on high-resolution CT, conventional tomography, or stereoradiography. May be due to osteoarthrosis, but the radiographic presence of osteoarthritis is not a sufficient criterion for the diagnosis to be declared. Zygapophysial joint pain may be caused by rheumatoid arthritis, ankylosing spondylitis, septic arthritis, or villo-nodular synovitis.

Sprains and other injuries to the capsule of zygapophysial joints have been demonstrated at post mortem and may be the cause of pain in some patients, but these types of injuries cannot be demonstrated in vivo using currently available imaging techniques.

Remarks
See also XXVI-17, Lumbar Segmental Dysfunction.

Code

Trauma	
533.X1kS/C	633.X1*R
Degenerative	
533.X6oS/C	633.X6aR

References

Bough, B., Thakore, J., Davies, M., and Dowling, F., Degeneration of the lumbar facet joints: arthrography and pathology, J. Bone Joint Surg., 72B (1990) 275–276.

Carette, S., Marcoux, S., Truchon, R., et al., A controlled trial of corticosteroid injections into facet joints for chronic low back pain, New Engl. J. Med., 325 (1991) 1002–1007.

Carrera, G.F. and Williams, A.L., Current concepts in evaluation of the lumbar facet joints, Crit. Rev. Diagn. Imaging, 21 (1984) 85–104.

Eisenstein, S.M. and Parry, C.R., The lumbar facet arthrosis syndrome, J. Bone Joint Surg., 69B (1987) 3–7.

Fairbank, J.C.T., Park, W.M., McCall, I.W. and O'Brien, J.P., Apophyseal injection of local anesthetic as a diagnostic aid in primary low-back pain syndromes, Spine, 6 (1981) 598–605.

Helbig, T. and Lee, C.K., The lumbar facet syndrome, Spine, 13 (1988) 61–64.

Lewinnek, G.E. and Warfield, C.A., Facet joint degeneration as a cause of low back pain, Clin. Orthop., 213 (1986) 216–222.

Lippit, A.B., The facet joint and its role in spine pain: management with facet joint injections, Spine, 9 (1984) 746–750.

Marks, R., Distribution of pain provoked from lumbar facet joints and related structures during diagnostic spinal infiltration, Pain, 39 (1989) 37–40.

Mooney, V. and Robertson, J., The facet syndrome, Clin, Orthop., 115 (1976) 149–156.

Moran, R., O'Connell, D. and Walsh, M.G., The diagnostic value of facet joint injections, Spine, 12 (1986) 1407–1410.

Twomey, L.T., Taylor, J.R. and Taylor, M.M., Unsuspected damage to lumbar zygapophyseal (facet) joints after motor vehicle accidents, Med. J. Aust., 151 (1989) 210–217.

Lumbar Muscle Sprain (XXVI-14)

Definition
Lumbar spinal pain stemming from a lesion in a specified muscle caused by strain of that muscle beyond its normal physiological limits.

Clinical Features
Lumbar spinal pain, with or without referred pain, associated with tenderness in the affected muscle and aggravated by either passive stretching or resisted contraction of that muscle.

Diagnostic Criteria
The following criteria must all be satisfied.

1. The affected muscle must be specified.
2. A history of activities consistent with the affected muscle having been strained.
3. The muscle is tender to palpation.
4. (a) Aggravation of the pain by any clinical test that can be shown to selectively stress the affected muscle, or
   (b) Selective infiltration of the affected muscle with local anesthetic completely relieves the patient's pain.

Pathology
Rupture of muscle fibers, usually near their myotendinous junction, that elicits and inflammatory repair response.

Remarks
This nosological entity has been included in recognition of its frequent use in clinical practice, and because "muscle sprain" is readily diagnosed in injuries of the limbs. However, in the context of spinal pain this entity

is only presumptive, since no clinical test for spinal muscle sprain has been validated.

Code
533.X1lS

References
Fairbank, J.C.T. and O'Brien, J.P., Iliac crest syndrome: a treatable cause of low-back pain, Spine, 8 (1983) 220–224.

Garrett, W.E., Saffrean, M.R., Seaber, A.V., et al., Biomechanical comparison of stimulated and non-stimulated skeletal muscle pulled to failure, Am. J. Sports Med., 15 (1987) 448–454.

Garrett, W.E., Nikoloau, P.K., Ribbeck, B.M., et al., The effect of muscle architecture on the biomechanical failure properties of skeletal muscle under passive tension, Am. J. Sports Med., 16 (1988) 7–12.

Ingpen, M.L. and Burry, H.C., A lumbo-sacral strain syndrome, Ann. Phys. Med., 10 (1970) 270–274.

Nikolau, P.K., MacDonald, B.L., Glisson, R.R., et al., Biomechanical and histological evaluation of muscle after controlled strain injury, Am. J. Sports Med., 15 (1987) 9–14.

Lumbar Trigger Point Syndrome (XXVI-15)

Definition
Lumbar spinal pain stemming from a trigger point or trigger points in one or more of the muscles of the lumbar spine.

Clinical Features
Lumbar spinal pain, with or without referred pain, associated with a trigger point in one or more muscles of the lumbar vertebral column.

Diagnostic Criteria
The following criteria must all be satisfied.

1. A trigger point must be present in a muscle, consisting of a palpable, tender, firm, fusiform nodule oriented in the direction of the affected muscle's fibers.
2. The muscle must be specified.
3. Palpation of the trigger point reproduces the patient's pain and/or referred pain.
4. Elimination of the trigger point relieves the patient's pain. Elimination may be achieved by stretching the affected muscle, dry needling the trigger point, or infiltrating it with local anesthetic.

Pathology
Unknown. Trigger points are believed to represent areas of contracted muscle that have failed to relax as a result of failure of calcium ions to sequestrate. Pain arises as a result of the accumulation of algogenic metabolites.

Remarks

For the diagnosis to be accorded, the diagnostic criteria for a trigger point must be fulfilled. Simple tenderness in a muscle without a palpable band does not satisfy the criteria, whereupon an alternative diagnosis must be accorded, such as muscle sprain, if the criteria for that condition are fulfilled, or spinal pain of unknown origin.

Schedule of Trigger Point Sites

XXVI-15.1(S)
    Multifidus
    Code 532.X1aS

XXVI-15.2(S)
    Longissimus Thoracis
    Code 532.X1bS

XXVI-15.3(S)
    Iliocostalis Lumborum
    Code 532.X1cS

XXVI-15.4(S)
    Lumbar Trigger Point Not Otherwise Specified
    Code 532.X1*S

References

Simons, D.G., Myofascial pain syndromes: Where are we? Where are we going? Arch. Phys. Med. Rehab., 69 (1988) 207–212.

Travell, J.G. and Simons, D.G., Myofascial pain and dysfunction. In: The Trigger Point Manual, Williams & Wilkins, Baltimore (1983).

Lumbar Muscle Spasm (XXVI-16)

Definition
Lumbar spinal pain resulting from sustained or repeated involuntary activity of the lumbar spinal muscles.

Clinical Features
Lumbar spinal pain for which there is no other underlying cause, associated with demonstrable sustained muscle activity.

Diagnostic Features
Palpable spasm is usually found at some time, most often in the paravertebral muscles.

Pathology
Unknown. Presumably sustained muscle activity prevents adequate wash-out of algogenic chemicals produced by the sustained metabolic activity of the muscle.

Remarks
While there are beliefs in a pain–muscle spasm–pain cycle, clinical tests or conventional electromyography have not been shown to demonstrate reliably the presence of sustained muscle activity in such situations. The strongest evidence for repeated involuntary muscle spasm stems from sleep-EMG studies conducted on patients with low-back pain, but although it is associated with back pain a causal relationship between this type of muscle activity and back pain has not been established.

Code
532.X1tS	Trauma
532.X2hS	Infection
532.X4aS	Neoplasm
532.X6aS	Degenerative
532.X7dS	Dysfunctional
532.X8fS	Unknown

References

Fischer, A.A. and Chang, C.H., Electromyographic evidence of paraspinal muscle spasm during sleep in patients with low back pain, Clin. J. Pain, 1 (1985) 147–154.

Garrett, W., Anderson, G., Richardson, W., et al., Muscle: future directions. In: J.W. Frymoyer and S.L. Gordon (Eds.), New Perspectives on Low Back Pain, American Academy of Orthopaedic Surgeons, Park Ridge, Ill., 1989, pp. 373–379.

Garrett, W., Bradley, W., Byrd, S., et al., Muscle: basic science perspectives. In: J.W. Frymoyer and S.L. Gordon (Eds.), New Perspectives on Low Back Pain, American Academy of Orthopaedic Surgeons, Park Ridge, Ill. 1989, pp. 335–372.

Roland, M.O., A critical review of the evidence for a pain-spasm-pain cycle in spinal disorders, Clin. Biomech., 1 (1986) 102–109.

Lumbar Segmental Dysfunction (XXVI-17)

Definition
Lumbar spinal pain ostensibly due to excessive strains imposed on the restraining elements of a single spinal motion segment.

Clinical Features
Lumbar spinal pain, with or without referred pain, that can be aggravated by selectively stressing a particular spinal segment.

Diagnostic Criteria
All the following criteria should be satisfied.

1. The affected segment must be specified.
2. The patient's pain is aggravated by clinical tests that selectively stress the affected segment.
3. Stressing adjacent segments does not reproduce the patient's pain.

Pathology
Unknown. Presumably involves excessive strain imposed by activities of daily living on structures such as the ligaments, joints, or intervertebral disk of the affected segment.

Remarks

This diagnosis is offered as a partial distinction from spinal pain of unknown origin in so far as the source of the patient's pain can at least be narrowed to a particular offending segment. Further investigation of a patient accorded this diagnosis might result in the patient's condition being ascribed a more definitive diagnosis such as discogenic pain or zygapophysial joint pain, but the diagnosis of segmental dysfunction could be applied if facilities for undertaking the appropriate investigations are not available, if the physician or patient does not wish to pursue such investigations, or if the pain arises from multiple sites in the same segment rendering investigation futile or meaningless.

For this diagnosis to be sustained it is critical that the clinical tests used be shown to be able to stress selectively the segment in question and to have acceptable interobserver reliability. To date, no studies have established validity for any techniques purported to demonstrate segmental dysfunction.

Code
533.X1hS
533.X7eS

Lumbar Ligament Sprain (XXVI-18)

Definition

Lumbar spinal pain stemming from a lesion in a specified ligament caused by strain of that ligament beyond its normal physiological limit.

Clinical Features

Lumbar spinal pain, with or without referred pain, aggravated by active or passive movements that strain the affected ligament.

Diagnostic Criteria

All the following criteria should be satisfied; otherwise the diagnosis can only be presumptive.

1. The affected ligament must be specified.
2. A history of an acute or chronic mechanical disturbance of the vertebral column which would be expected to have strained the specified ligament.
3. (a) Aggravation of the pain by any clinical test that has been shown to stress the specified ligament selectively, or
   (b) Aggravation of the pain by a combination of clinical tests each of which stresses several ligaments or other structures but which have only the specified ligament in common, or
   (c) Selective infiltration of the putatively symptomatic ligament with local anesthetic under radiographic control completely relieves the patients pain.

Pathology

Unknown and unstudied. Presumably partial rupture of the collagen fibers of the ligament at a microscopic or macroscopic level causes inflammation of the injured part. May involve sustained strain of the ligament at the limit of its physiological range at a length short of partial failure but sufficient to elicit nociceptive stimulation consistent with impending damage to the ligament.

Remarks

Any clinical tests or local anesthetic infiltration of the ligament must be shown to be specific for that ligament. Any conventional or otherwise established clinical tests must have been shown to have good interobserver reliability.

Ligament sprain is an acceptable diagnosis in the context of injuries of the joints of the appendicular skeleton because the affected ligament is usually accessible to palpation for tenderness and because the ligament can be selectively stressed by passive movements of the related limb segments. However, this facility does not pertain to the lumbar spine. Lumbar ligaments are either impalpable or difficult to stress selectively. Hence the diagnosis is somewhat conjectural.

Code
533.X1mS

Sprain of the Anulus Fibrosus (XXVI-19)

Definition

Lumbar spinal pain arising from a lesion in the anulus fibrosus of an intervertebral disk caused by excessive strain of the anulus fibrosus.

Clinical Features

Lumbar spinal pain, with or without referred pain, aggravated by movements that stress an anulus fibrosus, associated with a history compatible with singular or cumulative injury to the anulus fibrosus.

Diagnostic Criteria

The following criteria must be fulfilled.

1. The affected anulus fibrosus must be specified.
2. A history of activities or injury consistent with the affected anulus fibrosus having been strained.
3. (a) Aggravation of the pain by clinical tests that selectively stress the affected anulus fibrosus, or
   (b) Relief of the patient's pain upon selectively infiltrating the affected anulus fibrosus with local anesthetic.

Pathology

Analogous to ligament sprain. Partial or complete tears of the anulus fibrosus in a location consistent with the nature of the precipitating stress; typically: circumferential tears of the outer layers of the anulus fibrosus caused by excessive combined flexion and rotation of the affected segment. Pain arises either as a result of an inflammatory repair response to the injured collagen fibers or as a result of excessive strain imposed by activities of daily living on the remaining, intact collagen fibers of the anulus fibrosus, which alone are insufficient to sustain these loads within their accustomed, normal physiological limits.

Remarks

Any clinical test used to diagnose sprain of the anulus fibrosus should be shown to be valid and reliable. To date, no such test has been developed. Consequently, until this is done this entity must remain conjectural. Such clinical tests as have been advocated for this condition (Farfan 1985) have not been assessed for validity.

Code

533.X1nS

Reference

Farfan, H.F., The use of mechanical etiology to determine the efficacy of active intervention in single joint lumbar intervertebral joint problems, Spine, 10 (1985) 350–358.

Interspinous Pseudarthrosis (Kissing Spines, Baastrup's Disease) (XXVI-20)

Definition

Lumbar spinal pain stemming from a pseudarthrosis formed between consecutive lumbar spinous processes.

Clinical Features

Lumbar, lumbosacral, or sacral spinal pain associated with midline tenderness over the affected interspinous space, the pain being aggravated by extension of that segment of the vertebral column.

Diagnostic Criteria

The pseudarthrosis must be evident radiographically and must be shown to be symptomatic by having the pain relieved upon selective anesthetization of the pseudarthrosis, provided that the local anesthetic injected does not spread to affect other structures that might constitute an alternative source of the patient's pain.

Pathology

Periostitis as a result of repeated contact between the two bones, progressing to sclerosis of the contact sites of the two bones.

Remarks

The radiographic presence of a pseudarthrosis in a patient with spinal pain is insufficient grounds alone to justify the diagnosis. The pseudarthrosis must be shown to be symptomatic. Relief of pain following infiltration of local anesthetic into the lesion is not necessarily attended by relief following surgical treatment.

Code

533.X1oS

Reference

Beks, J.W.F., Kissing spines: fact or fancy? Acta Neurochir., 100 (1989) 134–135.

Lumbar Instability (XXVI-21)

Definition

Lumbar spinal pain ostensibly due to excessive or abnormal motion of lumbar motion segment that exhibits decreased stiffness (Pope and Panjabi 1985) or an increased neutral zone (Panjabi et al. 1989).

Clinical Features

Lumbar spinal pain, with or without referred pain, that can be aggravated by movements that stress the affected spinal segment, accompanied by radiographic evidence of instability.

Diagnostic Criteria

No universally accepted criteria exist for the clinical or radiographic diagnosis of instability, but for this classification to be used, one of the sets of criteria proposed in the literature must be satisfied, such as those of Posner et al. (1982), Kalebo et al. (1990), or Nachemson (1991).

Pathology

Loss of stiffness in one or more of the elements of a lumbar motion segment that resist translation, rotation, or both. The pain presumably arises as a result of excessive stresses being imposed by movement on structures such as the ligaments, joints, or anulus fibrosus of the affected segment.

Remarks

No studies have revealed exactly what the source of pain is in unstable lumbar motion segments nor what the mechanism of pain production is. This diagnosis is, therefore, offered only as one of association between lumbar spinal pain and demonstrable movement abnormalities. No studies have vindicated any clinical test for instability. Consequently, the diagnosis can be sustained only if the radiographic criteria are strictly satisfied. At the time of writing, although such criteria have been enunciated, reservations have also been raised about the internal and external reliability of measurements made on radiographs of the type used to demonstrate instability (Shaffer et al. 1990).

Code
533.X7jS

Reference

Kalebo, P., Kadzialka, R. and Sward, L., Compression-traction radiography of lumbar segmental instability, Spine, 15 (1990) 351–355.

Nachemson, A.L., Instability of the lumbar spine: pathology, treatment, and clinical evaluation, Neurosurgery Clinics of North America, 2 (1991) 785–790.

Panjabi, M., Abumi, K., Duranceau, J. and Oxland, T., Spinal stability and intersegmental muscle forces in a biomechanical model, Spine, 14 (1989) 194–200.

Pope, M.H. and Panjabi, M., Biomechanical definitions of spinal instability, Spine, 10 (1985) 255–256.

Posner, I., White, A.A., Edwards, W.T. and Hayes, W.C., A biomechanical analysis of the clinical stability of the lumbar and lumbosacral spine, Spine, 7 (1982) 374–389.

Shaffer, W.O., Spratt, K.F., Weinstein, J., Lehmann, T.R. and Goel, V. The consistency and accuracy of roentgenograms for measuring sagittal translation in the lumbar vertebral motion segment: an experimental model, Spine, 15 (1990) 741–750.

Clinical Features
Lumbar spinal pain, with or without referred pain, in association with a radiographically demonstrable pars interarticularis defect that has been shown to be the source of the patient's pain.

Diagnostic Criteria
The patient's pain should be fully or substantially relieved upon anesthetization of the pars interarticularis defect using a procedure that ensures that no other structure is anesthetized that might alternatively be the source of the patient's pain.

Remarks
This classification should not be used unless the diagnostic criterion is satisfied. The presence of a pars interarticularis defect on radiographs or nuclear scans in a patient with lumbar spinal pain is not sufficient evidence to justify this diagnosis, because pars interarticularis defects occur in about 7% of asymptomatic individuals (Moreton 1966) and therefore may be only a coincidental finding in a patient with lumbar spinal pain. For this classification to be used evidence must be brought to bear that the observed defect is not asymptomatic.

Code
53X.X0*S

References

Moreton, R.D., Spondylolysis, JAMA, 195 (1966) 671–674.

Suh, P.B., Esses, S.I. and Kostuik J.P., Repair of pars interarticularis defect: the prognostic value of pars infiltration, Spine, 16, Suppl. 8S (1991) S445–S448.

Spondylolysis (XXVI-22)

Definition
Lumbar spinal pain arising from a painful pars interarticularis defect.

Prolapsed Intervertebral Disk (XXVI-23)

Code
502.X1cS/C
602.X1aR

GROUP XXVII: SACRAL SPINAL OR RADICULAR PAIN SYNDROMES

Sacral Spinal or Radicular Pain Attributable to a Fracture (XXVII-1)

Definition
Sacral spinal pain occurring in a patient with a history of injury in whom radiography or other imaging studies demonstrate the presence of a fracture that can reasonably be interpreted as the cause of pain.

Clinical Features
Sacral spinal pain with or without referred pain.

Diagnostic Features
Radiographic or other imaging evidence of a fracture of the sacrum.

Code
533.X2lS/C

Sacral Spinal or Radicular Pain Attributable to an Infection (XXVII-2)

Definition
Sacral spinal pain occurring in a patient with clinical and/or other features of an infection, in whom the site of infection can be specified and can reasonably be interpreted as the source of the pain.

Clinical Features
Sacral spinal pain with or without referred pain, associated with pyrexia or other clinical features of infection.

Diagnostic Features
A presumptive diagnosis can be made on the basis of an elevated white cell count or other serological features of infection, together with imaging evidence of the presence of a site of infection in the sacrum or its adnexa. Absolute confirmation relies on histological and/or bacteriological confirmation using material obtained by direct or needle biopsy.

Schedule of Sites of Infection
XXVII-2.1(S)(R)
    Infection of the Sacrum (osteomyelitis)
    Code 533.X2aS/C 633.X2aR
XXVII-2.2(S)
    Septic Arthritis of the Sacroiliac Joint
    Code 533.X2bS
XXVII-2.3(S)
    Infection of a Paravertebral Muscle

(psoas abscess)
    Code 533.X2cS
XXVII-2.4(S)
    Infection of a Surgical Fusion-Site
    Code 533.X2dS
XXVII-2.5(S)
    Infection of a Retroperitoneal Organ or Space
    Code 533.X2eS
XXVII-2.6(S)(R)
    Infection of the Epidural Space
    (epidural abscess)
    Code 533.X2fS/C 633.X2bR
XXVII-2.7(S)(R)
    Infection of the Meninges (meningitis)
    Code 502.X2dS/C 602.X2dR

Sacral Spinal or Radicular Pain Attributable to a Neoplasm (XXVII-3)

Definition
Sacral spinal pain associated with a neoplasm that can reasonably be interpreted as the source of the pain.

Clinical Features
Sacral spinal pain with or without referred pain.

Diagnostic Features
A presumptive diagnosis may be made on the basis of imaging evidence of a neoplasm that directly or indirectly affects one or other of the tissues innervated by sacral spinal nerves. Absolute confirmation relies on obtaining histological evidence by direct or needle biopsy.

Schedule of Neoplastic Diseases
XXVII-3.1(S)(R)
    Primary Tumor of the Sacrum
    Code 533.X4tS/C 633.X4kR
XXVII-3.2(S)
    Primary Tumor of the Sacroiliac Joint
    Code 533.X4kS
XXVII-3.3(S)(R)
    Primary Tumor of a Parasacral Muscle
    Code 533.X4mS
XXVII-3.4(S)(R)
    Primary Tumor of Epidural Fat
    (e.g., lipoma)
    Code 533.X4nS/C 633.X4lR
XXVII-3.5(S)(R)
    Primary Tumor of Epidural Vessels
    (e.g., angioma)
    Code 533.X4oS/C 633.X4mR

XXVII-3.6(S)(R)
  Primary Tumor of Meninges
  (e.g., meningioma)
  Code 503.X4dS/C 603.X4dR
XXVII-3.7(S)(R)
  Primary Tumor of a Spinal Nerve (e.g.,
  neurofibroma, schwannoma, neuroblastoma)
  Code 533.X4eS/C 603.X4eR
XXVII-3.8(S)(R)
  Metastatic Tumor Affecting the Sacrum
  Code 533.X4pS/C 633.X4nR
XXVII-3.9(S)(R)
  Metastatic Tumor Affecting the Sacral Canal
  Code 533.X4qS/C 633.X4oR
XXVII-3.10
  Other Infiltrating Neoplastic Disease Affect-
  ing the Sacrum (e.g., lymphoma)
  Code 533.X4rS/C 633.X4pR

Sacral Spinal or Radicular Pain Attributable to Metabolic Bone Disease (XXVII-4)

Definition
Sacral spinal pain associated with a metabolic bone disease that can reasonably be interpreted as the source of the pain.

Clinical Features
Sacral spinal pain with or without referred pain.

Diagnostic Features
Imaging or other evidence of metabolic bone disease affecting the sacrum, confirmed by appropriate serological or biochemical investigations and/or histological evidence obtained by needle or other biopsy.

Schedule of Metabolic Bone Diseases
XXVII-4.1(S)(R)
  Osteoporosis of Age
  Code 532.X5gS/C 632.X5gR
XXVII-4.2(S)(R)
  Osteoporosis of Unknown Cause
  Code 532.X5hS/C 632.X5hR
XXVII-4.3(S)(R)
  Osteoporosis of Some Known Cause Other
  than Age
  Code 532.X5iS/C 632.X5iR
XXVII-4.4(S)(R)
  Hyperparathyroidism
  Code 532.X5jS/C 632.X5jR
XXVII-4.5(S)(R)
  Paget's Disease of Bone
  Code 532.X5kS/C 632.X5kR

XXVII-4.6(S)(R)
  Metabolic Disease of Bone Otherwise Not
  Classified
  Code 532.X5lS/C 632.X5lR

Sacral Spinal or Radicular Pain Attributable to Arthritis (XXVII-5)

Definition
Sacral spinal pain associated with arthritis that can reasonably be interpreted as the source of the pain.

Clinical Features
Sacral spinal pain with or without referred pain.

Diagnostic Features
Imaging or other evidence of arthritis affecting the sacroiliac joints.

Schedule of Arthritides
XXVII-5.1(S)
  Rheumatoid Arthritis of the Sacroiliac Joint
  Code 534.X3bS
XXVII-5.2(S)
  Ankylosing Spondylitis
  Code 532.X8aS
XXVII-5.3(S)(R)
  Seronegative Spondylarthropathy Otherwise
  Not Classified
  Code 523.X8aS/C 623.X8aR
XXVII-5.4(S)
  Sacroiliitis (evident on bone-scan)
  Code 532.X8gS
XXVII-5.5(S)
  Osteitis Condensans Ilii
  Code 532.X8uS

Reference
Bellamy, N., Park, W. and Rooney, P.J., What do we know about the sacroiliac joint? Sem. Arthritis Rheum., 12 (1983) 282–313.

Spinal Stenosis: Cauda Equina Lesion (XXVII-6)

Definition
Chronic pain usually experienced in the buttocks and legs, at times extremely severe. Usually deep and aching with "heaviness and numbness" in the leg from buttock to foot, associated with narrowing of the vertebral canal.

Site
Low back, buttocks, and lower extremities.

System
Musculoskeletal system.

Main Features
Patients usually have a long history of gradually increasing lumbar spinal with referred pain in the buttocks or lower limbs, with or without radicular pain, aggravated by extension of the lumbar spine, or by sustained postures that involve accentuation of the lumbar lordosis (like prolonged standing), and by walking. Walking also produces overt or subtle neurological features in the lower limbs that range from sensations of heaviness or clumsiness to paresthesias, numbness, weakness, and temporary paralysis of the lower limbs. The onset of these neurological features may be measured in terms of a "walking distance," which diminishes as the condition progresses in severity.

Associated Symptoms
There may be paresthesias and bowel or bladder disturbance, or impotence.

Aggravating Factors
Walking, standing.

Signs and Laboratory Findings
X-rays usually demonstrate diffuse severe degenerative disease with facet hypertrophy and a shallow anteroposterior diameter of the lumbar canal. Cystometrogram may be helpful in diagnosis. Myelography and CT scanning are helpful in showing narrowing of the spinal canal. Magnetic resonance imaging and electrodiagnostic studies can also be helpful in demonstrating the areas involved. The dilemma posed by this condition is the discrepancy between physical signs, which are usually not great, and the subjective complaints.

Etiology
Congenital factors, (e.g., lumbar spondylosis, lumbar spondylolisthesis; degenerative disease, osteoarthritis).

Pathology
Encroachment upon and narrowing of the vertebral canal as a whole or of multiple lateral recesses thereof by osteophytes of the zygapophysial joints or syndesmophytes of the intervertebral disks. Congenital narrowing of the vertebral canal may predispose to this condition insofar as symptoms may arise in the face of osteophytes and syndesmophytes that in other individuals would not cause significant encroachment. The mechanism of the neurological features is unknown but may involve constriction of the dural sac with obstruction of flow of the cerebrospinal fluid, or obstruction of venous blood flow in the vertebral canal, or direct compression of spinal nerve roots.

Radicular pain may arise as a result of compression or other compromise of one or more nerve roots but there is no evidence that the constrictive effects of spinal stenosis cause spinal pain and referred pain. These latter forms of pain ostensibly arise from the disorders of one or more of the disks or zygapophysial joints whose osteophytic overgrowth coincidentally causes the stenosis.

Spinal stenosis is characterized by an essentially global distribution of neurological symptoms in the lower limbs, and in this respect should be distinguished from radicular pain due to foraminal stenosis, in which the pathology is restricted to a single intervertebral foramen and as such does not encroach upon the vertebral canal as a whole.

Treatment
Surgical decompression.

Differential Diagnosis
Peripheral vascular claudication, sciatic nerve compression, osteoarthritis of hip or knee, retroperitoneal tumors, other tumor or abscess, prolapsed lumbar disk.

Code
533.X6*S/C   Back
633.X6*R   Legs

Sacral Spinal or Radicular Pain Associated with a Congenital Vertebral Anomaly (XXVII-7)

Definition
Sacral spinal pain associated with a congenital vertebral anomaly.

Clinical Features
Sacral spinal pain with or without referred pain.

Diagnostic Features
Imaging evidence of a congenital vertebral anomaly affecting the sacrum.

Remarks
There is no evidence that congenital anomalies per se cause pain. Although they may be associated with pain, the specificity of this association is unknown. This classification should be used only when the cause of pain cannot be otherwise specified, but should not be used to imply that the congenital anomaly is the actual source of pain.

Code
533.X0*S/C
533.X0*R
633.X0*R

Pain Referred from Abdominal or Pelvic Viscera or Vessels Perceived as Sacral Spinal Pain (XXVII-8)

Definition
Sacral spinal pain associated with disease of an abdominal or pelvic viscus or vessel that reasonably can be interpreted as the source of pain.

Clinical Features
Sacral spinal pain with or without referred pain, together with features of the disease affecting the viscus or vessel concerned.

Diagnostic Features
Imaging or other evidence of the primary disease affecting an abdominal or pelvic viscus or vessel.

Schedule of Diseases
XXVII-8.0   Classified elsewhere:
Dysmenorrhea (see XXIV-2 and XXIV-3)
Endometriosis (see XXIV-4)
Posterior Parametritis (see XXIV-5)
Retroversion of the Uterus (see XXIV-7)
Carcinoma of the rectum (see XXIX-5.1)
XXVII-8.1   Irritation of Presacral Tissues by Blood
Code 533.X6aS/C
XXVII-8.2   Irritation of Presacral Tissues by Contents of Ruptured Viscera
Code 533.X6bS/C

Sacral Spinal Pain of Unknown or Uncertain Origin (XXVII-9)

Definition
Sacral spinal pain occurring in a patient whose clinical features and associated features do not enable the cause and source of the pain to be determined, and whose cause or source cannot be or has not been determined by special investigations.

Clinical Features
Sacral spinal pain with or without referred pain.

Diagnostic Features
Sacral spinal pain for which no other cause has been found or can be attributed.

Pathology
Unspecified.

Remarks
This definition is intended to cover those complaints that for whatever reason currently defy conventional diagnosis. It does not encompass pain of psychological origin. It presupposes an organic basis for the pain but one that cannot be or has not been established reliably by clinical examination or special investigations, such as imaging techniques or diagnostic blocks.

This diagnosis may be used as a temporary diagnosis. Patients given this diagnosis could in due course be accorded a more definitive diagnosis once appropriate diagnostic techniques are devised or applied. In some instances, a more definitive diagnosis might be attainable using currently available techniques, but for logistic or ethical reasons these may not have been applied.

Code
5XX.X8*S

Sacroiliac Joint Pain (XXVII-10)

Definition
Spinal pain stemming from a sacroiliac joint.

Clinical Features
Pain perceived in the region of the sacroiliac joint with or without referred pain into the lower limb girdle or lower limb itself.

Diagnostic Criteria
The following criteria should all be fulfilled.

1. Pain is present in the region of the sacroiliac joint.
2. Stressing the sacroiliac joint by clinical tests that are selective for the joint reproduces the patient's pain, or
3. Selectively infiltrating the putatively symptomatic joint with local anesthetic completely relieves the patient of the pain.

Pathology
Unknown. Presumably the pain is caused by excessive stresses being imposed on the ligaments of the sacroiliac joint as a result of some structural fault in the joint itself or as a result of the joint as a whole being subject to inordinate stresses.

Remarks
This category does not encompass sacroiliitis, ankylosing spondylitis, or seronegative spondylarthropathies that may be demonstrated by radionuclide imaging other forms of imaging or diagnosed by other means. This category infers a mechanical disorder of the joint.

Mechanical disorders of the sacroiliac joint are the subject of controversy. While there are beliefs that such disorders can befall the sacroiliac joint, no clinical tests of laudable validity and reliability have been devised whereby this condition can be diagnosed. The presence of such a condition, however, in the absence of any overt inflammatory joint disease, is implied by a positive response to an intraarticular injection of local anesthetic. Until such time as appropriate clinical tests are demonstrated to be valid and reliable, any diagnosis of sacroiliac joint pain based exclusively on clinical examination must be held to be only presumptive.

Code
533.X6dS

Reference
Waisbrod, H., Krainick, J.U. and Gerbershagen, H.U., Sacroiliac joint arthrodesis for chronic low back pain, Arch. Orthop. Traum. Surg., 106 (1987) 238–240.

GROUP XXVIII: COCCYGEAL PAIN SYNDROMES

Coccygeal Pain of Unknown or Uncertain Origin (XXVIII-1)

Definition
Coccygeal pain occurring in a patient whose clinical features and associated features do not enable the cause and source of the pain to be determined, and whose cause or source cannot be or has not been determined by special investigations.

Clinical Features
Coccygeal pain with or without referred pain.

Diagnostic Features
Coccygeal pain for which no other cause has been found or can be attributed.

Pathology
Unspecified.

Remarks
This definition is intended to cover those complaints that for whatever reason currently defy conventional diagnosis. It does not encompass pain of psychological origin. It presupposes an organic basis for the pain but one that cannot be or has not been established reliably by clinical examination or special investigations, such as imaging techniques or diagnostic blocks.

This diagnosis may be used as a temporary diagnosis. Patients given this diagnosis could in due course be accorded a more definitive diagnosis once appropriate diagnostic techniques are devised or applied. In some instances, a more definitive diagnosis might be attainable using currently available techniques, but for logistic or ethical reasons these may not have been applied.

Code
5XX.X8hS

Posterior Sacrococcygeal Joint Pain (XXVIII-2)

Definition
Pain perceived in the coccygeal region, stemming from one or both of the posterior sacrococcygeal joints.

Clinical Features
Pain in the sacrococcygeal region.

Diagnostic Criteria
Complete relief of pain upon infiltration of the putatively symptomatic joint or joints with local anesthetic, provided that the injection can be shown to have been selective in that it has not infiltrated other structures that might constitute the actual source of pain.

Pathology
Unknown, but presumably involves sprain of the capsule of the affected joint.

Code
533.X1pS   Trauma
533.X6eS   Degenerative

GROUP XXIX: DIFFUSE OR GENERALIZED SPINAL PAIN

Generalized Spinal Pain Attributable to Multiple Fractures (XXIX-1)

Definition
Generalized spinal pain occurring in a patient with a history of injury in whom radiography or other imaging studies demonstrate the presence of multiple fractures that can reasonably be interpreted as the cause of their pain.

Clinical Features
Generalized spinal pain with or without referred pain.

Diagnostic Features
Radiographic or other imaging evidence of multiple fractures throughout the vertebral column.

Code
933.X1*S/C
933.X1*R

Generalized Spinal Pain Attributable to Disseminated Neoplastic Disease (XXIX-2)

Definition
Generalized spinal pain associated with widespread neoplastic disease of the vertebral column or its adnexa that can reasonably be interpreted as the source of the pain.

Clinical Features
Generalized spinal pain with or without referred pain.

Diagnostic Features
Imaging or other evidence of neoplastic disease that directly or indirectly affects multiple regions of the vertebral column or its adnexa.

Schedule of Neoplastic Diseases
XXIX-2.1(S)(R)
     Disseminated Primary Tumors Affecting the Vertebral Column or Its Adnexa (e.g., multiple myeloma)
     Code 933.X4aS/C   933.X4aR
XXIX-2.2(S)(R)
     Disseminated Metastatic Tumors Affecting the Vertebral Column or Its Adnexa
     Code 933.X4bS/C   933.X4bR
XXIX-2.3(S)(R)
     Infiltrating Neoplastic Disease of the Vertebral

Column or Its Adnexa, Other than Primary or Metastatic Tumors (e.g., lymphoma)
     Code 933.X4cS/C   933.X4cR

Generalized Spinal Pain Attributable to Metabolic Bone Disease (XXIX-3)

Definition
Generalized spinal pain associated with a metabolic bone disease that can reasonably be interpreted as the source of the pain.

Clinical Features
Generalized spinal pain with or without referred pain.

Diagnostic Features
Imaging or other evidence of metabolic bone disease affecting multiple regions of the vertebral column.

Schedule of Metabolic Bone Diseases
XXIX-3.1(S)(R)
     Osteoporosis of Age
     Code 933.X5aS/C   933.X5aR
XXIX-3.2(S)(R)
     Osteoporosis of Unknown Cause
     Code 933.X5bS/C   933.X5bR
XXIX-3.3(S)(R)
     Osteoporosis of Some Known Cause Other than Age
     Code 933.X5cS/C   933.X5cR
XXIX-3.4(S)(R)
     Hyperparathyroidism
     Code 933.X5dS/C   933.X5dR
XXIX-3.5(S)(R)
     Paget's Disease of Bone
     Code 933.X5eS/C   933.X5eR
XXIX-3.6(S)(R)
     Metabolic Disease of Bone Not Otherwise Classified
     Code 933.X5fS/C   933.X5fR

Generalized Spinal Pain Attributable to Arthritis (XXIX-4)

Definition
Generalized spinal pain associated with arthritis that can reasonably be interpreted as the source of the pain.

Clinical Features
Generalized spinal pain with or without referred pain.

Diagnostic Features
Imaging or other evidence of arthritis affecting the joints of multiple regions of the vertebral column.

Schedule of Arthritides
XXIX-4.1(S)(R)
    Rheumatoid Arthritis
    Code 932.X3aS/C 932.X3aR
XXIX-4.2(S)(R)
    Ankylosing Spondylitis
    Code 932.X3bS/C 932.X3bR
XXIX-4.3(S)(R)
    Osteoarthritis
    Code 932.X8*S/C 932.X8*R
XXIX-4.4(S)(R)
    Seronegative Spondylarthropathy Not
    Otherwise Classified
    Code 932.X8bS/C 932.X8bR

Ankylosing Spondylitis (XXIX-4.2)

Definition
Aching low back pain and stiffness of gradual development due to chronic inflammatory change of unknown origin.

Site
Low back.

System
Musculoskeletal system.

Main Features
Prevalence in 1–2% of the population. Males nine times more common than females. Peak onset in the third or fourth decades. More common in Caucasian populations, but some other ethnic groups, e.g., Haida Indians, have unusually high prevalence rates. Chronic, persistent low back pain of insidious onset, aching discomfort, and stiffness while sleeping that forces the patient to get up and move around; morning stiffness is usually greater than half an hour in duration, and stiffness occurs also after periods of inactivity ("gelling phenomenon").

Associated Symptoms
Peripheral joint disease in 20% of patients, conjunctivitis and iritis in 25% of patients, chronic pulmonary fibrosis and cardiovascular disease.

Aggravating Features
Inactivity.

Signs
Depressed spinal mobility and chest expansion with chest involvement.

Laboratory Findings
None specific; 90% of patients are HLA-B27 positive, but 8–10% of normal populations also are HLA-B27 positive.

Radiographic Findings
Bilateral symmetric sacroiliitis; syndesmophytes of lumbar thoracic spines.

Usual Course
Chronic lumbar pain often with acute exacerbations intermittently; pain diminishes as spine fuses.

Relief
Some severe morning stiffness or pain abates with activity. A good response to nonsteroidal anti-inflammatory drugs.

Complications
Spinal immobility, fracture of fused spine. Higher spinal disease may cause vertical odontoid subluxation or penetration with brain-stem compression.

Etiology
Unknown; may be immunological, with possible environmental factors, along with apparent genetic susceptibility.

Essential Features
Chronic aching lumbar pain and stiffness with "gelling" and with characteristic X-ray changes as described.

Differential Diagnosis
Psoriatic spondylitis; Reiter's spondylitis; mechanical back pain; discogenic back pain.

Code
932.X3bS/C
932.X3bR

Back Pain of Other Visceral or Neurological Origin Involving the Spine (XXIX-5)

Carcinoma of the Rectum (XXIX-5.1)

Code
Pelvic pain
753.X4*S/C 753.X4*R
Perineal pain
853.X4*S/C 853.X4*R

Tumor Infiltration of the Lumbosacral Plexus (XXIX-5.2)

Definition
Progressively intense pain in the low back or hip with radiation into the lower extremity.

Site
Lower back and leg.

System
Nervous system (lumbosacral plexus).

Main Features
Lumbosacral plexopathy occurs most commonly in patients with genitourinary, gynecological, and colonic cancers as a result of local tumor extension. The local pain is pressure-like or aching in quality. The referred pain varies with the site of plexus involvement and can be burning, crampy, or lancinating. Upper lumbar plexus involvement produces pain in the anterior thigh and groin, whereas pain in the L5–S1 distribution radiates down the posterior aspect of the leg to the heel. The pain is often worse at night and is usually aggravated by movement of the hip joint.

Associated Symptoms
Typically, leg weakness and numbness occur three to five months after the onset of pain. Sphincter disturbance is uncommon.

Signs and Laboratory Findings
There may be tenderness in the region of the sciatic notch. There is usually limitation of both direct and reverse straight leg raising. Focal weakness and sensory loss with depressed deep tendon reflexes may be evident. The cardinal feature is progressive weakness in a pattern involving more than one nerve root. There may be pedal edema due to lymphatic obstruction.

An intravenous pyelogram may show hydronephrosis. A CT scan through the abdomen and pelvis is the definitive study. It may show a paralumbar or pelvic soft tissue mass and there may be bony erosion of the pelvic side wall. Myelography may be positive if there is epidural extension of disease.

Usual Course
The course is inexorably progressive and leads to a wheelchair- or bedridden existence.

Summary of Essential Features and Diagnostic Criteria
Low back and hip pain radiating into the leg is followed in weeks to months by progressive numbness, paresthesias, weakness, and leg edema. The physical findings indicate that more than one nerve root is involved. CT scan of the abdomen and pelvis is the study of choice.

Differential Diagnosis
Myelography and cerebrospinal fluid analysis should rule out epidural and meningeal metastatic disease, respectively. Other entities to consider are radiation fibrosis, lumbosacral neuritis, and disk disease.

Code
502.X4dS/C
502.X4dR

Tumor Infiltration of the Sacrum and Sacral Nerves (XXIX-5.3)

Definition
Dull aching sacral pain accompanied by burning or throbbing pain in the rectum and perineum.

Site
Sacrum, rectum, and perineum.

Systems
Skeletal and nervous systems.

Main Features
Pain in a sacral distribution usually occurs in the fifth, sixth, and seventh decades as a result of the spread of bladder, gynecological, or colonic cancer. There is dull aching midline pain and usually burning or throbbing pain in the soft tissues of the rectal and perineal region. The pain is usually made worse by sitting and lying. The rectal and perineal component of the pain may respond poorly to analgesic agents.

Associated Symptoms
With bilateral involvement, sphincter incontinence and impotence are common.

Signs and Laboratory Findings
There may be tenderness over the sacrum and in the region of the sciatic notches. Sometimes there is limitation of both direct and reverse straight leg raising. Involvement of S1 and S2 roots will produce weakness of ankle plantar flexion, and the ankle jerks may be absent. There is usually sensory loss in the perianal region and in the genitalia, and this may be accompanied by hyperpathia. CT scan of the pelvis usually shows sacral erosion with a presacral mass.

Usual Course
The pain and sensory loss may be unilateral initially with progression to bilateral sacral involvement and sphincter disturbance.

Social and Physical Disability
The major disabilities are the results of intractable pain and loss of sphincter function. An in-dwelling urinary catheter may be required.

Summary of Essential Features

The essential features are dull aching sacral pain with burning or throbbing perineal pain. There is usually sacral sensory loss and sphincter incontinence. A CT scan of the pelvis may show sacral erosion and a presacral soft tissue mass.

Diagnostic Criteria

1. Dull aching sacral pain.
2. Burning or throbbing perineal pain.
3. Perineal sensory loss and sphincter dysfunction.
4. CT scan of pelvis may show sacral erosion and presacral soft tissue mass.

Differential Diagnosis

The differential diagnosis includes post-traumatic neuromas in patients with previous pelvic surgery, pelvic abscess, radiation fibrosis, and tension myalgias of the pelvic floor.

Code

Nerve infiltration
702.X4*S/C   702.X4*R
Musculoskeletal deposits
732.X4*S/C   732.X4*R

GROUP XXX: LOW BACK PAIN OF PSYCHOLOGICAL ORIGIN WITH SPINAL REFERRAL

The frequency of low back pain due solely to psychological causes is unknown but probably relatively low compared with low back pain overall, which of course is very common. Psychological causes may play an important part in protracted low back pain in a large number of patients. They will, however, rarely be seen to be the sole cause of the pain, nor will the diagnosis emphasize them in the first instance.

Low Back Pain of Psychological Origin with Spinal Referral (XXX-1)

(See also I-16)

Code

533.X7bS	Tension
51X.X9aS	Delusional
51X.X9bS	Conversion
51X.X9fS	Depression

H. LOCAL SYNDROMES OF THE LOWER LIMBS

GROUP XXXI: LOCAL SYNDROMES IN THE LEG OR FOOT: PAIN OF NEUROLOGICAL ORIGIN

Lateral Femoral Cutaneous Neuropathy (Meralgia Paresthetica) (XXXI-1)

Definition
Hypoesthesia and painful dysesthesia in the distribution of the lateral femoral cutaneous nerve.

Site
Upper anterolateral thigh.

System
Peripheral nervous system.

Main Features
Prevalence: more common in middle age, males slightly more often than females. Associated with obesity, pregnancy, trauma to inguinal region, diabetes mellitus, and possibly other factors. *Pain Quality:* all complaints are of pain or related sensations in the upper anterolateral thigh region; patients may describe burning, tingling, aching, numbness, hypersensitivity to touch, or just vague discomfort. *Time Pattern:* usually gradually abates over months to years without specific therapy.

Signs
Hypoesthesia and paresthesia in upper anterolateral thigh; occasionally tenderness over lateral femoral cutaneous nerve as it passes through iliacus fascia under inguinal ligament.

Relief
Reassurance is the first step. If pelvic tilt is a factor, it should be compensated with heel lift. Diabetes or any other systemic disease will be treated appropriately. In obese patients, the pain will benefit from loss of weight. Surgical decompression of the lateral femoral cutaneous nerve as it passes under the inguinal ligament is, on rare occasions, helpful in the patient who has failed conservative therapy.

Essential Features
Hypoesthesia and paresthesia in upper anterolateral thigh.

Differential Diagnosis
Radiculopathy of L2 or L3; upper lumbosacral plexus lesion due to infection or tumor; entrapment of superior gluteal nerve (piriformis syndrome); arthropathy of hip or rarely the knee.

Code
602.X1a

Obturator Neuralgia (XXXI-2)

Definition
Pain in the distribution of the obturator nerve.

Site
Groin and medial thigh as far distal as the knee; usually unilateral.

System
Peripheral nervous system.

Main Features
Constant pain in the groin and medial thigh; there may be sensory loss in medial thigh and weakness in thigh adductor muscles. Indefinite persistence if cause not treated.

Associated Symptoms
If secondary to obturator hernia, pain is increased by an increase in intra-abdominal pressure. If secondary to osteitis pubis, pain is increased by walking or hip motions. May be tender in region of obturator canal.

Signs
Hypoesthesia of medial thigh region, weakness and atrophy in adductor muscles.

Laboratory Findings
If the neuropathy is severe, there may be EMG evidence of denervation in the adductor muscles of the thigh.

Usual Course
Constant aching pain that persists unless the cause is treated successfully.

Complications
Progressive loss of sensory and motor functions in obturator nerve.

Social and Physical Disability
When severe, may impede ambulation and physical activity involving hip.

Pathology

Obturator hernia; osteitis pubis, often secondary to lower urinary tract infection or surgery; lateral pelvic neoplasm encroaching on nerve.

Essential Features

Pain in groin and medial thigh; with time the development of sensory and motor changes in obturator nerve distribution.

Differential Diagnosis

Tumor or inflammation involving L2–L4 roots, psoas muscle, pelvic side wall. Hip arthropathy.

Code

602.X6a	Obturator hernia
602.X1b	Surgery
602.X2a	Inflammation
602.X4a	Neoplasm

Femoral Neuralgia (XXXI-3)

Definition

Pain in the distribution of the femoral nerve.

Site

Anterior surface of thigh, anteromedial surface of leg, medial aspect of foot to base of first toe.

System

Peripheral nervous system.

Main Features

Constant aching pain in anterior thigh, knee, medial leg, and foot. The pain may involve only a portion of the sensory field due to pathology in only one branch of the nerve. There may be sensory loss in similar areas and weakness of the quadriceps femoris, sartorius, and associated hip flexor muscles.

Associated Symptoms

If the disorder is secondary to femoral hernia, pain is increased by increase in intra-abdominal pressure. Trauma to the saphenous nerve may result in an isolated sensory deficit in the knee or leg with local pain.

Signs

Hypoesthesia in anterior thigh, medial leg, and foot or portion thereof; weakness and atrophy in sartorius or quadriceps femoris muscles if lesion proximal to upper thigh. There may be local tenderness at the site of nerve injury.

Laboratory Findings

If the neuropathy is severe, there may be EMG evidence of denervation in sartorius and quadriceps femoris muscles.

Usual Course

Constant aching pain which persists unless cause is successfully treated.

Complications

Progressive sensory and motor loss in femoral nerve or its branches depending upon site of lesion.

Social and Physical Disability

Major gait disturbance if quadriceps femoris is paretic.

Pathology

Trauma to femoral nerve or its branches; femoral hernia.

Essential Features

Pain, weakness, and sensory loss in the distribution of the femoral nerve or its branches.

Differential Diagnosis

Neoplasm or infection impinging upon femoral nerve, L2–L4 roots, psoas muscle, or pelvic sidewall. Hip or knee arthropathy.

Code

602.X2b	Inflammation
602.X4b	Neoplasm
602.X6b	Arthropathy

Sciatica Neuralgia (XXXI-4)

Definition

Pain in the distribution of the sciatic nerve due to pathology of the nerve itself.

Site

Lower extremity; may vary from gluteal crease to toes depending upon level of nerve injury.

System

Peripheral nervous system.

Main Features

Continuous or lancinating pain or both, referred to the region innervated by the damaged portion of the nerve; exacerbated by manipulation or palpation of the involved segment of the sciatic nerve.

Associated Symptoms

Weakness and sensory loss in muscles and other tissues innervated by the damaged portion of the nerve; secondary changes due to denervation if there is major injury to the nerve.

Signs

Sensory loss; weakness, atrophy, and reduced reflexes in denervated muscles.

Laboratory Findings

Electromyographic and nerve conduction studies document nerve damage; roentgenograms or CT scans may reveal lesion causing nerve damage.

Usual Course

If a progressing lesion is the cause of the pain, the patient will have an increasing neurological deficit and pain may decrease. If a static intraneural lesion is the cause of the pain, the neurological deficit is fixed and pain is likely to persist indefinitely.

Relief

Remove offending lesion impinging upon nerve.

Complications

Progressive neurological deficit in the territory of the involved nerve.

Social and Physical Disability

Severe pain can preclude normal daily activities; a variable loss of function occurs due to nerve damage.

Pathology

Varying degrees of myelin and axonal damage within nerve. Compression of the sciatic nerve by the piriformis muscle can be a cause. The actual cause of the pain is unknown.

Essential Features

Pain in the distribution of the damaged nerve.

Differential Diagnosis

Myelopathy, radiculopathy, lumbosacral plexus lesion involving L4–S1 segments.

Code

602.X1c

Interdigital Neuralgia of the Foot (Morton's Metatarsalgia) (XXXI-5)

Definition

Pain in the metatarsal region.

Site

Usually in the area of the third and fourth metatarsal heads.

System

Peripheral nervous system.

Main Features

Constant aching pain, often lancinating; often worse at night or during exercise; perceived in the region of the metatarsal head. Most commonly involves third and fourth metatarsals.

Signs

Hypoesthesia of opposing surface of adjacent toes; focal tenderness between metatarsal heads when palpated.

Laboratory Tests

None

Usual Course

Pain initially when walking, relieved by rest. Progressively severe and frequent lancinating pain in the toes associated with constant metatarsal ache. May follow local trauma. Some cases spontaneously remit. Often associated with abnormal postures (narrow shoes or high heels) or deformities of the foot and alleviated by treatment of causative condition.

Relief

Orthotic devices to force plantar flexion, i.e., metatarsal bars or pads; local infiltration of steroids with local anesthetic; when conservative therapy fails, incision of transverse metatarsal ligament and excision of interdigital neuroma.

Pathology

Compression of interdigital nerve by metatarsal heads and transverse metatarsal ligament; development of interdigital neuroma.

Essential Features

Pain in region of metatarsal heads exacerbated by weight-bearing.

Differential Diagnosis

Sciatic or peroneal neuropathy, plantar fasciitis, metatarsal pathology, such as inflammation, march fracture, or osteoporosis of metatarsal head, Freiberg's infraction.

Code

603.X1d

Injection Neuropathy (XXXI-6)

Code

602.X5

Gluteal Syndromes (XXXI-7)

Definition

Aching myofascial pain arising from trigger points located in one of the three gluteal muscles.

Site

Gluteus maximus, medius, or minimus muscles.

System
Musculoskeletal system.

Main Features
Aching pain related to the gluteal muscles according to the following patterns. *Gluteus Maximus:* Trigger points in this muscle may refer pain to any part of the buttock or coccyx areas. *Gluteus Medius:* Trigger points in this muscle refer pain medially over the sacrum, laterally along the iliac crest, and occasionally downward to the mid-buttock level and upper portion of the posterior thigh. Sometimes it travels far down into the calf. When this occurs it mimics the pain pattern of "sciatica." *Gluteus Minimus:* Trigger points may arise in either the posterior or superior aspects of this muscle. Those in the posterior portion refer pain downward into the lower part of the buttock, the posterior part of the thigh, and rarely to the posterior part of the calf. The knee joint is spared in this distribution. Again, this pattern is similar to that of sciatica and also of other low back pain conditions involving the gluteal musculature. Trigger points located in the anterior portion refer pain similarly except that it is distributed along the lateral rather than posterior aspect of the thigh and calf.

Aggravating Factors
A foot with a long second and short first metatarsal bone. It can act as a perpetuating factor for all the gluteal muscles, especially the gluteus medius.

Signs
Pressure on the responsible trigger point will reproduce the referred pain pattern. Straight leg raising is usually restricted because of tightness in the hamstring and gluteus maximus muscles.

Pathology
See myofascial pain syndromes.

Etiology
Trigger points of the gluteal musculature very often function as satellite trigger points of those located in the quadratus lumborum muscle.

Differential Diagnosis
Sacroiliac joint dysfunction, sciatic neuritis, piriformis syndrome.

Code
632.X1e

Piriformis Syndrome (XXXI-8)

Definition
Pain in the buttock and posterior thigh due to myofascial injury of the piriformis muscle itself or dysfunction of the sacroiliac joint or pain in the posterior leg and foot, groin, and perineum due to entrapment of the sciatic or other nerves by the piriformis muscle within the greater sciatic foramen, or a combination of these causes.

Site
Buttock from sacrum to greater femoral trochanter with or without posterior thigh, leg, foot, groin, or perineum.

System
Musculoskeletal system.

Main Features
Sex Ratio: female to male 6:1. *Onset:* often occurs after severe or low grade chronic trauma in which the thigh medially rotates on the torso (stretching the piriformis) or in which the piriformis prevents excessive medial rotation by acting as a lateral rotator of the thigh during twisting and bending movements. The patient is often not aware of the injury until hours or days after the incident. Symptoms are particularly aggravated by sitting (which places pressure on the piriformis muscle) and by activity. Placing the hip in external rotation may decrease pain. *Course:* without appropriate intervention, persistent pain. Shortening of the piriformis muscle may occur, resulting in a lateral rotation contracture of the hip.

Associated Symptoms
Paresthesias in the same distribution as the pain; other myofascial pain syndromes in synergists of the piriformis muscle: iliopsoas, gluteus minimus, gluteus medius, tensor fascia lata, inferior and superior gemelli, obturator internus, as well as levator ani and coccygeus; dyspareunia, pain on passing constipated stool, impotence.

Signs
On external palpation through a relaxed gluteus maximus: buttock tenderness, medial and lateral piriformis trigger points, and frequently a myofascial taut band extending from sacrum to femoral greater trochanter. On internal palpation during rectal or vaginal examination: piriformis muscle tenderness and firmness (medial trigger point) on posterior palpation of the piriformis muscle on either side of the coccyx. Reproduction of buttock pain with stretching the piriformis muscle during hip flexion, abduction, and internal rotation while lying supine. Painful hip abduction against resistance while sitting (Pace Abduction Test). Leg length discrepancy. Weakness of hip abductors on the affected side. Sacroiliac dysfunction. Lateral rotation contracture of the hip.

Laboratory Findings
X-rays of lumbosacral spine, sacroiliac joints, hip joints, and pelvis usually normal or have unrelated findings. Bone scan (Tc-99m methylene diphosphonate) is usually normal but has been reported to show increased piriformis muscle uptake acutely. MRI may show atrophy of

the piriformis muscle. Selected nerve conduction studies may demonstrate nerve entrapment.

Usual Course
Persistent pain without appropriate intervention. Responds well to appropriate interventions, particularly in the early stages.

Relief
Correction of biomechanical factors (leg length discrepancy, hip abductor or lateral rotator weakness, etc.). Prolonged stretching of piriformis muscle using hip flexion, abduction, and internal rotation. Facilitation of stretching by: reciprocal inhibition and postisometric relaxation techniques; massage; acupressure (ischemic compression) to trigger points within piriformis muscle; intermittent cold (ice or fluorimethane spray); heat modalities (short wave diathermy or ultrasound). Injection (steroid, procaine/Xylocaine) to region of lateral attachment of piriformis on femoral greater trochanter (lateral trigger point), or to tender areas medial to sciatic nerve near sacrum (medial trigger point) with rectal/vaginal monitoring. If previous measures fail, surgical transection of piriformis tendon at greater trochanter with exploration of nerves and vascular structures within the greater sciatic foramen that may be entrapped by the piriformis muscle.

Pathology
Three main causes: (1) myofascial pain referred from trigger points in the piriformis muscle, (2) nerve and vascular entrapment by the piriformis muscle within the greater sciatic foramen, and (3) dysfunction of the sacroiliac joint. Myofascial injury to the piriformis muscle may be acute—blunt trauma, overstretch or overcontraction due to fall, motor vehicle accident, etc.—or chronic—repetitive low-grade activity, e.g., using a foot pedal with the hip in abduction while sitting. Vascular or nerve structures may be entrapped between the piriformis muscle and the rim of the greater sciatic foramen, or possibly by nerve entrapment within the muscle. Vulnerable structures include superior gluteal, inferior gluteal, and pudendal nerves and vessels; the sciatic and posterior femoral cutaneous nerves; and the nerves supplying the superior and inferior gemelli, the obturator internus, and the quadratus femoris muscles. Sacroiliac dysfunction may be due to contralateral oblique axis rotation of the sacrum with associated malalignment at the symphysis pubis.

Social and Physical Disabilities
Difficulty sitting for prolonged periods and difficulty with physical activities such as prolonged walking, standing, bending, lifting, or twisting compromise both sedentary and physically demanding occupations.

Essential Features
Buttock pain with or without thigh pain, which is aggravated by sitting or activity. Absence of low back or hip symptoms or pathology. Tenderness from sacrum to femoral greater trochanter externally. Posterolateral tenderness and firmness on rectal or vaginal examination. Aggravation by hip flexion, abduction, and internal rotation.

Differential Diagnosis
Lumbosacral radiculopathy, lumbar plexopathy, proximal hamstring tendinitis, ischial bursitis, trochanteric bursitis, sacroiliitis, facet syndrome, spinal stenosis (if bilateral symptoms). May occur concurrently with lumbar spine, sacroiliac, and/or hip joint pathology.

Code
632.X1f

References
Travell, J.G. and Simons, D.G.,. The lower extremities, piriformis, and other short lateral rotators. In: The Trigger Point Manual. Myofascial Pain and Dysfunction, Vol. 2., Williams & Wilkins, Baltimore, 1992, pp. 197–214.

Barton, P.M., Piriformis syndrome: a rational approach to management, Pain, 47 (1991) 345–352.

Fishman, L.M., Electrophysiological evidence of piriformis syndrome-II, Arch. Phys. Med. Rehab., 69 (1988) 800.

Karl, R.D., Jr., Yedinak, M.A., Harshorne, M.F., Cawthon, M.A., Bauman, J.M., Howard, W.H. and Bunker, S.R., Scintigraphic appearance of the piriformis muscle syndrome, Clin. Nucl. Med., 10 (1985) 361–363.

Kipervas, I.P., Ivanov, L.A., Urikh, E.A. and Pakhomov, S.K., Clinico-electromyographic characteristics of piriformis muscle syndrome (Russian), Zh. Nevropatol. Psikhiatr., 76 (1976) 1289–1292.

Nainzadeh, N. and Lane, M.E., Somatosensory evoked potentials following pudendal nerve stimulation as indicators of low sacral root involvement in a postlaminectomy patient, Arch. Phys. Med. Rehab., 68 (1987) 170–172.

Synek, V.M., Short latency somatosensory evoked potentials in patients with painful dysaesthesias in peripheral nerve lesions, Pain, 29 (1987) 49–58.

Synek, V.M., The piriformis syndrome: review and case presentation, Clin. Exper. Neurol., 23 (1987) 31–37.

Shin, D.Y. and Mizuguchi, T., Entrapment sciatic neuropathy in piriformis muscle syndrome: fact or myth, Arch. Phys. Med. Rehab., 73 (1992) 991.

Painful Legs and Moving Toes (XXXI-9)

Definition
Deep pain, often gnawing, twisting, or aching in an extremity, with involuntary movements of the extremity, especially the digits.

Site
Pain in lower leg and foot, and sometimes toe. It may be unilateral or bilateral, or start unilaterally and spread to the other limb.

System
Nervous system. In some cases peripheral causes have been described; the spinal cord is probably also involved.

Main Features
Pain is usually severe, deep, and poorly localized. It is often described as gnawing, twisting, aching. It is more severe in the leg than in the periphery. Sometimes relieved by activity, though it may be worse following exercise. It occurs in the second half of life. The movements may be florid or almost imperceptible, and in the latter case, the patient may never have noticed them. They consist of irregular, involuntary, and sometimes writhing movement of the toes, and they cannot be imitated voluntarily. They can be suppressed for a minute or two by voluntary effort and then return when the patient no longer attends to them. There can also be movements of the feet. There is not usually a relation between the pain and the movements.

Usual Course
It continues indefinitely.

Relief
No consistently effective measures have been found.

Pathology
Precise pathology unknown, but nerve root lesions have been described, and spinal cord damage.

Code
602.X8

(See XI-5 for Painful Arms and Moving Fingers)

References
Spillane, J.D., Nathan, P.W., Kelly, R.E. and Marsden, C.D., Painful legs and moving toes, Brain, 94 (1971) 541–556.

Nathan, P.W., Painful legs and moving toes: evidence on the site of the lesion, J. Neurol. Neurosurg. Psychiatry, 41 (1978) 934–939.

Montagna, P., Cirignotta, F., Sacquegna, T., Martinelli, P., Ambrosetta, G. and Lugaresi, E., Painful legs and moving toes: associated with polyneuropathy, J. Neurol. Neurosurg. Psychiatry, 46 (1983) 399–403.

Metastatic Disease (XXXI-10)

Definition
Pain in the hip joint and thigh region due to tumor infiltration of bone.

Site
Acetabulum, head of the femur, femoral neck, and femoral shaft.

System
Skeletal system.

Main Features
Metastases to the hip joint region produce continuous aching or throbbing pain in the groin with radiation through to the buttock and down the medial thigh to the knee. The pain is made worse by movements of the hip joint and is especially severe on weight-bearing. A metastatic deposit to the femoral shaft produces local pain, which is also aggravated by weight-bearing.

Associated Symptoms
Pain at rest due to tumor infiltration of bone usually responds reasonably well to nonsteroidal anti-inflammatory drugs and narcotic analgesics. Pain due to hip movement or weight-bearing responds poorly to analgesic agents.

Signs and Laboratory Findings
There may be tenderness in the groin and in the region of the greater trochanter. Internal and external rotation of the hip are especially painful. There is usually no deformity unless a pathological fracture has occurred. Plain films and bone scan may be positive.

Complications
The major complication is a pathological fracture of the femoral neck or the femoral shaft. This of course puts the patient to bed. Hip replacement or internal fixation of the femur produces dramatic pain relief.

Summary of Essential Features and Diagnostic Criteria
The essential features for disease in the hip joint are severe pain in the groin with radiation into the buttock and down the medial thigh. There is usually tenderness in the groin and increased pain on internal and external rotation. Plain films and bone scan may be positive.

Differential Diagnosis
The differential diagnosis includes upper lumbar plexopathy, avascular necrosis of the femoral head, and septic arthritis and radiation fibrosis of the hip joint.

Code
633.X4

Peroneal Muscular Atrophy (Charcot-Marie-Tooth Disease) (XXXI-11)

Definition
Pain in the limbs, usually constant and aching in the feet, in association with peroneal atrophy.

Site
The distal portion of the limbs, more often in the feet than in the hands, and across the joint spaces.

System
Peripheral nervous system.

Main Features
The pain arises in association with peroneal muscular atrophy. *Sex Ratio:* the male to female ratio is 1:1.6. *Age of Onset:* the illness normally appears in childhood and adolescence, with a reported age range for prevalence from 10–84 years. It is an inherited disorder, sometimes an autosomal dominant, sometimes an autosomal recessive, and sometimes a sex linked dominant genetic disorder. The sex linked form is less common than the other types. *Pain Quality:* pain is relatively rare in the disease, and has two patterns. The pain is usually aching in quality. It may be continuous or intermittent but is aggravated by activity, stress, cold, and damp. This aching pain appears most often as a complication of surgical foot corrections by triple arthrodesis. Pain and cramps in the muscle occasionally occur following activity. This pain is described as a burning discomfort. Anxiety and fatigue appear in association with the pain.

Signs
Features of the primary disease are evident. There is distal muscle wasting with the "classical" inverted "champagne bottle" legs. Deformity and subluxation of the distal joints occur. There are demonstrable sensory losses in a significant proportion of patients, predominantly affecting light touch and proprioception.

Usual Course
Unremitting.

Pathology
Degenerative changes appear in the dorsal root ganglion cells or motor neurons of the spinal cord with resulting axonal degeneration.

Relief
Cold, damp, and changes in the weather appear to cause an increase in the symptom. Tension, stress, fatigue, and movement all increase the pain. Rest, simple analgesics such as paracetamol (acetaminophen) and nonsteroidal anti-inflammatory drugs, and transcutaneous electrical stimulation help to ease the pain. Relief is also associated with warmth, massage, lying down, sleep, and distraction.

Laboratory Findings
Conduction velocities in motor nerves may be decreased, or denervation may be evident.

Essential Features
Pain in the relevant distribution in patients affected by the typical muscle disorder.

Code
Pain affecting joints only
203.X0
603.X0
(most often 203.60 and 603.60)

Pain affecting the belly of the muscle
205.X0
605.X0
(most often 205.60 and 605.60)

Note: Where pain affects both locations, code 203.X0 and 603.X0.

GROUP XXXII: PAIN SYNDROMES OF THE HIP AND THIGH OF MUSCULOSKELETAL ORIGIN

Ischial Bursitis (XXXII-1)

Definition
Severe, sharp, or aching pain syndrome arising from inflammatory lesion of ischial bursa.

Site
Buttock.

System
Musculoskeletal system.

Main Features
Uncommon. There is often severe sharp or aching pain while sitting or lying. With coexistent sciatic irritation, the pain may be acute, radiating in the sciatic distribution. Attacks may last weeks or months without treatment. Cases are often secondary to systemic inflammatory disease, such as ankylosing spondylitis, rheumatoid arthritis, or Reiter's syndrome.

Signs
Tenderness deep in buttock over ischial tuberosity that reproduces the patient's symptoms.

Relief
Injection into the ischial bursa with local anesthetic and steroid; "doughnut" cushion as used for treatment of hemorrhoids.

Complications
None.

Pathology
Inflammatory process of ischial bursa usually occurring with repeated trauma.

Essential Features
Recurring pain in ischial region aggravated by sitting or lying, relieved by injection.

Differential Diagnosis
Acute sciatica, spondylarthropathy, prostatitis.

Code
533.X3

Trochanteric Bursitis (XXXII-2)

Definition
Aching or burning pain in the high lateral part of the thigh and in the buttock caused by inflammation of the trochanteric bursa.

Site
Thigh and buttock.

System
Musculoskeletal system.

Main Features
Very common condition, especially in those over 40 years of age, marked by severe aching or burning pain usually perceived by the patient to be "in the hip" but which is localized to the high lateral thigh and low buttock, often radiating to the knee. The patient characteristically finds it impossible to sleep on the affected side. The acute episode may last weeks to months and may recur. Often associated with mild "hip" stiffness, somewhat relieved by activity.

Aggravating Factors
Aggravated by climbing stairs, extension of the back from flexion with knees straight.

Signs
Tenderness usually 2.5 cm posterior and superior to the greater trochanter that reproduces the patient's symptoms.

Usual Course
Usually of sudden onset. The pain tends to be severe and persistent. If untreated it may last for several months. Repeated attacks occur at variable intervals.

Relief
Local infiltration of local anesthetic and steroid into the area of the greatest tenderness produces excellent pain relief.

Complications
None.

Pathology
Inflammatory process of bursa caused by repeated trauma or generalized inflammation such as rheumatoid arthritis.

Essential Features
Local pain aggravated by climbing stairs, extension of the back from flexion with knees straight.

Differential Diagnosis
Disorders of the hip joint, referred pain from diseases of lumbosacral spine.

Code
634.X3d

Osteoarthritis of the Hip (XXXII-3)

Definition
Pain due to primary or secondary degenerative process involving the hip joint.

Main Features
As for osteoarthritis. Often felt deep in the groin, sometimes buttock or thigh, reproduced on passive or active movement of hip joint through a range of motion. As disease progresses, range of motion declines. Other features as for osteoarthritis (I-11).

Code
638.X6b

GROUP XXXIII: MUSCULOSKELETAL SYNDROMES OF THE LEG

Spinal Stenosis (XXXIII-1)

See section XXVII-6.

Code
633.X6

Osteoarthritis of the Knee (XXXIII-2)

Definition
Pain due to a degenerative process of one or more of the three compartments of the knee joint.

System
Musculoskeletal system.

Main Features
As for osteoarthritis but localized to the knee. Epidemiology, aggravating and relieving features, signs, usual course, physical disability, pathology, and differential diagnosis as for osteoarthritis (I-11).

Code
638.X6c

Night Cramps (XXXIII-3)

Definition
Painful nocturnal cramps in the calves.

Site
Lower limbs.

System
Musculoskeletal system.

Main Features
Severe aching cramps in the calves of the legs, often preventing the patient from sleep or waking him or her from sleep. Nightly pain for variable intervals which recur frequently in clusters. Experienced especially by children and the elderly, but can occur at any age.

Aggravating Factors
Aggravated by prolonged walking or standing on concrete floor. May be provoked by sudden dorsiflexion of ankle or knee joint.

Relief
Walking, moving the legs, elevation of the legs, or calf stretching provide occasional relief. Treatment with quinine, calcium supplements, diphenhydramine, diphenyl hydantoin, or vitamin E (alpha-tocopherol) may be helpful.

Differential Diagnosis
Electrolyte disorder, hypothyroidism.

Code
634.X8

Plantar Fasciitis (XXXIII-4)

Definition
Pain in the foot caused by inflammation of the plantar aponeurosis.

Site
Foot.

System
Musculoskeletal system.

Main Features
Pain with insidious onset in the plantar region of the foot, especially worse when initiating walking. Worse with prolonged activity. The patient may describe shooting or burning in the heel with each step.

Signs
Tenderness along the plantar fascia when ankle is dorsiflexed.

Radiographic Findings
Often associated with calcaneal spur when chronic.

Relief
Arch supports, local injection of corticosteroid, oral nonsteroidal anti-inflammatory agents. Surgery as a last resort.

Pathology
Fifteen percent have some form of systemic rheumatic disease, usually a seronegative form of spondylarthritis.

Differential Diagnosis
Reiter's syndrome, ankylosing spondylitis, rheumatoid arthritis, psoriatic arthritis.

Code
633.X3

PART III

PAIN TERMS

A CURRENT LIST WITH DEFINITIONS AND NOTES ON USAGE

Revisions prepared by an Ad Hoc Subcommittee of the IASP Task Force on Taxonomy

Harold Merskey (Chair)
Ulf Lindblom
James M. Mumford
Peter W. Nathan
and
Sir Sydney Sunderland

First Version published in *Pain*, Vol. 6, 1979, pages 249–252.
Updated in *Pain*, Supplement 3, 1986, pages S215–S221.
Reprinted 1991
Minor Revisions 1994

INTRODUCTION TO THE 1986 LIST

A list of pain terms was first published in 1979 (*Pain*, 6, 249–252). Many of the terms were already established in the literature. One, *allodynia,* quickly came into use in the columns of *Pain* and other journals. The terms have been translated into Portuguese (*Rev. Bras. Anest.*, 30, 5, [1980] 349–351,) into French (H. Dehen, Lexique de la douleur, *La Presse Médicale* 12, 23, [1983] 1459–1460), and into Turkish (as *Agri Terimlëri*, translated by T. Aldemir, *J. Turkish Soc. Algology*, 1 [1989] 45–46). A supplementary note was added to these pain terms in *Pain* (14 [1982] 205–206).

The original list was adopted by the first Subcommittee on Taxonomy of IASP. Subsequent revisions and additions were prepared by a subgroup of the Committee, particularly Drs. U. Lindblom, P.W. Nathan, W. Noordenbos, and H. Merskey. In 1984, in particular response to some observations by Dr. M. Devor, a further review was undertaken both by correspondence and during the 4th World Congress on Pain of IASP. Those taking part in that review included Dr. Devor, the other colleagues just mentioned, and Dr. J.M. Mumford, Sir Sydney Sunderland, and Dr. P.W. Wall. Following that review, it was agreed to take advantage of the publication of the draft collection of syndromes and their system for classification, to issue an updated list of terms with definitions and notes on usage.

The versions now presented are based upon some subsequent discussions by correspondence. The form of the definitions and notes at this point has been the responsibility of the editor (H.M.). It would be difficult now to single out individual contributions, but the editor remains heavily indebted to those five members of the original Subcommittee on Taxonomy who sustained this work in the form of an Ad Hoc group and whose names are listed at the beginning of this report. Their knowledge and patience was repeatedly provided freely and with good will.

The revised current list follows. The original comments provided as an introduction to the terms are given in the following two paragraphs, which indicate both the process by which the terms were first delivered and the justification for them.

"The usage of individual terms in medicine often varies widely. That need not be a cause of distress provided that each author makes clear precisely how he employs a word. Nevertheless, it is convenient and helpful to others if words can be used which have agreed technical meanings. Following correspondence and meetings during the period 1976–1978, the present committee agreed on the definitions which follow, and the notes have been prepared by the chairman in the light of members' comments. The definitions are intended to be specific and explanatory and to serve as an operational framework, not as a constraint on future development. They represent agreement between diverse specialties including anesthesiology, dentistry, neurology, neurosurgery, neurophysiology, psychiatry, and psychology. A starting point for some of these definitions was provided by the reports of a workshop on Oro-Facial Pain held at the U.S. National Institute of Dental Research in November 1974.

"The terms and definitions are not meant to provide a comprehensive glossary but rather a minimum standard vocabulary for members of different disciplines who work in the field of pain. We hope that they will prove acceptable to all those in the health professions who deal with pain. Not only are they a limited selection from available terms, but it is emphasized that except for pain itself, *they are defined primarily in relation to the skin and the special senses are excluded.* They may be used when appropriate for responses to somatic stimulation elsewhere or to the viscera. Except for Pain, the arrangement is in alphabetical order."

It is important to emphasize something that was implicit in the previous definitions but was not specifically stated: that the terms have been developed for use in clinical practice rather than for experimental work, physiology, or anatomical purposes.

CHANGES IN THE 1994 LIST

There was substantial correspondence from 1986 to 1993 among members of the Task Force and other colleagues. The previous definitions all remain unchanged, except for very slight alterations in the wording of the definitions of Central Pain and Hyperpathia. Two new terms have been introduced here: Neuropathic Pain and Peripheral Neuropathic Pain.

The terms Sympathetically Maintained Pain and Sympathetically Independent Pain have also been employed; however, these terms are used in connection with syndromes I-4 and I-5, now called Complex Regional Pain Syndromes, Types I and II. These were formerly labeled Reflex Sympathetic Dystrophy and Causalgia, and the discussion of Sympathetically Maintained Pain and Sympathetically Independent Pain is found with those categories.

Changes have been made in the notes on Allodynia to clarify the fact that it may refer to a light stimulus on damaged skin, as well as on normal skin. Also, in the tabulation of the implications of some of the definitions, the words *lowered threshold* have been removed from the features of Allodynia because it does not occur regularly. Small changes have been made to better de-scribe Hyperpathia in the definition and note. A sentence has been added to the note on Hyperalgesia to refer to current views on its physiology, although as with other definitions, that for Hyperalgesia remains tied to clinical criteria. Last, the note on neuropathy has been expanded.

PAIN TERMS

Pain

An unpleasant sensory and emotional experience associated with actual or potential tissue dam-age, or described in terms of such damage.

Note: Pain is always subjective. Each individual learns the application of the word through ex-periences related to injury in early life. Biologists recognize that those stimuli which cause pain are liable to damage tissue. Accordingly, pain is that experience we associate with actual or po-tential tissue damage. It is unquestionably a sensation in a part or parts of the body, but it is also always unpleasant and therefore also an emotional experience. Experiences which resemble pain but are not unpleasant, e.g., pricking, should not be called pain. Unpleasant abnormal experi-ences (dysesthesias) may also be pain but are not necessarily so because, subjectively, they may not have the usual sensory qualities of pain.

Many people report pain in the absence of tissue damage or any likely pathophysiological cause; usually this happens for psychological reasons. There is usually no way to distinguish their ex-perience from that due to tissue damage if we take the subjective report. If they regard their experience as pain and if they report it in the same ways as pain caused by tissue damage, it should be accepted as pain. This definition avoids tying pain to the stimulus. Activity induced in the nociceptor and nociceptive pathways by a noxious stimulus is not pain, which is always a psychological state, even though we may well appreciate that pain most often has a proximate physical cause.

Allodynia

Pain due to a stimulus which does not normally provoke pain.

Note: The term *allodynia* was originally introduced to separate from hyperalgesia and hyperes-thesia, the conditions seen in patients with lesions of the nervous system where touch, light pressure, or moderate cold or warmth evoke pain when applied to apparently normal skin. *Allo* means "other" in Greek and is a common prefix for medical conditions that diverge from the expected. *Odynia* is derived from the Greek word "odune" or "odyne," which is used in "pleurodynia" and "coccydynia" and is similar in meaning to the root from which we derive words with -algia or -algesia in them. Allodynia was suggested following discussions with Pro-fessor Paul Potter of the Department of the History of Medicine and Science at The University of Western Ontario.

The words "to normal skin" were used in the original definition but later were omitted in order to remove any suggestion that allodynia applied only to referred pain. Originally, also, the pain-provoking stimulus was described as "non-noxious." However, a stimulus may be noxious at some times and not at others, for example, with intact skin and sunburned skin, and also, the boundaries of noxious stimulation may be hard to delimit. Since the Committee aimed at provid-ing terms for clinical use, it did not wish to define them by reference to the specific physical characteristics of the stimulation, e.g., pressure in kilopascals per square centimeter. Moreover, even in intact skin there is little evidence one way or the other that a strong painful pinch to a normal person does or does not damage tissue. Accordingly, it was considered to be preferable to define allodynia in terms of the response to clinical stimuli and to point out that the normal response to the stimulus could almost always be tested elsewhere in the body, usually in a corre-sponding part. Further, allodynia is taken to apply to conditions which may give rise to sensiti-zation of the skin, e.g., sunburn, inflammation, trauma.

It is important to recognize that allodynia involves a change in the quality of a sensation, whether tactile, thermal, or of any other sort. The original modality is normally non-painful, but the response is painful. There is thus a loss of specificity of a sensory modality. By contrast, hyperalgesia (q.v.) represents an augmented response in a specific mode, viz., pain. With other cutaneous modalities, hyperesthesia is the term which corresponds to hyperalgesia, and as with hyperalgesia, the quality is not altered. In allodynia the stimulus mode and the response mode differ, unlike the situation with hyperalgesia. This distinction should not be confused by the fact that allodynia and hyperalgesia can be plotted with overlap along the same continuum of physical intensity in certain circumstances, for example, with pressure or temperature.

See also the notes on hyperalgesia and hyperpathia.

Analgesia

Absence of pain in response to stimulation which would normally be painful.

Note: As with allodynia (q.v.), the stimulus is defined by its usual subjective effects.

Anesthesia dolorosa

Pain in an area or region which is anesthetic.

Causalgia

A syndrome of sustained burning pain, allodynia, and hyperpathia after a traumatic nerve lesion, often combined with vasomotor and sudomotor dysfunction and later trophic changes.

Central pain

Pain initiated or caused by a primary lesion or dysfunction in the central nervous system.

Dysesthesia

An unpleasant abnormal sensation, whether spontaneous or evoked.

Note: Compare with pain and with paresthesia. Special cases of dysesthesia include hyperalgesia and allodynia. A dysesthesia should always be unpleasant and a paresthesia should not be unpleasant, although it is recognized that the borderline may present some difficulties when it comes to deciding as to whether a sensation is pleasant or unpleasant. It should always be specified whether the sensations are spontaneous or evoked.

Hyperalgesia

An increased response to a stimulus which is normally painful.

Note: Hyperalgesia reflects increased pain on suprathreshold stimulation. For pain evoked by stimuli that usually are not painful, the term allodynia is preferred, while hyperalgesia is more appropriately used for cases with an increased response at a normal threshold, or at an increased threshold, e.g., in patients with neuropathy. It should also be recognized that with allodynia the stimulus and the response are in different modes, whereas with hyperalgesia they are in the same mode. Current evidence suggests that hyperalgesia is a consequence of perturbation of the nociceptive system with peripheral or central sensitization, or both, but it is important to distinguish between the clinical phenomena, which this definition emphasizes, and the interpretation, which may well change as knowledge advances.

Hyperesthesia

Increased sensitivity to stimulation, excluding the special senses.

Note: The stimulus and locus should be specified. Hyperesthesia may refer to various modes of cutaneous sensibility including touch and thermal sensation without pain, as well as to pain. The word is used to indicate both diminished threshold to any stimulus and an increased response to stimuli that are normally recognized.

Allodynia is suggested for pain after stimulation which is not normally painful. Hyperesthesia includes both allodynia and hyperalgesia, but the more specific terms should be used wherever they are applicable.

Hyperpathia   A painful syndrome characterized by an abnormally painful reaction to a stimulus, especially a repetitive stimulus, as well as an increased threshold.

Note: It may occur with allodynia, hyperesthesia, hyperalgesia, or dysesthesia. Faulty identification and localization of the stimulus, delay, radiating sensation, and after-sensation may be present, and the pain is often explosive in character. The changes in this note are the specification of allodynia and the inclusion of hyperalgesia explicitly. Previously hyperalgesia was implied, since hyperesthesia was mentioned in the previous note and hyperalgesia is a special case of hyperesthesia.

Hypoalgesia   Diminished pain in response to a normally painful stimulus.

Note: Hypoalgesia was formerly defined as diminished sensitivity to noxious stimulation, making it a particular case of hypoesthesia (q.v.). However, it now refers only to the occurrence of relatively less pain in response to stimulation that produces pain. Hypoesthesia covers the case of diminished sensitivity to stimulation that is normally painful.

The implications of some of the above definitions may be summarized for convenience as follows:

Allodynia:	lowered threshold:	stimulus and response mode differ
Hyperalgesia:	increased response:	stimulus and response mode are the same
Hyperpathia:	raised threshold: increased response:	stimulus and response mode may be the same or different
Hypoalgesia:	raised threshold: lowered response:	stimulus and response mode are the same

The above essentials of the definitions do not have to be symmetrical and are not symmetrical at present. Lowered threshold may occur with allodynia but is not required. Also, there is no category for lowered threshold and lowered response—if it ever occurs.

Hypoesthesia   Decreased sensitivity to stimulation, excluding the special senses.

Note: Stimulation and locus to be specified.

Neuralgia   Pain in the distribution of a nerve or nerves.

Note: Common usage, especially in Europe, often implies a paroxysmal quality, but neuralgia should not be reserved for paroxysmal pains.

Neuritis   Inflammation of a nerve or nerves.

Note: Not to be used unless inflammation is thought to be present.

Neurogenic pain   Pain initiated or caused by a primary lesion, dysfunction, or transitory perturbation in the peripheral or central nervous system.

Neuropathic pain Pain initiated or caused by a primary lesion or dysfunction in the nervous system.

Note: See also Neurogenic Pain and Central Pain. Peripheral neuropathic pain occurs when the lesion or dysfunction affects the peripheral nervous system. Central pain may be retained as the term when the lesion or dysfunction affects the central nervous system.

Neuropathy   A disturbance of function or pathological change in a nerve: in one nerve, mononeuropathy; in several nerves, mononeuropathy multiplex; if diffuse and bilateral, polyneuropathy.

Note: Neuritis (q.v.) is a special case of neuropathy and is now reserved for inflammatory processes affecting nerves. Neuropathy is not intended to cover cases like neurapraxia, neurotmesis, section of a nerve, or transitory impact like a blow, stretching, or an epileptic discharge. The term *neurogenic* applies to pain due to such temporary perturbations.

Nociceptor

A receptor preferentially sensitive to a noxious stimulus or to a stimulus which would become noxious if prolonged.

Note: Avoid use of terms like pain receptor, pain pathway, etc.

Noxious stimulus

A noxious stimulus is one which is damaging to normal tissues.

Note: Although the definition of a noxious stimulus has been retained, the term is not used in this list to define other terms.

Pain threshold

The least experience of pain which a subject can recognize.

Note: Traditionally the threshold has often been defined, as we defined it formerly, as the least stimulus intensity at which a subject perceives pain. Properly defined, the threshold is really the experience of the patient, whereas the intensity measured is an external event. It has been common usage for most pain research workers to define the threshold in terms of the stimulus, and that should be avoided. However, the threshold stimulus can be recognized as such and measured. In psychophysics, thresholds are defined as the level at which 50% of stimuli are recognized. In that case, the pain threshold would be the level at which 50% of stimuli would be recognized as painful. The stimulus is not pain (q.v.) and cannot be a measure of pain.

Pain tolerance level

The greatest level of pain which a subject is prepared to tolerate.

Note: As with pain threshold, the pain tolerance level is the subjective experience of the individual. The stimuli which are normally measured in relation to its production are the pain tolerance level stimuli and not the level itself. Thus, the same argument applies to pain tolerance level as to pain threshold, and it is not defined in terms of the external stimulation as such.

Paresthesia

An abnormal sensation, whether spontaneous or evoked.

Note: Compare with dysesthesia. After much discussion, it has been agreed to recommend that paresthesia be used to describe an abnormal sensation that is not unpleasant while dysesthesia be used preferentially for an abnormal sensation that is considered to be unpleasant. The use of one term (paresthesia) to indicate spontaneous sensations and the other to refer to evoked sensations is not favored. There is a sense in which, since paresthesia refers to abnormal sensations in general, it might include dysesthesia, but the reverse is not true. Dysesthesia does not include all abnormal sensations, but only those which are unpleasant.

Peripheral neurogenic pain

Pain initiated or caused by a primary lesion or dysfunction or transitory perturbation in the peripheral nervous system.

Peripheral neuropathic pain

Pain initiated or caused by a primary lesion or dysfunction in the peripheral nervous system.

INDEX